Innovating Minds

Innovating Minds

Rethinking Creativity to Inspire Change

WILMA KOUTSTAAL

AND

JONATHAN T. BINKS

OXFORD
UNIVERSITY PRESS

OXFORD

UNIVERSITY PRESS

Oxford University Press is a department of the University of
Oxford. It furthers the University's objective of excellence in research,
scholarship, and education by publishing worldwide.

Oxford   New York
Auckland   Cape Town   Dar es Salaam   Hong Kong   Karachi
Kuala Lumpur   Madrid   Melbourne   Mexico City   Nairobi
New Delhi   Shanghai   Taipei   Toronto

With offices in
Argentina   Austria   Brazil   Chile   Czech Republic   France   Greece
Guatemala   Hungary   Italy   Japan   Poland   Portugal   Singapore
South Korea   Switzerland   Thailand   Turkey   Ukraine   Vietnam

Published in the United States of America by
Oxford University Press
198 Madison Avenue, New York, NY 10016

Library of Congress Cataloging-in-Publication Data
Koutstaal, Wilma.
Innovating minds: rethinking creativity to inspire change/Wilma Koutstaal
and Jonathan T. Binks.
pages cm
Includes bibliographical references and index.
ISBN 978-0-19-931602-1
1. Thought and thinking.   2. Creative thinking.   3. Divergent thinking.
4. Adaptability (Psychology)   I. Binks, Jonathan T.   II. Title.
BF441.K5863 2015
153.3'5—dc23
2014037832

9 8 7 6 5 4 3 2 1
Printed in the United States of America
on acid-free paper

This book is dedicated to the memory of Cyril Binks, a consummate craftsman, and to Willemina Koutstaal, a noticer par excellence.

CONTENTS

This book invites us to discover how we can all become more creative thinkers and doers. A central question at the heart of this book is: How can we more flexibly and responsively bring about positive change in our world and in ourselves?

We will ask you to actively work through ideas as, together, we explore a new way of understanding our own and others' thinking. The science-based "thinking framework" that we will learn can help each of us—as individuals and as groups, teams, or organizations—to be more creative, innovative, and mentally agile.

A primary message of this book is that positive change and creativity can be encouraged through gaining a better understanding of the ways in which our thinking *really* works. Thinking emerges not just from our brains, our minds, or our environments in isolation but from an ongoing dynamic interaction of brain, mind, and environment. By gaining a better understanding of our thinking (our own and that of others across time) we can optimize our "innovating minds"—minds that continually creatively adapt themselves, flexibly building on what they have learned, helping others to do so, and shaping environments that sustain and spur further innovation.

We will learn about the processes of generating and testing ideas and how ideas lead to yet other ideas. We will see that there is not as sharp a divide as might be supposed between thinking and action or between creating and innovating but that these cycle together, each informing the other. Creativity and innovation—changing the ways in which we and other people think about, listen to, look at, or do things and helping to solve problems (large or small)—rarely happen in a single step or a single moment.

In creativity, our actions bootstrap our thinking and our thinking bootstraps our actions. We perceive, act, and perceive again. This is what we call *making* and *finding*. In our efforts to discover and create we repeatedly alternate between making (guided by what we intend) and finding (responding to what emerges as a consequence of our intentions). Although many propose distinctions between creativity and innovation, such as suggesting that creativity involves the generation of ideas and that innovation involves the application or realization of ideas (including also adapting ideas in use elsewhere), the view of creativity that we develop throughout this book does not propose such a sharp distinction. Making and finding and the perception-action cycle apply to both creativity and innovation.

The thinking framework that we introduce in this book asks us to approach creativity and change—whether as individuals, teams, or organizations—through a unique combination of five questions. First: What ideas are competing for your attention and awareness, and how are you helping to form and *re*-form them? Second: Should you be zooming out to a bigger picture, a more abstract perspective, or zooming in to a more detailed and specific view? Adjusting where we should be in our level of abstraction (what we refer to as *detail stepping*) is an often overlooked but pervasive contributor to creativity. Third: Are you allowing sufficient room for both spontaneity and deliberateness in your creative process? Do you know when to trust your routines? Fourth: Are you receptive to the interplay of motivation, emotions, and perception in your thinking? How are you choosing your goals and keeping them in mind? Fifth: How are your physical, symbolic, and social thinking spaces (including your working tools) spurring or spurning creative insights?

Our science-based thinking framework is rooted in research from many different fields that share an interest in achieving a better understanding of how we newly imagine and work through opportunities and problems. We traverse research findings from neuronal ensembles and brain networks to individuals in interacting groups and to organizations that span continents. We explore the science of thinking in our minds and brains in ongoing dynamic interaction with our richly symbolic social and physical environments. We scout a rich world of research that illuminates the real-world creative challenges of people in all walks of life. We meet architects, choreographers, composers, and musicians and learn of their creative obstacles and opportunities. We encounter, too, the innovative struggles and successes of dancers, designers, engineers, film crews, nurses, and physicians. We gain insight into the creative realizations of manufacturers, teams of scientists, software developers, and theater companies. We chart change and innovation in a variety of organizations, from design companies to hospitals to nonprofits dedicated to preserving and protecting our environment.

We discover early that innovative ideas are not only about "concepts" and are not just "in our heads." Ideas are in our minds but are also deeply intertwined with motivation and emotion, perception and action, and in continual interplay with our environments in all their physical, social, and symbolic complexities. We soon discover, too, that creativity and innovation are profoundly iterative. Bursts of creativity involve much more than sudden insight and often emerge from acting on and in the world in an ongoing interchange of making, finding, and making once more.

Our thinking framework provides a widely integrative perspective that asks us to always see ourselves and others as in a changing "idea landscape" in which thoughts and possibilities are continually forming, emerging, disappearing, and resurfacing into our awareness. Although we sometimes deliberately evoke ideas, at other times thoughts arise more spontaneously or even automatically. It is our ability to aptly modulate between these processes of cognitive control that offers us the greatest opportunities for mental agility and creative change.

Ideas crucially differ, too, in their degree of abstractness or specificity. We gain the most power and reach from our experiences when we can aptly and effectively move up and down in our level of detail. Sometimes we need to delve deeply into concrete particulars, with all their rich specificity and context. At other times, it is essential that we nimbly climb up and across those rich particulars, using abstractions that select, summarize, generalize, or extract some features of our experiences and set aside others. We need to be able to draw on modes of thinking that are closely tied to our immediate experiences but also on those modes that provide us with distance and perspective.

There are six main parts to this book. These are interlocking and mutually reinforcing. To highlight overarching themes, each part begins with a set of brief "thinking prompts." Each part closes with a series of more personally directed "cross checks and queries" designed to encourage your reflection and suggest various connections to your own work and practice. Throughout we use diagrams and schematic illustrations to convey key concepts. Many parts also include separate "research highlights" and "thought boxes" that selectively extend ideas introduced in the main text. Words or phrases placed in boldface italics are further explained at the end of the book, in our "Concepts Guide."

In Part 1 we invite you to think about what an idea is. We introduce what we call "idea landscapes" as a way of helping you to think about when and how ideas come to mind and the pivotal role of our environments in prompting or precluding good ideas. We outline our science-based thinking framework—the integrated Controlled-Automatic, Specific-Abstract framework (iCASA)—for mental agility and creativity. We also introduce the importance of goals, especially open goals, in sculpting and shaping our idea landscapes.

Parts 2 and 3 develop the core ideas of what we call *detail stepping* (modulating our level of abstraction) and *control dialing* (varying our degree of cognitive control). Detail stepping and control dialing are metaphorical expressions coined to more tangibly and easily convey two central aspects of our thinking. Detail stepping refers to the level of abstractness of the content of our thinking, or *what* we are thinking about, and our ability to move up or down in levels of detail. Control dialing refers to the degree of cognitive control we are experiencing in the process of our thinking—the *how* of our thinking—and our ability to increase or decrease our degree of control. In Part 2, we illustrate the many ways in which we can capture and express our ideas at differing levels of abstraction. We explore how our environments and actions change our level of detail and impact our creative directions. Part 3 looks at how differing degrees of cognitive control shape creativity. At different times and in different ways we can benefit from varying our degrees of cognitive control—being more defocused or focused, more spontaneous or more deliberate.

In Part 4 we concentrate on the cyclical contributions of perception and action to innovative thinking and doing in our making-finding processes. We explore how constraints are both made and found, how we can introduce novelty into our worlds by learning to vary, and how we improvise collectively.

Part 5 expands our consideration of idea landscapes to groups and organizations. We underscore the importance not only of seeking novelty but also of recognizing when to wisely rely on already tested and proven approaches. We introduce the creatively significant concepts of adaptive expertise and of absorptive capacity for organizations in facilitating innovation and change.

In Part 6, the final part, we emphasize the temporal dimensions of organizational change and creativity in both the longer and the shorter term. We draw cross connections between autobiographical memory and organizational memory and knowledge. We walk through the key components of goal tuning—crucial for selecting and updating our goals and having them come to mind in our idea landscapes when and if we need them. This concluding part focuses again on the surprising ways in which our environments and shared idea landscapes may foster our efforts to initiate positive change and carry forward our creative ideals. We close by weaving together broader themes of the book with the five "thinking framework" questions, inviting you to draw further connections going forward—as together we rethink creativity to inspire change.

Our own generative and making/finding processes in researching and writing have been creatively cued by the generosity of readers of varying drafts of the manuscript. Joan Bossert, our editor at Oxford University Press, has been an ever-thoughtful and stalwart champion of the ideas behind and for the book from the beginning and has deftly guided us in ways large and small; for responsively and adeptly shepherding the manuscript process at OUP we thank Louis Gulino. Ben Denkinger and Shane Hoversten were receptive and envisioning readers, recognizing strengths and aptly calling for further strengths; John Kruse, of 3M user experience and product design, offered multiple insights and an expert practitioner's perspective; Chip Pitts offered bolstering words and valuable leads to sources we might otherwise have overlooked; our anonymous reviewers gave us incisive pointers and inspiring support. We thank our copyeditor Heidi Thaens for her watchful eye and attentive ear.

Our colleagues and students have been a source of explicit and implicit wisdom and intellectual sustenance across many years. We are grateful to so many creative exemplars—artists, scientists, thought leaders—who daily inspire and sustain us through their dedication, perseverance, and pioneering reach for promising newness.

For specific comments relating to our discussion of their research and thinking, for reading portions of our manuscript, or for permission to cite their work that is in progress, we thank Professor Jonathan Cagan, Department of Mechanical Engineering, Carnegie Mellon University; Professors Shawn Cole, Amy Edmondson, Karim Lakhani, and Ryan Raffaelli of the Harvard Business School; Alice Foxley, landscape architect at Studio Karst, earlier with Vogt Landscape Architects; Professor Liane Gabora, Department of Psychology, University of British Columbia; Professor David Kirsh, Department of Cognitive Science, University of California, San Diego; Alex Olson, a Los Angeles–based visual artist; Dr. Alonso Vera at NASA Ames Research Center; Professor Glenn Voss, Cox School of Business; and Professor Zannie Voss, Meadows School of the Arts, Southern Methodist University.

The artwork emerging through the book's front cover, and also animating the lettering, is called *Transitions*. Painted and photographed by Jon, the book's coauthor, the work was chosen to convey a sense of the ongoing interplay of thinking and acting in our experience, with the multiple variations and gradations of color suggesting dynamic continua and change.

Innovating Minds

Part 1

What Are Ideas, and Where Do They Come From?

Thinking prompts

- What is an idea?
- What are "open goals" and how can they help us to be more creative?
- How do our emotions, motivations, perceptions, and concepts work together?
- How do our various environments shape and guide innovative thinking?
- What forms of experience lead to enduring newness in our brains and our worlds?

We all at various times in our lives want or need to accomplish something creative or innovative. But where do good—or potentially good—new ideas come from? How do we manage our ideas and hold on to them? How do we capture them? How do we make or recognize promising ideas and skillfully revise them to become powerfully innovative, in order to promote positive change in the world, in ourselves, and in others? How can we as individuals and as organizations be more *innovative thinkers and doers*? How can we rethink creativity to inspire change?

OUR IDEA WORLDS, OUR IDEA LANDSCAPES

At the broadest level, all of our ideas occur in a set of three entwined and continuously changing worlds: our minds, our brains, and our environments. These are our "idea worlds." The dynamic interplay of these ever-present players in our thinking is pictured in Figure 1.1.

At the center of our idea worlds are our minds. This is where we perceive, categorize, remember, imagine, and reconceptualize what we experience. In our minds, we register the effects of our actions in the world and the progress we are making in the pursuit of our individual and collective endeavors. Here we also become aware of new aspirations and potential new directions,

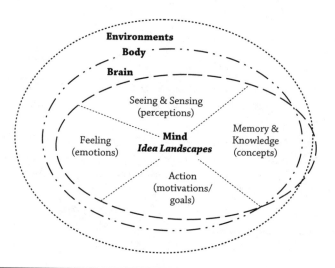

| OUR MINDS, BRAINS, AND ENVIRONMENTS ARE EQUALLY POWERFUL AND ALWAYS PRESENT PLAYERS IN PROMOTING CREATIVE IDEAS. | OUR IDEA WORLDS. Creative ideas are generated and realized at the dynamic intersections of our mind with our brain and our environments. The dotted and dashed lines are meant to represent the many permeable and reciprocally interacting relations of our environments (physical, social, symbolic) with our brains and minds across time. Our minds and thinking encompass more than our memory and knowledge; they also include seeing and sensing, feeling, and our intentions and motivations for action; we later refer to these four constituents of our thinking as concepts, perceptions, emotions, and motivations/goals. |

Figure 1.1

and experience the diverse emotions and motivations that accompany our efforts to act, learn, and change in the world. Within our minds some ideas are always reaching awareness and others are subsiding or still being formed. We will see later that these ongoing fluctuations in our thinking and awareness—what we call our *idea landscapes*—are at the core of our creative work.

Supporting and sustaining our minds is our immensely complex and dynamically changing brain—itself in close and continual interchange with our bodies as we think and act in our environments. Just like our selves, our brains are never the same from moment to moment. Our brains are ever eager to anticipate and predict. Based on what we sense and do, earlier predictions and anticipations are constantly being updated and fine-tuned. In our brains, learning and relearning is always "on."[1]

It is sometimes said that "the mind is what the brain does." This is, in good measure, true. Our minds emerge from the activity of our brain: neurons firing, integrating information, and communicating with one another across synapses, nodes, and networks. But this simple expression doesn't convey the whole picture. Our minds are supported, too, and constantly cued and called by our physical, social, and symbolic environments: words on a page or spoken to us, visual images, numbers or formulas, sounds and signals. And our ability to produce and interpret words, visual images, or numbers is not something we entirely accomplished individually in our lifetimes. It rests on and emerges from a sociocultural and linguistic heritage and forms of social organization that extend far beyond our individual brains.

The most direct and immediate environments for our minds and brains are our bodies. It is with our bodies that we physically encounter other objects, ourselves, and each other in an ongoing cycle of perceiving and acting. Our bodies influence both how we navigate and interact with the world and how we think. Through physically reworking forms, gesturing, glancing, moving through space, and turning our heads in shared attention we bring new information into our idea worlds and use this information to act once again.

Beyond our bodies, our environments extend in both time and space, encompassing symbolic and social interactions in all their rich complexity. The things we choose to see and do, the places we go, the people we know and return to, the tools we use, what we listen and attend to, what we ignore and what we are drawn to—these all dynamically inform and form our environments. Our environments carry memory and ideas forward. Think of the jottings that we scribble in the margins of our books, or the sketches and notes on our desks or desktops, or the assorted potential ingredients that we may survey before beginning to prepare a new culinary dish. We generate creative ideas not only individually but also collectively—as teams or in groups—based on our shared direct and indirect experiences. We elaborate on each other's ideas; one idea dovetails with another as we prompt and prod each other's thinking.

We cannot understand creativity or identify potential barriers to the generation of novel and innovative ideas and methods if we isolate our minds or brains from our environments. Our minds, brains, and environments are in perpetual interplay. It is at their intersections that new ideas emerge and can be realized.

A CREATIVE THINKING SCENARIO— TIMEKEEPING WITHOUT CLOCKS

Let's take part in a thinking exercise—drawn from the scientific research literature[2]—that will make these ideas more concrete and give us the opportunity to work through them closely. We will spend some time on this example and then revisit it in various parts of this book. We will draw on our experiences from this exercise to explore and connect the fundamental building blocks of our thinking framework.

Before we begin, please gather several sheets of blank paper and a pen or pencil so that you'll be able to capture and explain your ideas.

Imagine that you are asked to bring to mind multiple ways of keeping track of time. Your goal is to find ways of measuring out comparatively short periods of time—analogous to seconds, minutes, or hours—rather than longer periods such as days, weeks, or months.

You are by yourself, without a watch, clock, or any form of conventional timekeeping device, in a large windowless room with a 10-foot ceiling. There is a door with a doorknob and a hanging light fixture. The room also features a sink and drain with a working tap. The only other items available to you in the room are three rolls of adhesive tape and one each of the following:

A box of matches
A 1-quart plastic kitchen container (with lid)
A 1-gallon metal can of black latex paint (with lid)
A 2-inch-wide paintbrush with wooden handle
A 7-foot aluminum ladder
A 6-inch serrated hunting knife
A blue click-type ballpoint pen
A 12-inch wooden ruler
A 6-pound lead weight with hook
An 8-inch-tall candlestick with holder

A roll of twine
A thermometer
A large bottle of vodka

Your task is to think of as many different ways or processes as possible whereby you could use these materials to measure shorter periods of time. The time unit that you generate does not have to be any known unit except that it must be repeatable at a later point with a conventional clock.

Before reading further, please review the scenario above. Take about 10 minutes to try to generate some ideas for measuring the passage of short periods of time using the materials listed. For example, you might generate an idea such as lighting the candle by using one of the matches from the box of matches and then placing the thermometer a premeasured distance from the candle flame until the thermometer reached a designated temperature. Your unit of time would then be the time required for the burning candle to cause the thermometer to reach your chosen temperature.

Describe or draw your ideas on a piece of paper. Be patient and persistent. When you think that you have generated as many different ideas as you can, turn this page.

What came to your mind? What range of ideas did you explore? Did you think about counting a drip rate or the rate of flow of a liquid? Or did you consider the period of a pendulum, or the rate of an object falling freely or rolling downward owing to the force of gravity? Did you perhaps think about using your own actions in relation to one or more of the objects, such as rapidly clicking the ballpoint pen a certain number of times or rhythmically unrolling 12-inch sections of one of the rolls of adhesive tape, using the ruler as a guide?

Whatever ideas you had, where did they come from? How do possible novel approaches or actions come to mind in a situation such as this?

As you reflect on your own thinking processes, you may well find that there is no single or simple answer to these questions. Ideas may have come to you as you visualized the objects or imagined yourself handling and using them or grouping objects with each other. Or you may have remembered something from your own experiences or from something that you had read or been taught that you then connected to the task. Also, how you worked through and captured or expressed your ideas in sketches or diagrams may have prompted new ideas: the process of sketching or explaining your ideas may have automatically and with little effort "associatively cued" yet other ideas or possibilities. Perhaps you may have found yourself thinking of analogies or parallels from other situations.

The design scenario you just took part in was, in fact, actually used in a published experiment conducted with 71 senior undergraduate engineering students at Carnegie Mellon University. The study was designed to test the ways in which our creative and problem-solving goals influence how—and if—we use potentially relevant information that we may encounter in our environments. To explore this question, the published experiment included two additional twists.

The first twist was that different students were given different types of additional reading material. Some of the students were provided with detailed information about the mechanisms of various types of clocks (a grandfather clock, a windup clock, and a quartz wristwatch). Other students were, instead, given detailed information about the mechanisms and functions of various devices that were not clocks and thus only related by distant analogy to the problem (a water meter, a heart-rate monitor, and a cassette-tape recorder). The remaining students were given information that was entirely unrelated and not relevant to the problem (three current news stories or "filler material").

The second twist was that the additional information was presented at different *times* during the design task. Some of the engineering students were given additional information either before they had started working on the timekeeping problem or later, during a break, after they had already been thinking about it and begun to generate ideas. Specifically, some students read about clocks before beginning the design task (*clocks before group*). Other students read about other devices before they encountered the scenario (*devices before group*). Still other students read about other devices during their break, after they had already begun to work on the design problem (*devices during group*). Finally, the remaining students read only filler material, both initially and during the break, providing a baseline comparison group (*control group*).

The groups and the types of reading material they encountered before beginning the design task and later during the break are summarized in Table 1.1.

Which of the four groups do you think generated ideas of the greatest variety, or the most novel ideas? In thinking about your answers, imagine yourself in the place of someone proceeding through each sequence of events. Note what that person would have read and when he or she would have read it.

Do you think that being provided with a detailed description of the mechanisms and functions of clocks *before* the design task would help or instead hinder the generation of creative ideas? One possibility is that encountering the clock descriptions at the outset would lead people to focus more narrowly on accepted mechanisms of timekeeping. Another possibility, though, is that the richly detailed characterization of the different sorts of clocks and their mechanisms or functions would help to associatively trigger useful ideas.

And for those who read about other devices—unrelated to clocks—what effects might that have had on generating alternative ways to keep time?

Table 1.1 THE PROCEDURE FOR THE EXPERIMENT
ON TIMEKEEPING WITHOUT CLOCKS

Group	Initial reading	Begin design	Break reading	Resume design
Clocks before	Clocks	→	Filler	→→
Devices before	Devices	→	Filler	→→
Devices during	Filler	→	Devices	→→
Control	Filler	→	Filler	→→

Students in each of the four groups proceeded through the steps as shown, starting with the initial reading and then moving into the first phase of idea generation, (Begin design), followed by a break with designated readings and then returning back to their idea generation (Resume design).[3]

How could reading about a cassette-tape player or a water meter, for example, help one to think of timekeeping approaches? Are such examples too far removed or remote from the problem at hand to be useful? Or is the distance of the example itself beneficial? Would it matter if the students read about other devices before they began the design task, or rather later, during their break after they had begun working and had a fuller understanding of what the task required? Why do you think so?

Let's first take the group who started out by reading the detailed descriptions of the mechanisms and functions of three different kinds of clocks. How did they do compared with the students who started out by reading about the other kinds of devices before they began the design task? The students who at the outset read about the functions and mechanisms of clocks generated a similar number of ideas, but those ideas were rated as *higher in novelty* than those of the group who started out by reading about the more distantly related water meter, cassette-tape player, and heart-rate monitor. This suggests that the rich descriptions of different timepieces and how they worked helped to prime or associatively trigger new ideas. In contrast, encountering the descriptions of comparatively distantly related devices before starting the task did not help promote novel thinking.

But what if, instead, the detailed functions and mechanisms of distantly related devices were encountered during the break—*after* the students had already been thinking about and working through, for a short time, the problem-solving exercise? The results for this group were different. When the group received the distant examples—such as those of the heart-rate monitor and the cassette-tape player—after they had already been thinking about the design problem, these distant examples significantly boosted the novelty of their ideas and suggestions. The novelty of their solutions was significantly greater than that of the group which encountered the distant analogies only at the outset. Why would this be so? Why would the *timing* of reading identical materials make such a difference in the students' creative performance?

A key difference between the groups is that only those who had been thinking about the design problem had reason or motivation to notice the potential *relevance* of the functional descriptions of the apparently unrelated devices. Students who had already been introduced to the problem and were actively struggling with it were likely sensitized to and *ready* for any ideas or connections of ideas that might possibly help them. These students would also encode, process, and categorize potentially relevant information in a more goal-guided way. For these students, reading about such remotely associated ideas and functions as the displacement of water and the measurement of water flow or the idea of a magnetic tape moving through a recording head with tension or traction helped spark new creative approaches for measuring time as they linked these ideas to the materials at hand. Upon reading about the cassette-tape player they might, for example, suddenly imagine successively unwinding 12-inch units of adhesive tape.

In contrast, this was not the case for those who had not yet been introduced to the design problem and had no particular goals in mind when they read the apparently unrelated device descriptions. For these participants, the relevance of the descriptions at the time that they read them was not clear, so they likely encoded and mentally processed the material in a more generic and less problem-focused way. Distant analogies or distant information can facilitate creative conjunctions, but such far-removed comparisons or relations have to come to mind in the first place, and they also need to be accessible to our minds when we need them.

There are always many things and ideas competing for our awareness. What, then, determines which of these many possibilities gain entry into our awareness? Major contributors are the *open goals* that we have and that we are striving to achieve.

Generally, "a goal can be [conceptualized] as a future-oriented image of an ideal occurrence, stored in memory for comparison with actual occurrences."[4] Open goals, or pending goals, are aims or intentions that we have but that are not yet met or that are incompletely realized. They are aims that we are still working toward, either in the foreground or in the background of our awareness. Such open goals tend to remain more highly neurally activated and so help to guide our perception, what we notice, and where our attention is drawn. Our ongoing goals or projects can lead us to notice the possible connections and relevance of even quite distant information.[5]

Open goals increase the likelihood that distantly related [ideas] become incorporated into problem solving. These distantly related ideas may spur innovative or creative solutions.[6]

—*Engineering and design researchers Ian Tseng, Jarrod Moss, Jonathan Cagan, and Kenneth Kotovsky on their "timekeeping without clocks" experiment*

Information is helpful only if it is mentally accessible to us at the right time. Open goals allow us to notice selectively and purposively. Ongoing, unfulfilled, as yet unmet aspirations change what we see as relevant, so that what might otherwise escape attention draws our attention because it is connected to our pending goals. Encountering a piece of scrap metal along a bike path may evoke a very different response from a sculptor who uses everyday objects in her work than it would from a cyclist enjoying his new bicycle. Even simply reminding ourselves of our broader goal of being creative can attune us to new possibilities and lead us to draw unexpected and surprising associations.[7]

Open goals are related to the process of "brooding" on an unsolved ("unhatched") problem known as **incubation**. After reaching an impasse or block in our prolonged deliberate problem-solving efforts, we may turn our attention elsewhere, and suddenly experience an "aha!" or "Eureka!" moment.[8] Unlike incubation, open goals are relevant to all phases of our thinking and creative endeavors, not just at times of impasse. In Part 3, we take up the topic of incubation and the closely related ideas of times in between and the importance of taking the right types of breaks.

Our open goals, in combination with direct and indirect promptings and constraints from our environment, shape the unfolding progress of our idea repertoires. Consider the results of a field study with an expert practitioner of traditional Chinese ink painting. Researchers asked the painter to create two sets of large paintings on the theme of the four seasons: one set of paintings on completely blank surfaces and a second set on surfaces each already containing 15 random lines drawn by the experimenters. The painter devoted more time to the paintings in which he had to incorporate the random lines, and the paintings were found to be livelier and more interesting both by the painter and as judged by others who had no knowledge of how the paintings had been created.[9] Like everyday found objects, the random lines introduced their own features and their own unique specificity, which initiated and permitted fresh approaches within the painter's habitual expertise.

Ideas and cross-connections among ideas are always forming and fluctuating in and out of our awareness, prompted by what we are seeing and doing. We use the term **idea landscape** to refer to the relative ease of bringing to mind ideas (or intimations of ideas) from the past, present, or anticipated future. As we will see in the upcoming section, our idea landscapes consist of "peaks and valleys" with information at the peaks currently within our conscious awareness and information in the valleys not currently readily accessible to us.

At any one moment, some of our experiences may be available in our long-term knowledge but not necessarily easily brought to mind. Take, for example, the "tip of the tongue" phenomenon. Sometimes we know a given fact or name but are temporarily unable to effectively retrieve it. But if we recollect where we may have met someone, his or her name may suddenly pop into our awareness. We usually have one thing as the focus of our attention, with several other things not currently in our focal awareness but in our peripheral awareness. In our short-term working memory—that smaller set of ideas that we are currently most directly and intentionally working with in our minds—often one or two ideas may be especially accessible to us.[10]

If we are to optimize our **creativity** and **innovation** as individuals and teams, we need to understand how our goals and environments interplay with our idea landscapes. The ways in which we initially select, activate, and responsively update our goals based on the progress and obstacles we may encounter are discussed in depth in Parts 4 and 6, where we introduce the processes that we call *making and finding* and *goal tuning*. Before that, though, we first need to develop a broader perspective on our thinking framework, beginning with the core concept of idea landscapes.

INTRODUCING OUR THINKING FRAMEWORK

Several years ago we encountered a deceptively simple single-panel newspaper cartoon. In the cartoon, two individuals are standing before a company bulletin board upon which is tacked a large one-word notice in bold letters: **Think!** The two look at each other quizzically and one asks, "What do you suppose it means?"[11]

What *does* "thinking" mean? That question is at the heart of this book.

Having asked this question, we find that there is a tangle of things that need to be considered. There's how ideas prompt other ideas, there's how objects (like cartoons) and people (conversations, passing remarks) turn our thinking in new directions, there's how our efforts are met with success or obstacles and how we feel about that, there's whether pen and paper or a digital device will be ready to hand as we develop an idea, there's how people in groups and groups of groups meet and share thoughts. No one of these alone is "thinking"—thinking is all of these and more in dynamic interplay. So how can we understand and talk about thinking? This is where the thinking framework comes in.

Our thinking framework is a way of orienting ourselves and keeping ourselves oriented in that tangle of things that we need to consider. A framework is not a solid block but more of a lattice or support. Once we have a framework, we can understand how the varied pieces fit together and relate one to another. Applied to creativity and change, our framework allows us to move from just a "listing" or cataloguing of discrete items to seeing how what seems unconnected is, in fact, connected.

Even though each thought and every creative thought is singular, there are patterns. We can learn the patterns, and understanding the patterns can help us to get "unstuck" in our thinking and prevent us from getting stuck in the first place. By understanding the thinking framework we may find reasons to be more patient with our own and others' thinking. We may become more tolerant of the apparent indirection and waywardness of our thinking and more ready to notice when we should just let thinking "run" by itself and when we should deliberately intervene. We may become more sensitive to moments when we should zoom out or zoom in or when, instead, we should adopt a midlevel of **abstraction**, setting aside some details but highlighting others. Thinking itself changes as we learn more about our own thinking.

There are many factors that, together, contribute to the successful generation and iterative realization of good ideas. The integrative thinking framework for creativity and change that we develop in this book encompasses five key, interrelated factors: idea landscapes; levels of detail/abstraction; degrees of mental control; the interplay of concepts, emotions, motivations/goals, and perception; and our dynamic environments/dynamic brains. We discuss each of these five factors in turn before bringing them all together in what we call our **integrated Controlled-Automatic, Specific-Abstract (iCASA) thinking framework**.

1. Idea Landscapes

Thinking Framework Question 1:

What ideas are competing for your attention and awareness, and how are you helping to form and *re*-form them?

We can think of our thoughts, or mental representations of ideas, as continually moving in and out of our awareness in an ongoing, changing mental landscape. Ideas are mental representations or "*re*-presentations" in our minds of one or more aspects of external or internal things, events, relations, or processes. Mental representations that are accessible are ideas that are readily brought into our awareness or into our thinking processes. That is, we can access or reach them when—and if—we need them. We use the metaphor of "idea landscapes" to refer to these ongoing undulations in how readily we can access or bring ideas to mind. Ideas need time to emerge and to configure and reconfigure; they need time and space to take form, to connect, and reconnect.

At any one time some ideas are in peak or focal awareness and others are in our peripheral awareness. Still other ideas are not currently in our conscious awareness but are potentially available if we attempt to recall them or if they are brought to the forefront of our awareness because of something or someone we encounter. These ongoing fluctuations as ideas surface and recede from our awareness are conveyed schematically in Figure 1.2. We can both shape and be shaped by our idea landscapes.

Imagine for a moment that you happen to overhear someone say the word "green." This simple auditory event might associatively prompt or cue thoughts in your mind about plants and nature, about freshness, or about unripeness. It might also, either instead or concurrently, elicit thoughts

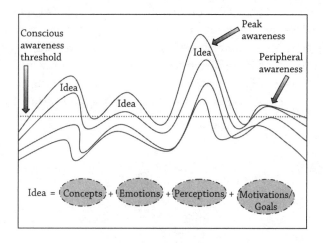

OUR IDEAS CAN BE THOUGHT OF AS RISING AND FALLING ABOVE AND BELOW OUR AWARENESS, AS IF IN A MENTAL LANDSCAPE OF PEAKS AND VALLEYS.	OUR IDEA LANDSCAPES. In this highly schematic depiction, ideas are continually arising, subsiding, and recombining in our conscious awareness, with some ideas in peak or focal awareness and others in peripheral awareness. Ideas that are readily reached and brought to mind are accessible to us. Ideas are admixtures of concepts, emotions, perceptions, and motivations/goals: These are the four interrelated constituents of our ideas and of our thinking. The dashed lines around the ovals indicate that concepts, emotions, perceptions, and motivations/goals frequently interact and intermingle in our thinking. The multiple flowing lines represent the many threads and fluctuating paths of our moment-to-moment ideas and their changing combinations.

Figure 1.2

about environmentalism, or (by way of common analogies) connections to inexperience and naivete, to money, or even envy. Which of these many possibilities occur or co-occur to you is shaped by your immediately prior, current, and longer-term experiences. Your experiences are carried in mental representations—and neural connections between representations—that vary in how readily they can be accessed and recombined.

Our mental ***representations*** are multiple and overlapping neuronal ensembles that code and encode our sensory, conceptual, and emotional experiences of the world and our actions. These highly interconnected interacting groups of neurons are made up of many nodes, synapses, and networked pathways that register and store different kinds of information. They combine, cull, contrast, and encapsulate features and relations from our experiences. A few partially overlapping neuronal ensembles with their shared and distinct features are depicted abstractly in Figure 1.3.

Mental representations can differ widely in how stable or robust they are to disruption. Some representations (and relations among representations) are comparatively fleeting or transient and may require ongoing attention, cognitive effort, or support from our immediate environment to be maintained in our awareness. Support—and also potentially disruption, interference, or derailment—may come from our physical and social environment

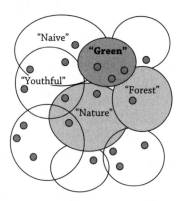

PREVIOUSLY ASSOCIATED IDEAS CAN CUE ONE ANOTHER, PROMPTING SIMILAR OR MORE DISTANT CONNECTIONS IN OUR MINDS.	MENTAL REPRESENTATIONS AS NEURONAL ENSEMBLES. Ideas are highly interconnected and overlapping in our brain, with shared features and also distinct features (small filled circles) that potentially can lead to the activation of associated representations. For example, here the concept of green is activated (dark gray) and leads to the activation of the associated concepts of nature and forest (light gray).[12]

Figure 1.3

and our individual and varied interactions with it. Notes, sketches, maps, gestures, prototypes, video and audio recordings, as well as our shared memories all may help us to form, capture, and elaborate ideas.[13]

Much of our knowledge and prior learning is stored within distributed regions of our brains through connected patterns of neurons that are not currently actively firing. These latent representations (synaptic weightings and connectivity among neurons and neuronal assemblies) of what we know and can imagine or reexperience are not currently in the forefront of conscious awareness or within our awareness at all. Yet these concepts and memories can be brought actively into mind and *reconstructed* in the present through a change of our internal or external context or changes in our needs and goals. We have vast amounts of information stored and potentially available in our memory that is not accessible until it is reactivated through an environmental, emotional, physiological, or other trigger. Such triggers or cues are constantly shifting and sifting our awareness; they are essential partners in our idea landscapes.[14]

Returning to our example of your chancing to overhear someone say the word "green" and the varied thoughts it brought to mind, what mental representations may have been called upon? First let's begin with the sound of the word that you heard. The sound of the word "green" unfolded in time. After processing the initial sounds "gr" or "gre," your brain may already have anticipated a number of possible completions to the sounds—such as "great," "greet," or "group"—with one or more of these words momentarily becoming more readily accessible to you even if it didn't fully reach your conscious awareness.

Based on our past experiences, our brains will rapidly anticipate—on the order of about a quarter of a second—what the multiple possible words that we are hearing or reading may turn out to be. Once we have heard the full word, our brains focus in on that word alone and suppress the incorrect anticipations.[15] Upon hearing the entire word "green," your brain may have accessed additional sensory-perceptual and conceptual-categorical information. You may have identified the word as related to color and also possibly to a narrower or wider range of hues such as emerald green or lime green. At the same time or soon after, your notion of green may have become associatively linked to emotional and evaluative responses such as the positive connotations of green, suggesting freshness or spring or youthfulness. ***Associative cuing*** is a pervasive presence in our idea landscapes, encompassing sound or visually based promptings as well as semantic or meaning-based associations.

More generally, mental representations can be spatial, action-like, or object-like. They can carry information about concepts, emotions or affect, motivations, and perceptions. Mental representations enable us to have an internal *mental model* of the world and of our relations to the environment and to one another. Crucially, our mental representations allow us to think about things, events, and people even when they are not physically present. Variations in the ease with which we can access and use our mental representations are fundamental to our ability to draw on prior learning and experiences and to imagine and create possible futures.

Our idea landscapes can be shared. They can overlap, to differing degrees, with those of other individuals or groups with whom we interact or organizations to which we belong. Such sharing of ideas across groups, large and small, is portrayed in Figure 1.4. Our idea landscapes are influenced by those with whom we communicate, whether we are physically in the same space, and how often we communicate with one another or even if we know one another. Groups and organizations, just like individuals, may form collective idea landscapes across times and spaces, developing group memories,

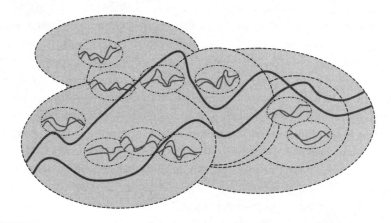

WE CONTINUALLY SHARE—AND DRAW UPON—THE IDEA LANDSCAPES OF OTHERS.	IDEA LANDSCAPES ARE SHARED ACROSS INDIVIDUALS, GROUPS, AND ORGANIZATIONS. Individuals (smallest ovals) simultaneously share membership in multiple concurrent and partially overlapping teams or groups (clusters of ovals) within an organization (largest ovals). Within groups, as in individuals, there may be multiple streams of ideas and connections among ideas fluctuating in and out of conscious awareness (represented by the flowing lines). Groups and organizations dynamically form and change their idea landscapes through their interactions and communications.

Figure 1.4

emotions, and knowledge for acting together through routines or established procedures.

The collective knowledge of a team or organization can take shape in different and interrelated ways: shared, complementary, or embedded in artifacts. Collective knowledge can be experiences, beliefs, or expertise held in common (shared) by each group member. In addition, collective knowledge might be distributed among and across the members of a group, with individuals offering differing complementary types of expertise and experience that is then combined, coordinated, and integrated—leading to a whole that is greater than the sum of its parts. Collective knowledge may also, in parallel, be captured and carried forward in physical and symbolic artifacts created or used by a group. Documented procedures, intranet resources or databases, organizational structures, and formal or informal routines are all forms of collective knowledge.[16]

With experience, we gain mutual understanding of how we think and how we think together. We form *shared mental models* of where we are and where we want to go. A mental model is our understanding of the relations between events, objects, or people. Mental models are cognitive representations that help us reason about the world and how things and tasks are configured and interrelated. When we have a shared mental model we have a common basic understanding about how events or processes will likely unfold. With a shared mental model we can efficiently coordinate our efforts and step in to help each other in the face of both surprise *and* the fully expected.

Shared mental models, by ensuring that we "are on the same page," allow us to act proactively to help each other because we understand what we each are facing. Many well-performing teams may communicate directly with each other *less often* because their communication needs are reduced given their shared mental model. Think of a baseball or basketball team or the members of a jazz quartet who have long played and worked together.[17] Shared mental models can enable us to move beyond simple cooperation toward full collaboration as we work toward our creative goals. As we will see in Part 5, we can be prompted to develop team mental models through a process of individually and then collectively clarifying our goals, identifying and selecting feasible approaches, recognizing explicit and implicit constraints, and coordinating shared knowledge.[18]

Interpreting and making meaning of our collective experiences is a multidirectional process whereby we attempt to understand and act together into the future. In sensemaking we aim to evaluate events, what they mean, and arrive at shared team, group, or organizational understandings and plans of action.[19] The widely integrative process of **sensemaking** is "a motivated, continuous effort to understand connections (which can be among people, places, and events) in order to anticipate their trajectories and act effectively."[20] In sensemaking we continually strive to interpret where we are in the ongoing streaming of experience and what it means. We try to incorporate a range of perspectives to arrive at an overarching sense of organizational meaning and identity. We iteratively ask, "What's going on here?" and "What do I do next?"[21] Both individually and collectively, we strive to act and anticipate with informed foresight.[22]

Evolving, shepherding, and successively realizing our ideas for creativity and change critically depends on how our individual idea landscapes interact with those of others and the shared idea landscapes that we build together. Our idea landscapes are stretched and pulled in promising new directions by the individuals and groups we encounter.

People who are in idea contact—both formally and informally—with different groups and subgroups have the potential for novel and creative idea intersections arising from diverse perspectives and experiences. We can generate new ideas more readily when we and our ideas bridge many different idea cultures with their divergent approaches, expertise, and receptivities.[23]

2. Levels of Detail

Thinking Framework Question 2:

Are you aptly zooming in and zooming out?

Imagine that we see two children playing with a ball. We could think of the color of the ball, the children's clothing, their heights, their movements through space, the concept of gravity, cooperative and collaborative play, the fleetingness of childhood, or the hope and promise of new generations. These various ideas differ in their level of abstraction, with some more specifically focused on the current scenario and others more cross-situational or general. The children's ball could have its own unique history of scuffs and dents and smudges, and from this perspective it is one of a kind. The children's ball could also remind us, and them, of the many times they had spent together on warm summer evenings and cool, misty autumn mornings, playing and sharing, competing and learning new skills, in deepening friendship.

We can think of our experiences at multiple levels of generality and detail, from unique, one-of-a-kind and one-of-a-time and one-of-a-space occurrences to clusters of similar but not identical experiences. The categories we choose and how we conjoin them may also vary in how narrow or broad they are and the particular dimensions on which they are based: playing in summer or autumn, playing baseball or soccer. No one level of generality or detail is necessarily a more accurate, informative, or useful characterization. All of the levels may be valuable at different times and for different purposes. Maximizing our mental agility and creativity across times and situations requires us to flexibly span the full extent of possible levels of specificity.

> You don't really want to say "the tree," you want to say "the sycamore".... We seem to be able to relate to detail. We seem to have an appetite for it.[24]
>
> —Poet and musician Leonard Cohen

> But as to all the detail, I think that's almost something I have to curb. I cannot tell a story without wanting to say what kind of house people lived in, if it was brick, what color of brick, what there was in the kitchen, and all sorts of things that can become too much of a weight, and sometimes I do consciously try to cut them down a bit.[25]
>
> —Nobel Laureate in Literature Alice Munro

Our thinking about events and objects and their interrelations can take place at many levels of detail or **abstraction**. Sometimes our thinking can be comparatively more concrete or specific. At other times it can be relatively more abstract or general. From moment to moment and across time our concepts vary in their level of detail, as do our motivations/goals, emotions, and perceptions. There is, as shown in Figure 1.5, a continuum of abstraction in all of our thinking, ranging from the specific and detailed to the highly general and abstract, with many midlevel abstractions in between.

In the course of any given creative or design project, research shows that we move up and down and in between numerous levels of abstraction and specificity. Prompted by what we see and find in our efforts at discovering or making—or as we are revising and realizing an emergent creative intention—we may ascend and descend in the level of abstraction in our thinking. We may repeatedly climb or jump from the specific to the abstract and the abstract back to the specific, going from detail to midlevel to abstract and multiple intervening levels.[26]

Moving up and down in our levels of abstraction and specificity enables us to progressively guide and constrain our creative, **design**, and problem-solving

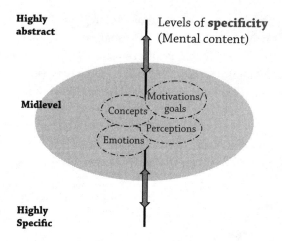

Highly abstract

Levels of **specificity**
(Mental content)

Midlevel

Concepts   Motivations/ goals

Emotions   Perceptions

Highly Specific

OUR CONCEPTS, PERCEPTIONS, EMOTIONS, AND MOTIVATIONS/ GOALS VARY IN THEIR LEVEL OF SPECIFICITY FROM HIGHLY ABSTRACT TO MIDLEVEL TO HIGHLY SPECIFIC.	THINKING TAKES PLACE AT MANY AND VARYING LEVELS OF ABSTRACTION. Here the vertical dimension or axis represents varying levels of specificity in each of the four interrelated constituents of our thinking. The large oval represents our momentary idea landscape, with its peaks and valleys of ideas entering, forming, and receding from awareness. Optimizing our creativity and mental agility requires adaptively moving across a wide range of levels of abstraction or specificity, with no one level of detail always best.

Figure 1.5

efforts, capturing and refining ideas in our continually changing idea landscapes. We may have a "big picture" or "in the large" understanding of what we hope and need to achieve. But we also need to work through the many concrete "in the small" steps needed to reach that overarching goal.

Gaining insight into the concrete particulars may inform our big-picture goals and vice versa, with each mutually advancing our creative progress. In working through a complex issue, identifying a given problem may require us to step down and notice another even more concrete problem that is contributing to the one we first identified; stepping down may also lead us to notice an opportunity we had not previously recognized. In our thinking we are repeatedly moving and "branching" between problem and subproblem identification, solution identification, and noticing new opportunities for acting.[27]

Researchers asked two highly experienced computer programmers to think aloud as they thought through an open-ended, design problem that was not clearly defined. Analyses of what the programmers said revealed that their thinking moved frequently back and forth from higher-level abstractions to more concrete or midlevels of detail. Although across the entire design session the overall level of the engineers' thinking moved from highly abstract to very concrete, there were many micromoments where they "stepped down" a level or two and then back up one or more levels, only then to step down again.

The precise thinking patterns differed between the two designers, but both showed repeated steps up and down, ascending and descending in their levels of abstraction. "The designers expanded their solutions by rapidly shifting between levels of abstraction and developing low-level partial solutions prior to a high-level [problem] decomposition. . . . The designers interleaved problem specification, that is the inference of new requirements, with solution development throughout the session."[28]

A simplified depiction of one designer's thinking process as he worked through the design problem is shown in Figure 1.6.

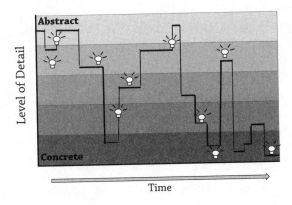

WE MOVE UP AND DOWN IN OUR LEVELS OF ABSTRACTION AS WE DEVELOP AND EXPAND OUR UNFOLDING IDEAS.	DESIGNERS FLEXIBLY CHANGE THEIR LEVELS OF ABSTRACTION. Across time, designers worked through potential solutions at many levels of detail. They experienced insights (here represented by lightbulbs) at varying levels of abstraction in response to emerging opportunities or difficulties.[29]

Figure 1.6

The level of abstraction that is right for us at any given time is influenced by many features of our situation, such as our or our team's level of experience in the field of endeavor or task at hand as well as our or our group's particular ways of best learning and creating. Ideally we can adroitly move up or down in our level of detail in our idea landscapes as our goals and changing contexts require. We need deep and close immersion in particulars and concreteness. Equally we need conceptual distancing to extract, see, and pursue larger patterns, categories, and goals.

Flexibly moving between differing levels of detail or abstraction is what we metaphorically refer to as **detail stepping**. Across time and our changing situations we are continually adjusting our levels of detail or specificity in our concepts, emotions, perception, and motivations/goals. Some of those adjustments or changes may be intentionally selected by us. Others may be indirectly or directly induced through our environments.

Often we may overvalue abstraction.[30] To counteract an excessive emphasis on abstraction and to underscore the remarkable contributions of concrete particulars throughout our creative processes, we use the term "detail stepping" rather than "abstraction stepping." It is possible to be too abstract as well as to be too detailed, and we need to move repeatedly between greater and lesser levels of specificity during our creative pursuits.

Detail stepping, as we will see in Part 2, is a crucial but often overlooked contributor to both sparking and adaptively carrying forward creativity and change.

3. Degrees of Control

Thinking Framework Question 3:

Do you allow room for both spontaneity *and* deliberateness in your thinking?

Not all of our thinking is deliberate. Some of our thinking, including sometimes our most creative thinking, appears to simply "happen" or "occur" to us rather than being intentionally generated. Our thinking and acting can vary across multiple degrees of cognitive control. Sometimes we can be exceedingly "top-down" and intentionally directed in our thinking. At other times we may be relatively spontaneous or improvisational. At still other moments we may find ourselves following thought patterns that are quite automatic, habitual, or routine. All of these degrees of mental control may interweave in our thinking as we pursue creativity and positive change.

Consider, for example, a simple type of word problem. You are given three apparently unrelated words and are asked to think of a fourth word that is associatively related to all three words and that can form a phrase with each of those words. For example, the apparently unrelated words "age," "mile," and "sand" all share an association with "stone": "Stone Age," "milestone," and "sandstone." What single word is associated with "reading," "service," and "stick"? Or what word is common to "baby," "spring," and "cap"? How can you access or identify the word that can be combined with each of the other three words in the group to meet the requirements?

One approach might be through spontaneous insight: the solution word may seem to automatically and suddenly pop into your mind. Another approach, though, could be more deliberate and systematic. No sudden insights occur, but you instead successively seek out and try out different alternatives for pairs of the unrelated words until you find a solution that works.

Researchers using such simple word problems (sometimes called remote associate problems, compound remote associate problems, or word triplets) have found that, for different problems, participants sometimes find solutions by insight and sometimes by deliberate search. Research has shown that highly creative individuals can flexibly move between different degrees of cognitive control, varying their degree of deliberateness and top-down control. At times creative individuals persistently search for an idea and at other times they flexibly allow themselves more spontaneous and undirected thinking. Both deliberate and spontaneous thinking have a key role in creative and agile thought and action.[31] (Incidentally, the answers for the two remote associate problems given earlier are "lip" and "shower.")

The abstractness versus concreteness of our thinking involves the "what" of our thought—that is, the representational *content* of our thinking. Degrees of control, instead, are about the "how" of our thinking, the *manner of our thinking process*, rather than the what.

Our levels of deliberate attention, effort, and planfulness form a continuum, admitting of many variations. Alterations in our degree of cognitive control, whether induced by us or by our circumstances, are what we refer to as **control dialing**. We believe it may be easier to understand degrees of control through the metaphor of a dial—a dial that we ourselves can turn toward greater or lesser degrees of cognitive control or that our circumstances may adjust toward deliberateness, spontaneity, or habit. A dial can be turned in a single sweep, through gradual increments, or held at a particular setting.

The problem is this: you don't want to be working completely in the dark, but if you have too much control, then nothing works out well. . . . I try to let in the unexpected as I'm working like mad to control it.[32]

—*Contemporary photographer James Welling*

Just as for our levels of detail or abstraction, no one of these degrees of control is necessarily more productive, valuable, or effective. Rather, to optimize our creative potential we need to be able to contextually adjust our degree of cognitive control. Sometimes we need to move toward greater deliberateness or, instead, toward greater spontaneity or reliance on well-learned procedures or associations. As we see in Figure 1.7, our thinking may occur at any one of multiple points on a continuum of cognitive control, influencing how

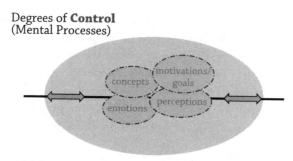

Degrees of **Control**
(Mental Processes)

Highly Controlled   Spontaneous   Highly Automatic

| WE CAN USE AND ACCESS OUR CONCEPTS, PERCEPTIONS, EMOTIONS, AND MOTIVATIONS/ GOALS THROUGH VARYING DEGREES OF CONTROL, RANGING FROM HIGHLY CONTROLLED TO SPONTANEOUS TO HIGHLY AUTOMATIC. | THINKING INVOLVES MANY AND VARYING DEGREES OF COGNITIVE CONTROL. Here the horizontal dimension or axis represents varying degrees of control in each of the four interrelated constituents of our thinking. The large oval represents our momentary idea landscape, with its peaks and valleys of ideas entering, forming, and receding from awareness. Optimizing our creativity and mental agility requires adaptively moving across a wide range of degrees of mental control, with no one degree of control always best. |

Figure 1.7

we generate concepts and the degree of spontaneity or automaticity of our motivations, emotions, and perceptions.

Adjustments or changes in our degree of cognitive control may be deliberately selected by us or indirectly or directly induced by our environments. Upon encountering an unexpected obstacle, we may often increase our effort and attention, focusing more intently and purposively on the task at hand. If, though, the situation continues to unfold as we expect, we may ease back into a more habitual mode of responding.

Observing experienced surgeons in the operating room, researchers found that the surgeons frequently adapted their degree of control on a moment-by-moment basis. The surgeons would speed up or slow down in response to emerging cues and constantly monitor their changing situation. When they slowed down, they were not necessarily physically slowing down in their movements but rather deepening their focus and regrouping their mental effort. The diverse ways in which the surgeons modulated their cognitive control are outlined in the research highlight in Part 3, titled "Varying Degrees of Control in the Operating Room."[33]

No one point on the continuum of cognitive control (deliberate to spontaneous to automatic) is invariably appropriate across all situations, and in any one situation we may often rapidly shuttle between many degrees of control. It is possible to be overcontrolled as well as undercontrolled. Depending on our changing contexts and goals, we need, as we will see in Part 3, to move repeatedly between greater and lesser degrees of cognitive control during our creative pursuits and problem solving.

4. The Intermingling of Concepts With Feeling, Perceiving, and Motivations/Goals

Thinking Framework Question 4:

As you think, are you using the full interplay not only of concepts but also of sensing, feeling, and well-chosen action goals?

Although we have separate words for concepts, perception, emotions, and motivations and these do, to some extent, refer to different aspects of our experience, the boundaries between them are not closed but rather are permeable and interpenetrating. Perceiving, feeling, acting, and categorizing often blend seamlessly in our thinking.

Think about your idea of an elephant. What comes to mind when you think of an elephant? Some of what you bring to mind is sensory or perceptual in nature—the sheer size and immense weight of an elephant, its exquisitely maneuverable trunk and the leathered and weathered texture of its skin, or its distinctively affecting trumpeting call. You might also know where elephants are likely to live, how long they live, their diet, and their long gestation period; you might be aware of their intelligence and complex social structure. These conceptual or encyclopedic forms of knowledge meld with the sensory-perceptual information you have acquired about these magnificent animals. Removing either form of knowledge would substantially impair your understanding of everything that the word "elephant" means.

Now think about your idea of anger. What comes to mind in this case? You may perhaps think of actions and ways of acting or intending to act when you see someone who is angry, one who is sulking in quiet fury or explosively slamming doors. You may then experience a flood of ideas relating to frustration and pent-up energy, impediments, and obstacles to goals. Here our sense of the feelings associated with anger and our notions of angry-like actions and angry-like motivations are closely intertwined and mutually cohering. A notion of anger devoid of any suggestions of action or motivation would scarcely qualify as a concept of anger at all.

We also have ideas about relations and relations of relations, such as cause and effect or a domino effect in which one event sparks a series of subsequent events. These ideas also carry perceptual-motor information, as when we imagine a domino falling forward onto another and then another, and then another again. Other relations are more visual-perceptual, as when we think of similar items as nearer to one another, inside of one another, as clustered together, or of bridging, bordering, bolstering, or branching.

Each of the four major constituents of our thinking (concepts, perceptions, emotions, and motivations/goals), as illustrated in Figure 1.8, are continually represented and intermingling in our multidimensional idea landscapes.

This intermingling is also occurring in our brains. Based on our previous experiences, our brains have formed extensive overlapping, interconnected, distributed neural networks that continually help us to make sense of, interpret, and remember new information. These interconnections dynamically link and interrelate our perception to concepts, our concepts to emotion, our emotion to our concepts, and our concepts to action. Changes in any one of these constituents can influence the others in a reciprocal and mutually interactive manner.[34]

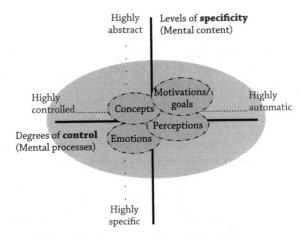

Figure 1.8

CREATIVE THINKING DRAWS NOT ONLY ON OUR CONCEPTS BUT ALSO ON OUR PERCEPTIONS, EMOTIONS, AND MOTIVATIONS/GOALS. THESE FOUR CONSTITUENTS OF OUR THINKING DYNAMICALLY INFLUENCE AND INTERACT WITH ONE ANOTHER.	THINKING INVOLVES MORE THAN CONCEPTS. Although we have separate words for perceiving, feeling, acting, and categorizing, and these do, to some extent, refer to different aspects of our experience, the boundaries between them are not closed but instead are permeable—as shown here by the porous and overlapping smaller ovals. The large oval represents our momentary idea landscape, with its peaks and valleys of ideas entering, forming, and receding from awareness.

Research Highlight: *Getting Creative—Thinking Warm-ups*

Our idea landscapes and thinking processes often implicitly carry over from one situation to another. Simply asking people to think about different ways to use a familiar object, such as a paper clip or a chair, for as little as 10 minutes improved their ability to later solve entirely unrelated insight problems and other novel visuospatial reasoning problems. The participants who thought of novel uses for objects outperformed those who were asked simply to generate the first words that came to their minds in a word-association task. The "novel uses" participants also were more insightful and more flexible problem solvers than were another group of control participants who were given no task at all.[35]

Why might engaging in this "novel uses" activity increase insight and problem-solving flexibility? Generating new and unconventional uses for objects relies on many different mental and imaginative processes but especially invites us to think in more concrete and perceptually specific ways. This may help us to see beyond a standard or conventional response, attuning us to new possibilities. We know that perceptual noticing is important in creative thinking and the generation of hypotheses.[36]

The generating of alternative uses for objects also invites us to use different mental categories, including goal-related categories, and to use differing degrees of mental control, ranging from spontaneous thinking to deliberate strategic thinking. Indeed, other researchers have found that asking people to engage in verbal or musical improvisation exercises subsequently increased the fluency, originality, and flexibility of their thinking on the novel uses task.[37] Engaging in a divergent thinking activity, such as the alternative uses task, which encourages a wide and varied range of responses without any one single correct answer, may alter the level of stringency or tightness of our cognitive control. Such divergent thinking tasks may induce "a less focused, more 'integrative' control mode that reduces top-down control."[38]

Recent brain imaging results show that when someone even briefly generates novel ways to use various common objects, such as a tin can or an umbrella, there is increased collaborative cross-talk between areas of the brain that are part of the brain's "default-mode network." As we will see later, the default-mode network is a key player when we imagine the future or mentally reconstruct possible scenarios.[39]

Playfully engaging in the imaginative reconstruction of previously unthought of uses of objects may provide a type of "thinking warm-up" that better readies us mentally for the forms of thinking that are called upon in creative thought.

As a first example of the interplay of the four constituents of thought, consider two characteristics that undergird creative search and exploration: curiosity and having a healthy respect for and tolerance of ambiguity.[40] Neither of these characteristics is only about concepts. Each has some aspects that are about concepts, but the cognitive aspects (how we approach and assimilate information) meld with emotion, motivation, and perception. Curiosity is, indeed, about searching for information, but it is much more. Curiosity is feeling intrigued (emotion), being energized or inclined or disinclined to act (motivation), and actively questioning what we notice and sense (perception).

As a second, more extended example, let's focus next on the interrelationship between emotions and concepts. Emotions in all their varied and intermixed forms provide us with essential information. They keep us alert and alive to our level of progress toward our goals and help to signal discrepancies, divergences, or obstacles. Our emotions and also our moods (which are often more diffuse and extended in time than are emotions) are part of our idea landscape and may themselves change it.[41]

Many forms and shades of emotion may contribute to our creative processes. No one single emotional state is always conducive to creativity.[42] Across time, the experience of an admixture of emotions—but with positive mood or affect more frequent than negative affect and buoyed throughout with some optimism—may best foster creativity in individuals and groups. Although over time and on average a somewhat higher frequency of positive rather than negative emotions contributes to creativity, there is no "magic number" or precise ratio, and negative emotions or moods also provide crucial information.[43]

Mild and temporary boosts in our positive affect may influence the flexibility of our thinking and categorization. Research has shown, for example, that individuals in a mildly positive mood are more willing to extend the notion of "vehicle" to include less typical examples of that category—such as "camel," "elevator," and "feet"—than are individuals in a neutral mood.[44] Mild positive emotion can enhance the likelihood of our noticing associations among ideas that are more remote or further afield.[45] People in a mildly positive mood may also be more willing to explore and test various ideas or hypotheses beyond what might be strictly required by the task at hand.

In one study, third-year medical students were given positive feedback regarding their performance on an incidental anagram task. These students later generated a correct diagnosis for a hypothetical patient more quickly than did those who were not given such positive feedback. In addition, they were more inquisitive and broadly integrative in their thinking about the possible contributing factors to that patient's diagnosis and what differentiated the hypothetical patient's case from apparently similar cases.[46] More generally, the experience of mildly pleasurable reward-like states often enhances the ease and speed with which different ideas come to mind, with positive affect increasing the fluency of idea generation and the identification of possible new avenues to pursue.[47]

The influence can also occur in the opposite direction. Changing where we are in our conceptual or cognitive space concurrently tends to change where we are in emotional space. The very process of flexibly bringing to mind multiple alternatives and thinking exploratively and playfully can itself sometimes induce positive mood.[48]

Each of our thoughts and behaviors reflects a unique cognitive–affective blend, and it is usually not possible to fully separate concepts and emotion. All thoughts and behaviors are interminglings of these (and of perception and motivation) to varying degrees. Our thoughts and creative efforts never arise in a vacuum. Rather, they emerge in and from within an already existing dynamic landscape of ideas and feelings. If we are, for example, already feeling moderately positive and are aptly cognitively flexible, then additional positive affect may have little benefit. Likewise, emotions that are motivationally highly intense, whether they are positive (e.g., excessive enthusiasm) or negative (e.g., fear), often lead to a narrowing rather than a broadening of our conceptual scope.[49]

We very much need, too, to take account of changes in our emotions over time. When we initially encounter obstacles or setbacks, we often experience frustration or other negative emotions. But these negative feelings may prompt us to focus our attention and problem solving more closely on the situation at hand—opening new perspectives and options for us.[50]

Consider two groups of students asked to propose novel ideas to improve university teaching. Before generating their ideas, one group was first encouraged to write about and vividly remember a situation that made them feel distressed or nervous and then to write about and clearly remember a situation that made them feel inspired or enthusiastic. Students in a second group first wrote about what they did the previous day (inducing a neutral emotional state) and then about a situation that, as in the first group, made them feel inspired or enthusiastic. Students in both groups experienced shifts in their emotions, but the first group experienced a comparatively more dramatic shift. Both groups generated the same number of ideas for improving teaching, but the first group generated ideas of higher novelty that spanned a wider range of topics. These findings suggest that, beyond deriving creative momentum from positive feelings, we can also benefit from the dynamic shiftings in our emotions, as varied emotions furnish us with different perspectives.[51]

Although here we have focused on the effects of emotion largely on our individual thinking, our emotions are highly socially influenced and may be shared across individuals or groups or teams. Individuals involved in an interpersonal bargaining exercise who had earlier been encouraged to experience mild positive emotion (through evaluating several dozen cartoons as very funny or less funny and receiving a small incidental gift) negotiated more effectively and achieved solutions that had higher joint benefits than did persons in a control group.[52] Organizations also have histories of emotion—including positive emotion—that may influence their creative processes and outcomes. Groups that have a history of more frequently experiencing positive than negative emotions are more innovative, pointing to the interactive relations between emotion and cognition not only within individuals but also among individuals and teams across time.[53] Just as for individuals, no single emotional state is always conducive to group or organizational creativity; a combination that somewhat favors positive emotion may be best.[54]

Our varied emotions both channel and are channeled by our equally varied and dynamic motivational states. Just as it is difficult to sharply separate cognition from emotion, it may be equally challenging to clearly separate cognition from motivation. How we envision and anticipate what it is that we would like to accomplish shapes the ideas that we notice and bring to mind. At times we focus on what it is that we wish to avoid or to prevent. At other times we concentrate on what it is that we hope to move toward or to advance. The same situation can give rise to either approach-oriented or avoidance-oriented motivation in different individuals or in ourselves at different times. When we are in an *approach-oriented* motivational state, our attention is concentrated on the positive steps needed to move toward and realize an anticipated outcome. When, though, we are in an *avoidance-oriented* motivational state, our attention is concentrated on avoiding mistakes and circumventing or minimizing obstacles or setbacks.[55]

Our creative endeavors rely on a balancing of both motivations: approach (promotion) and avoidance (prevention). We need to focus on positively and actively promoting our creative goals but equally we need to balance this with a consideration of anticipated difficulties and an evaluation of possible missteps while still keeping our creative goals in mind. Periodically pausing to imagine that we did not succeed in an important project can help alert us to ways of addressing obstacles before they become overwhelming or no longer surmountable. Such "pre-mortems," or forms of future-focused hindsight, may helpfully alter our mental idea landscapes, preempting misguided directions.[56]

Similarly, at times the constraints on a particular project—such as a deadline, budget, or written specifications—might be seen as obstacles to be surmounted. Yet at other times the same constraints might be embraced as welcome guidelines to channel our innovative efforts. It may be easier to productively vary our ideas and actions within well-specified constraints than it would be if we had only overly generalized notions of what is required. A poet may be vexed by the constraints imposed by a poetic form or rhyming scheme, but those same constraints may ignite intense individuality of expression. We might even, as we will see in Part 4, purposefully introduce self-imposed requirements in an effort to narrow the range of possibilities open to us, enabling us to explore more deeply within a subset of options.[57]

Each of us may have a general predisposition to either a promotion or a prevention focus. However, our focus may change depending on context and can be induced through how our goals are framed. Before giving a public talk, singing, or acting in a play, we may often experience anxiety about how well we will do and have vivid concerns about what could go amiss. But what if we were to recharacterize or recategorize our feelings of arousal and anticipation not just as anxiety but also as positive excitement?[58]

University students were given two minutes to prepare a short (two- to three-minute) persuasive speech. In the speech, delivered in front of an experimenter and videotaped, the student was asked to explain why he or she was a good work partner. The students were told that the videotape of their speech would later be judged by their peers. Just before giving their speeches, some of the students were instructed to say "I am excited." Other students were instructed to say "I am calm."

Students who were randomly assigned to state "I am excited" right before giving their speeches were rated by three independent raters, who watched videotapes of their performance, as significantly more persuasive, more competent, more confident, and more persistent than were students who were asked instead to state "I am calm." Self-reports by the students showed that the speech-related anxiety did not go away. Instead, the students reinterpreted their physiological arousal as excitement. The reinterpretation may have changed the student's orientation from being on the vigilant "lookout" for threats to a more opportunity-focused perspective.

Our physical actions, too, influence the intermingling of our thoughts with feelings and sensations. Walking, for instance, has long been associated with the releasing of associations, memories, and opportunities for putting our thoughts together. At his home in rural England, Charles Darwin "walked everyday on the Sand-walk, his thinking path, and was constantly alert both for the regular patterns that might have meaning and for exceptions that might point to another story."[59] Recent research findings also point to the clear value of moving in space, whether walking or in a wheelchair, to opening us up to new ideas.[60] We'll see later, in Part 2, how the physical act of gesturing often becomes part of our thinking spaces and, in Part 6, how the creation of a new dance piece simultaneously relied on touch, intonation, words, and other vocalizations alongside movement in space.

Neither emotion nor cognition, neither motivation nor perception, exclusively prevail in our creative projects: we need them together and in all their varied combinations.

5. Our Dynamic Brains, Our Dynamic Environments

Thinking Framework Question 5:

How do you invite your environments and your "thinking tools" to creatively partner with you?

Imagine trying to develop an innovative new product or process entirely in your head, without the benefit of any intermediate physical support or prototypes and without any form of response from others. Or think of writing a poem or song lyrics without the tangible support offered by words written on a page and in the absence of any written or oral tradition or artistic culture. Consider how often and how deeply our creative explorations are guided and informed by procedures and structures developed by others (or by our earlier selves) that have been captured and preserved across time in words, objects, diagrams, equations, or other symbols. Our **environments**—not only physical but also symbolic, procedural, social, and extending over time—support, sustain, and sculpt our generative thinking and problem solving, enhancing or impeding our creative progress.

The use of diagrams, words, and communicative tools of all forms to share information with others and to test possibilities early in the development of an idea is often critical to successful innovation. Externalizing our ideas in the physical world—whether in the form of drawings, sketches, diagrams, notes, or prototypes—deeply impacts our thinking and creating. By forming a physical record of our internal ideas, we free up what's called short-term working memory—a limited space in our immediately accessible mental awareness—providing room for new combinations and possibilities.[61]

Tangibly expressing our ideas can help us to better see how things interrelate and encourage us to imaginatively play out in our minds how and if something might actually work. Realizing our ideas in a physical form, even if tentative or partial, additionally can promote creative understandings with others and shared mental models of what we are thinking. By physically recording and keeping track of our evolving ideas we decrease demands on our individual and collective memory and attention, better allowing for the revisiting, revising, and reconfiguration of those ideas. We both make and find: we intend to "make" and attempt to bring into being realizations of our ideas; along the way we "find"—encountering unanticipated pathways, obstacles, opportunities. Then, with the new information we've discovered, we make once more, in an ongoing cycle of ***making and finding***.

> I think initial "concepts" or ideas are always over-rated. My starting points are usually quite simple—the fun and skill is in the making. . . . What I love is the physical process of making a machine. It's partly drawing—not pretty drawings but drawing as a way of thinking through problems. . . . The making process also involves lots of prototypes—there are many problems drawings can never solve.[62]
>
> —*Inventor and cartoonist Tim Hunkin*

Both the *timing* and the *form* in which we capture our emerging thoughts sculpt our idea landscapes. In one study, more than 40 design teams, with three to five engineering students per team, were given several months to develop products and implementation plans for industry-sponsored projects. The teams were asked to design mechanical/electrical objects that met clear constraints. One team, for instance, was asked to design a wireless device for measuring power consumption with an ideal cost of less than $100.[63]

How the teams used their environments mattered. Design teams that created products that best met the client requirements more often used physical three-dimensional prototypes and electronic whiteboards to share information and emerging plans within the team than did the less successful teams. The less successful teams tended to use physical prototypes primarily only *late* in the design process, during the refinement of ideas, rather than earlier, during the generation and gathering of ideas. Less successful teams also relied more extensively on individual computers rather than team-based thinking-working spaces. The early and extensive use of communally shared and accessible notes and prototypes enhanced design team performance on multiple dimensions, including cost, functional performance, reliability, manufacturing requirements, and ease of use.

Beyond the physical realization or capturing of ideas, the other members of a team bring individual storehouses of knowledge and skill to a team. In this case, no one person in the group needs to know everything with equivalent specificity or expertise. Social interactions and communications between people in a group can extend, strengthen, and productively complicate our idea worlds, both through the sheer range of knowledge and information they introduce and the varied levels of detail with which people have mastered such knowledge.

> When each team member learns in a general sense what other team members know in detail, the team can draw on the detailed knowledge distributed across members of the collective.[64]
>
> —*Experts on team dynamics Steve Kozlowski and Daniel Ilgen*

The shared knowledge or memory of a group that is working together to further a creative enterprise can enable effective exploration of ideas at a midlevel of abstraction, comfortable in the recognition that the group has access to more grounded details as well as relevant abstractions if needed.[65] Flexibly adaptive change may be distinctively propelled by teams with both inside knowledge and outside expertise. Extension of our idea landscapes beyond our team or internal organization through innovation contests or prize-based competitions can also, as we will see in Part 5, provoke insightful problem solving.[66]

All of our thinking and creating involves repeated cycles between perception and action. Our perceptions of the external environment guide our actions, and our actions lead to consequences, which in turn change what we perceive and what our next moves might be. Cycling between acting and perceiving our environments (physical, social, symbolic) is fundamentally built into the ways our brains use, process, and extend our understandings and insights.[67] Rather than a single and sudden breaking forth, much of our thinking arises within "inextricable tangles of feedback, feedforward, and feed-around loops: loops that promiscuously criss-cross the boundaries of brain, body, and world."[68]

Our brains, too, are widely interconnected, communicating and exchanging information at multiple scales. There is a continual interchange between the right and left cerebral hemispheres (side to side) and anterior to posterior regions (front to back, and back to front). Broadly speaking, there is a division of labor in the brain with the frontal (anterior) regions of our brain largely devoted to the encoding and processing of *actions* (including language, goals, and planning), with the posterior (rearward) regions largely devoted to the encoding and processing of *perceptual* information. As schematically depicted in Figure 1.9, the frontal regions of the brain interact extensively and reciprocally with the posterior regions toward the back of the brain, in a continual perception-action cycle.

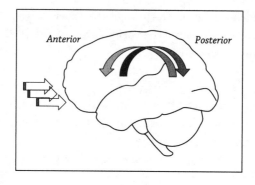

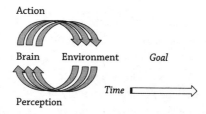

| INCOMING INFORMATION FROM THE ENVIRONMENT IS REGISTERED IN OUR BRAINS THROUGH PERCEPTION AND ITERATIVELY GUIDES OUR ACTIONS. | THROUGH OUR PERCEPTION-ACTION CYCLES WE CONTINUALLY LINK BRAIN AND ENVIRONMENT. As we move toward our goals we repeatedly cycle between action and perception, perceiving the effects of our actions on the environment and adjusting and responding accordingly.[69] |

Figure 1.9

The perception-action cycle is a basic biological principle that governs the functional relationships of the organism with its environment. As a process, it is the cybernetic circle of sensing and acting that guides the organism to its goals. . . . The perception-action cycle . . . engages neural networks at every hierarchical level of the neocortex, following processing paths that course through the environment and through connections between cortical areas.[70]

—*Neuroscientist and cognitive network theorist professor Joaquin Fuster*

There are complex interconnected networks within both the anterior and the posterior regions of the brain. Smaller and more local neural networks or subnetworks specialize in the representation and processing of information of different types and at varying levels of abstraction. These neural networks span both the gray matter of the cortex (the thin, intricately folded outer layer of neural tissue of the brain, consisting mostly of "gray" neurons) and white matter (the underlying axons that support longer range connections between brain regions, mostly coated with white myelin sheaths).

Beginning in the middle of the brain and moving forward (in the anterior direction, toward the prefrontal cortex), there is a gradual progressive increase in the level of abstractness of the action, goal, and planning information that is represented.

A similar gradual progressive increase of abstractness is found in the posterior half of the brain, but in this case with respect to perception. Moving forward from the very back of the brain toward the middle of the brain, there is a continuum or gradient of abstraction. In the most rearward areas of the brain (in occipital cortex) populations of neurons are only responsive to simple visual features, such as lines or contours in very specific orientations. As we move increasingly forward in the brain, away from the earliest visual processing regions, neuronal populations become receptive to ever more complex conjunctions of lines and shapes, eventually including neuronal ensembles that respond to entire objects or scenes such as faces or houses. These regions, nearer to the middle of the brain (moving forward into the temporal cortex), are devoted to the processing of integrated forms of information, interlinked with our prior conceptual knowledge about objects. Similar gradients of abstraction occur at a number of further, more fine-grained levels in several other regions of the brain.[71]

Given that our brains are in continual active interchange with our environments, the environments that we work and play within have a profound and pervasive impact on our creative potential and realizations. Our acquired experiences are represented in our brains through the formation, strengthening, and inhibiting of synaptic connections between neurons and coalitions of neurons. These coalitions interlink in broad far-reaching complex cognitive-perceptual and action-related neural networks that, in turn, help us to further interpret and understand what we see, hear, sense, and experience.

Changes in our experiential environments—particularly the introduction of newness or novelty—may be especially crucial in providing the stimulus for the generation of new neurons (a process called neurogenesis) deep within the inner brain, in regions such as the hippocampus (a brain region highly important to memory and to our encoding of the relations among objects and events).[72] Our daily and ongoing activities, including the new challenges that we take up and pursue, are continually changing our brains and the representations and processes that we can draw upon to meet new challenges. Learning to juggle, play a musical instrument, or use a new computer programming language continually changes neurons and synaptic connections (gray matter) and potentially also the larger-range connectivity of how one brain region may communicate with others (white matter).[73]

Not only physical juggling but "mental juggling" too may lead to structural changes in our brains. Among students who spent three months studying intensively for the Law School Admission Test (LSAT), for example, there were changes in the level of ongoing communication between brain regions involved in complex reasoning and analogy. These changes were observed during brain scanning when the students were not given any particular task to perform (what is known as resting-state functional connectivity). Compared with a matched group of students who planned to take the exam but who had not yet studied for it, students who studied for and took the LSAT showed increased correlations between resting-state activity in the left parietal cortex (a posterior region of the brain important in cognitive control) and both the left and right prefrontal cortex (anterior regions of the brain also important in cognitive control). These changes in resting-state connectivity, in turn, correlated with the amount of improvement the students showed in their scores from an initial LSAT practice test to later practice tests.[74] Other brain imaging measures further showed changes in the functional white matter (axonal) connectivity of the LSAT-taking students. Together, these findings suggest that extensive training on the complex reasoning exercises may have led to structural changes in the long-range white matter connections of the frontoparietal networks of their brains.[75]

There is a continual dynamic loop between our brains and our behavior: our brains are the source of our behavior, but our brains, in turn, are continually modified by our behavior. We all understand the need for athletes to train regularly and exert themselves to keep their skills at the highest caliber and not become rusty. The same applies to our brains and our thinking.

Thought Box: *Seeing, Sensing, and Our "Guy-Wires of Perception"*

Guy-wires are cables under tension used to support and add stability to physical structures that need extra support and bracing, such as high towers, roof antennas, newly planted trees, or tents. So too our ideas and creative endeavors need to be continually grounded and stabilized through our perception of our changing environment. The multiple "guy-wires of perception" anchor us and our brains in the perception-action cycle of thinking, where we continually perceive the world, act on the world, and then reevaluate the consequences of our actions based on what we now perceive.

Much more of our progress toward our goals is due to the environment than we give it credit for. Although the goals we hold in mind are essential, the external environment often helps us to successively form, refine, and articulate what we want to achieve. Our external environment provides us with support throughout the goal-pursuit process by reminding us of our goals and their current status, helping to sustain their activation level, and providing opportunities for unlooked for forms of convergent advance toward multiple goals.

Picture a sculptor in his or her studio, perhaps a sculptor who uses welded metal, such as David Smith, with many metal fragments and partial sculptural forms surrounding him. David Smith "ran his studio like a factory, stocked with large amounts of raw material. He claimed it was a way of liberating himself, of avoiding being precious with materials. Large sculptures were begun on the floor, steel arranged on a flat, white-painted background, then tack-welded and hauled up to be worked in the round."[76]

The white-painted backgrounds that were at first entirely incidental to his work later cued an entirely new direction. Smith developed a unique drawing process based on how his welding of a sculpture would burn a negative image of the sculpture into the surrounding white-painted floor. Noticing and intrigued by these unintended marks of his welding process, Smith reproduced the welding effect by deliberately spraying paint or enamel around objects placed on paper. His novel "sprays," or sprayed drawings, were "contrived with a wily stencil technique that cushions crisp white silhouettes in clouds of color."[77]

Sometimes when we are unsure of where to go next, it may greatly help to reimmerse ourselves back into a context related to our goals or subgoals. The external context or environment carries some of our memory and cognitive burden for us—typically in much richer and interconnected ways than may be true of our abstract thinking about it. Actually reexposing ourselves to the material or symbolic world of the problem—rather than just trying to think about it in our heads—can allow the promptings of the situation to emerge and help guide us toward possible next moves.

~~~~~~

We need to engage in *challenging* interactions with our perceptual and conceptual worlds, especially ones that call on us to make difficult fine-grained differentiations between otherwise similar-appearing procedures, ideas, or stimuli. Such challenging forms of learning, perceiving, and attending call on, reinforce, and *extend* our existing neural connections.[78]

Working together, newly formed and well-established neurons may enable our brains to encode experiences at a level of "memory resolution" that allows us to see subtle relevant similarities and also necessary distinctions. Well-established neurons readily allow us to encode features of objects and events that are similar to those we have previously experienced. New neurons may be more plastic or trainable and so may prove especially helpful in encoding novel, less familiar features.[79]

As we will see in Part 5, our neural and cognitive flexibilities are at their peak when we both explore new things and keep the skills we have already mastered well honed.

6. Bringing It All Together: The iCASA Thinking Framework

We have now introduced each of the five factors in our thinking framework: idea landscapes; levels of detail/abstraction; degrees of control; the intermingling of concepts with emotion, perceiving, and motivation; and the dynamic interaction of our brains and environments through making and finding and the broader perception-action cycle. The five factors can be compactly visualized in our *iCASA thinking framework*,[80] as shown in Figure 1.10.

Let's start with the center of the diagram. There, represented by the large oval, is our idea landscape. Our idea landscape—with its peaks and valleys of ideas entering, forming, and receding from our awareness—consists of ideas or representations that we can access and bring into our awareness. The content of our mental representations encompasses all four of the interrelated constituents of our thinking—concepts, perception, motivations, and emotions. The four constituents of our thinking are shown as partially overlapping ovals, with dashed lines symbolizing the permeable boundaries across and among them.

The vertical dimension symbolizes the level of specificity of our mental representations. On this dimension, the content of our mental representations

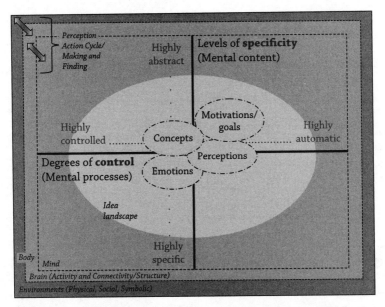

Figure 1.10 THE iCASA THINKING FRAMEWORK FOR CREATIVITY AND CHANGE. Our ideas (interminglings of concepts, emotions, perceptions, motivations/goals) vary in levels of specificity and degrees of control—and live in our broader physical, social, and symbolic environments, which are, in turn, supported by our dynamically changing brains. We continually perceive, act, and then perceive again, in an ongoing cycle of perception and action, of making and finding. The large oval represents our momentary idea landscape, with its peaks and valleys of ideas entering, receding from, and forming in our awareness.[81]

in each of the four constituents of our thinking ranges across a number of levels of specificity or detail from midlevels of abstraction to the very abstract or general or to the very concrete or specific. The horizontal dimension symbolizes the degree of cognitive control in our mental processes. Our degree of cognitive control varies from, on the one side, exceedingly controlled and deliberate thinking, to spontaneity or improvisational thinking in the middle portions, to automatic or habitual thinking on the other side. These idea landscapes occur within our dynamically changing, always learning brains and our changing experiential environments—physical, social, and symbolic.

Across time and contexts our idea landscapes continually change, with our relative placement in the levels of specificity and degrees of control in each of the four interrelated constituents of our thinking also fluctuating. At one moment we may intently and purposively scrutinize an object for subtle highly specific perceptual features; at another moment we may rely on more habitual or abstract perceptual processes. Similarly, we may sometimes carefully control or differentiate among

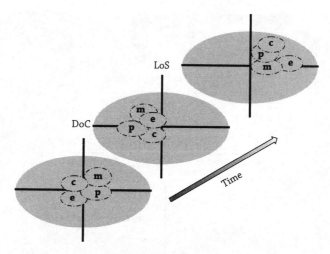

Figure 1.11 ACROSS TIME OUR IDEA LANDSCAPES DYNAMICALLY CHANGE. With changing contexts, across time we vary our degrees of control (DoC) and also our levels of specificity (LoS) in each of the four interrelated constituents of our thinking: concepts (c), emotions (e), perceptions (p), and motivations (m).[82]

our emotions, while at other times we may be more spontaneous or impressionistic. Likewise, with changing time and circumstances, we may be more or less deliberate and more or less specific in our motivations and categorizations. Three of the many possible configurations of the four constituents of our thinking at different moments in time are diagrammed in Figure 1.11.

With the introduction to our iCASA thinking framework now complete, we next—more deeply, concretely, and extensively—explore how it applies to innovation, creativity, and change. In Part 2, we will see how apt and adroit detail stepping can help us to be more agile thinkers, makers, and doers.

 Creativity Cross Checks and Queries

Questions to encourage reflection and connections to your own work and practice:

⇒ Are you trying to do everything in your head, or could your physical or social environments help you with some parts of your creative problem-solving endeavors?
  • Could you "offload" some of the mental work that you're doing onto your environment instead?

- Are you sharing ideas or prototypes or sketches with your team members, using whiteboards or shared digital working spaces so as to free up more of your idea landscape space for the melding and conjunction of novel ideas?
- Do you share your developing ideas often enough, soon enough, and widely enough with your colleagues? Do you bounce ideas off of one another to rapidly redirect or test the course of your explorations?
- Do you have tools or materials at hand that enable fast and flexible initial testing of ideas?
- Are you letting your actions fluidly "cycle" with perception, capitalizing on the way our brains naturally move between perception and action?
- Do you reimmerse yourself in your project, allowing particular words on the page, images, lines of code, equations, or other materials in the environment to get you started again and to readily suggest your next moves?

⇒ What objects or events in your creative/working environment may be cuing you and your thinking?

- How are sparks of freshness and triggers to novel ideas introduced into your creative spaces? Are there enough opportunities for chance encounters or new conjunctions produced by your own active explorations and those of others?
- Do you recognize emotional and motivational states as valuable contributors to your thinking processes and actions?

⇒ Are you preserving and storing potentially fruitful ideas whether in snippets or in more formal and elaborate ways?

- How do you capture and retain your ideas?
- How do you enable your ideas to newly combine and connect with one another?
- What drafts or notes or recordings or objects allow you to revisit emerging thoughts or connections at different times and in different orders, across different idea landscapes?

⇒ What are you doing and learning that stretches or surprises you or unsettles your assumptions and categories in a challenging way?

- How do you mix up some of your routines with new variations and divergences?
- Do you introduce brief breaks, pauses, or interludes into your day and your project time to allow alternative ideas to emerge into awareness and changing levels of deliberation versus spontaneity, using the full range of your "control dial"?

- How and when are you drawing on the experiences and diverse perspectives and "takes" of others?
⇒ Do you know and understand the guiding constraints in your creative endeavors?
  - What are your open goals?
  - Are you prepared and readied for happy serendipitous finds that could edge or guide you forward?
  - Are you patient through both the bursts and lulls in your own thinking and that of others? Do you give yourself time to let your ideas configure and reconfigure?
  - Do you welcome and respect your creative constraints as an impetus to new directions of thought?
  - Are you allowing yourself to be contextually nimble in traversing different levels of abstraction in your thinking ("detail stepping") — changing your focus and moving up, down, and across at different times and in response to different prompts or cues?

Part 2

Seeing the Forest
and the Trees: Varying Our
Levels of Abstraction

Thinking prompts

- What are abstractions? Why are midlevel abstractions often especially useful?
- Why and how are successive drafts, sketches, and prototypes so important?
- How are we being helped and hindered by the examples we encounter?
- How might we make more "creativity friendly" environments for ourselves and for others?
- When is something (relevantly) the same and when is it (relevantly) different?

Think of a simple action such as folding a piece of paper.

We can think of this action at many levels of abstraction. Thought of in more particular or specific terms, our action of folding the paper might be described as a half-fold or as folding into thirds. Folding is also—at more abstract levels—changing the surface as well as the shape and the size of the paper.

Any action can be thought of at differing levels of abstraction. Increasingly abstract terms encompass a wider range of possible actions; there are many ways in which we might change the surface and shape of a piece of paper besides folding it. For example, we might compact it by crumpling it into a ball or tearing it into smaller pieces. As shown in Figure 2.1 for this simple example, actions become increasingly differentiated or distinctive as we step downward in the hierarchy of abstraction.

Characterizing our actions at a midlevel of abstraction can often convey necessary specificity without either excessive detail or excessive abstraction. This provides us and others with concise and considerable information while still permitting flexibility. If, for example, you are asked to make a note to remind someone of an upcoming event, this request could be fulfilled in many ways: you might jot a reminder on a calendar, send an e-mail message, or add it to a to-do list. Each of these actions is an appropriate way of

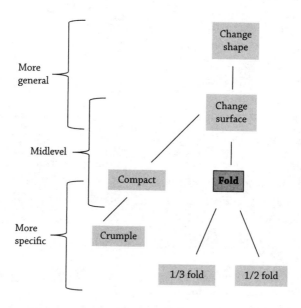

WE CAN THINK OF OUR ACTIONS IN MORE ABSTRACT OR MORE SPECIFIC WAYS, ALSO INCLUDING MIDLEVELS OF ABSTRACTION.	OUR ACTIONS CAN BE THOUGHT OF AT MANY LEVELS OF ABSTRACTION. Any given action can be represented at a number of different levels of abstraction, ranging from highly general and cross-situational characterizations to more specific and context-dependent characterizations. Midlevel abstractions encompass aspects of both generality and specificity and so can be simultaneously highly informative and flexible.[1]

Figure 2.1

meeting the request. Yet sometimes, depending on our context or goals, we may need to step up toward higher generality or step down toward greater specificity.

Now let's think of a more extended creative activity such as writing or drawing. We can think of the process of writing in terms of our overall goals of perhaps aiming to capture a fleeting impression, to evoke new sociocultural sensitivities, or to present a coherent and persuasive case. Or we can think of writing from the point of view of structure, organization, and logical flow, asking ourselves if a given paragraph fits best earlier or later and how to bridge from one paragraph to another. At the same time we can also think of writing at increasingly finer and more detailed levels, such as finding apt words or fluent phrasings.

The activity of writing is not confined to any one of these levels, since our focus and attention vary from midlevel to abstract to more detailed throughout the process. Experienced writers may show a wider range in the "zoom" of their focus during writing and revising. Experienced writers are able to zoom out and in, considering the global meaning and structure of their writing as well as the meanings of individual words and word sequences.[2]

Similarly, if we are drawing, we can begin with a global sense of the overall composition and then move to a more local or detailed consideration of mark making. Or we might proceed in the reverse order, beginning with a set of particular lines or strokes and building out from there to a larger whole. The process of drawing is not restricted to any one of these or intermediate levels but fluently moves between and across multiple levels of the local and the global.

> I sometimes begin drawing with no preconceived problem to solve, with only a desire to use pencil on paper and only to make lines, tones and styles with no conscious aim. But as my mind takes in what is so produced a point arrives where some idea becomes conscious and crystallizes.[3]
>
> —*Sculptor and artist Henry Moore*

> The main characteristic [that I seem to have somehow acquired] is an ability to understand many levels of abstraction simultaneously, and to shift effortlessly between in-the-large and in-the-small.[4]
>
> —*Computer scientist, mathematician, and author Donald Knuth*

When artists and nonartists in a research study were asked to "think aloud" as they set about choosing the objects they might draw from among a set of 30 possible items, artists made significantly more descriptive statements than did the nonartists—indicating a closer examination of concrete and specific artistic opportunities offered by the particular objects. After they had begun drawing, however, artists showed a different approach to detail. Having embarked on drawing, they now made significantly more statements about their larger-scale goals for the emerging artwork than did the nonartists. These changes in the primary focus of the artists' thinking, from in-the-small to in-the-large, point to situationally responsive detail stepping across their creative process.[5]

The aim of this Part is to help us become more aware of how detail stepping permeates and propels our creative and innovative efforts. What prompts us to move up or down in detail steps in our own thinking? How do our physical and social environments spur us to change our level of abstraction? How do we sometimes get stuck at a level of detail that's unpromising? How can we time or pace ourselves in our movements up and down in abstraction to best capture ideas as they happen?

Changes in our level of detail or abstraction occur regularly, not only in our concepts and perceptions but also in relation to our emotions, goals, and actions. When we are creatively agile, we move up and down in our levels of abstraction. As suggested in Figure 2.2, across time we step up or down in

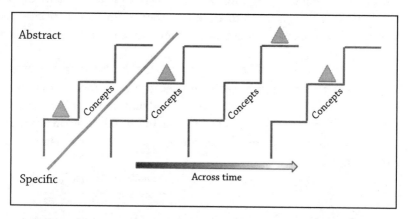

Figure 2.2 FLEXIBLY ALTERING OUR LEVELS OF ABSTRACTION ACROSS TIME. To be optimally mentally agile and creative across time and situations, we need to flexibly step up and down in our levels of abstraction. At certain points greater detail may be called for; at other points a higher level of abstraction may best provide new insights and clarity. We may think of detail stepping as moving up or down stairs, one or several steps at a time, or, perhaps, as taking longer or shorter steps along an inclined ramp.

our level of detail within any one of the constituents of our thinking. Equally important, as seen in Figure 2.3, at any one single moment in time we may be at differing levels of abstraction in each of the four interrelated constituents of our thinking (concepts, emotions, motivations/goals, and perceptions).

We begin with a broader exploration of detail stepping in relation to our idea landscapes and experience. This section provides us with a big-picture understanding of what abstraction is and why it matters. Next, we focus on detail stepping or changes in our levels of abstraction that arise in response to our immediate or incidental environments. Our environments enter into our thinking and creating through physically present or available objects and materials, such as sketches and prototypes. The selective alteration of these aspects of our environment can itself be a potent tool for triggering our thinking.

Then we turn to the ways in which our bodies and our own actions may move us in detail-abstraction space. We consider the role of gesturing and forms of mental or perceptual simulation. Mental or perceptual simulations are the imagined "workings through" of possible future situations or actions, visually or through other senses such as hearing or touch. We also unpack the vital role of affordances. **Affordances** are the possibilities for action and interaction that objects or their representations offer us. A handle may "afford" opportunities for grasping, or for pulling or lifting. A small space may afford the opportunity for hiding to a young child but not for an adult. Similarly, our tools and spaces for creating may offer us promising openings for action or problem solving.

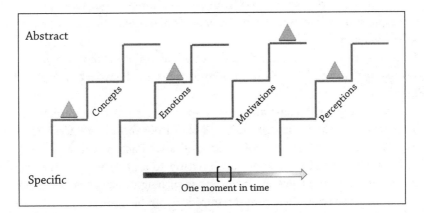

Figure 2.3 OUR LEVELS OF ABSTRACTION AT A SINGLE MOMENT IN TIME. At any one moment of our creative and problem-solving process our level of detail may differ within each of the four interrelated constituents of our thinking (concepts, emotions, motivations, and perceptions).

In the later sections of this Part we look at detail stepping in what might be termed our "thinking about thinking" and our modes of thinking. Here we explore levels of abstraction in our use of analogical or figurative thought. We also look at how different forms of physical, social, and temporal distance influence the level of detail in our thinking. We close by looking at levels of abstraction of mental representations in our brains, especially "detail steps" in the neural bases of our goals and concepts.

ABSTRACTION, PARTICULARITY, AND EXPERIENCE

Densely packed, crowded, profusely overlapping—our immediate sensory, emotional, and other experiences may engulf us in particulars that allow little "give" for spanning and connecting ideas. Abstractions here come to our rescue. Abstractions allow us to move up from the particulars and to flexibly connect and interrelate our experiences across times and spaces and varying contexts. Abstract concepts—such as our ideas of swiftness, opaqueness, or generosity—allow us to group, classify, or single out our experiences in generalized or more particularized and finely differentiated ways. We continually encode and form representations of objects and events at differing levels of abstraction.[6]

Some of our representations are highly specific, detailed, and what has been called **"experience near"**; these are richly embedded in the one-of-a-kind (one- place, one- time) particulars of our immediate experience. Other representations are more abstract or **"experience far."** These abstract representations are also derived from and anchored in our experience, but they capture only selected or isolated aspects of our experience while setting aside other aspects.[7]

One way in which we might think of our mental representations in relation to our experiences and our idea landscapes is schematically depicted in Figure 2.4.

Abstract representations allow us to extract aspects of experience from the contexts in which they occur. Think of our notions of blueness, smoothness, fleetness, malleability, loftiness, and awe. Each of these singles out a different aspect of our experience relating to a particular color, texture and touch, rapidity of movement or sense of height, elevation, or majesty. Once abstracted from their context, our ideas can be more readily and freely recombined; we might think, then, of "blue awe" or "malleable fleetness."

Our abstract representations can also characterize *relations* between and among things and events or people. We have representations not only for objects or events but also for ways in which objects or events might relate to

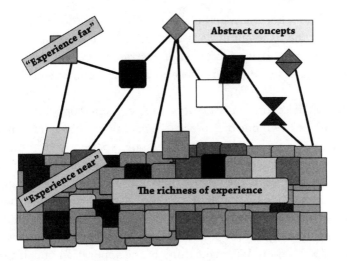

ABSTRACTIONS ARE ANCHORED IN OUR "RAW" OR "EXPERIENCE NEAR" REPRESENTATIONS AND CAN THEMSELVES BE RECOMBINED IN DIFFERENT WAYS.	THE POWER OF ABSTRACT CONCEPTS IN OUR EXPERIENCE. As shown in this highly schematic diagram, our immediate experience is tremendously rich, densely packed, and interlocking (analogically shown by the closely overlapping squares in the lower half of the diagram). Abstract concepts extract or isolate selected aspects, or portions, of our rich immediate experience (analogically shown by the lines connecting the overlapping squares in the lower half of the diagram to the shapes in the upper half of the diagram). Abstract concepts enable us to flexibly regroup and interrelate ideas without requiring a complete reimmersion in our immediate experience (shown by the lines connecting shapes to shapes within the upper half of the diagram). Traversing varying levels of abstraction introduces new possibilities and connections into our idea landscapes.

Figure 2.4

one another, such as contrasting or complementing, increasing or decreasing, and connecting or disconnecting. Abstractions allow us to compare and contrast by singling out sameness and difference as something to be attended to, enabling us to evaluate an immense range of other relations such as stability, harmony, and inclusion. They may also characterize relations across time, as in our ideas of immersion or of dissolving, or blending. These and the productive profusion of abstract terms allow us to traverse and capture facets of our experience in a highly compressed and efficient manner.

We have a choice in the abstractions we use. From moment to moment we can move up or down one or more levels, or stay at a given level of abstraction, moving along a level laterally. Often our experiences in themselves do not conclusively indicate which abstractions we might best use. Exchanging or alternating between the abstractions we are using can help us to see events—and relations between events—in a new way. Trying out a new abstraction may reveal connections to previously overlooked concrete particulars and also significant cross-connections between our more abstract readings of a situation. We might think of the application of paint to a canvas as gesturing, but alternatively as layering, shaping, or melding. Whereas gesturing evokes notions of motion and communication, layering and shaping may bring to mind construction and emergence. Opting to think about our own creative processes in one of these ways highlights certain possibilities over others. Have you ever thought of abstractions themselves as a type of locomotion in which we move through the spaces of our experience? But what if, instead, we think of abstractions as containers, or sets of circles, or even as clothing? What might it mean, for instance, to think of abstractions as clothing, that cloak, envelop, or display some portions of our experience but not others?

A common and often effortless way that we form abstractions is through analogical thinking. Take, for example, an industrial design studio team tasked with developing a movable x-ray stand. Although there are many alternative ways in which this design challenge might be approached, one of the design team members drew on knowledge of the steering mechanism of a small ferryboat pulling itself along a cable across a river. Recalling a much earlier summer he had spent working alongside a ferryman, his recollection evolved into a novel approach for steering and moving the x-ray stand in a long, steady, linear motion. Creativity here emerged through an analogy that abstracted one key component of a much earlier experience and introduced it into a new creative problem-solving context.[8]

Aside from analogy, there are many other routes to changing our level of abstraction in order to spark our creativity and instructive noticing. Caricatures and idealizations of forms or systems are one option. Or we could appeal to exemplary cases that epitomize a given idea. Alternatively, we might construct hypothetical situations that imaginatively draw out unforeseen or unexpected implications or imagine limit cases at the boundaries of our categories. These all are ways in which we can adjust our abstraction level.

Each of these options provides a pathway for our attention, making it easier for us to single out relevant or constant features or relations. Caricature and idealization, for instance, exaggerate central essential features and downplay comparatively incidental, accidentally variable features. Once we have extracted these more central features, we develop a generalized or "gist-like" mental representation that then can be applied more broadly and more flexibly because it is less tied to coincidental or unrelated aspects of a situation.

Think of Matisse's supple renditions of the human form or of Cézanne's planar evocations of landscape. Or think of Shakespeare's searing portrayals of the jealousy of Othello or the loyalty of Cordelia, or the deep play and dynamism of a Calder mobile. What do these works give us? In part they heighten and instruct our noticing by pointing us to overlooked aspects of a situation that were always there but that we didn't have the representational resources or vocabulary to draw upon. Physical embodiments of new exemplary abstractions instantiated in visual, verbal, or symbolic forms help us to better recognize more ambiguous, subtle, and novel instances of a similar kind. They bootstrap our ability to comprehend and recombine and cross connect our densely packed immediate experiences.

Finding new and more purpose-fitting (apt) abstractions is a pervasive contributor to innovative thinking and acting in many fields and subfields—spanning science and technology to medicine and law and beyond. Advances in computer science, for example, often hinge on the discovery and development of new abstractions that provide a different way of configuring how one thinks about what needs to be done and how to do it. Rather than seeing a computer program as a list of tasks, commands, or a "recipe," the form of computer programming known as object-oriented programming, for instance, reconstrues computer programs as involving entities (objects) that carry with themselves certain capabilities or ways of acting. By giving objects a degree of independence and unique responsibilities, programmers can "hand off" some of the details to those objects. Such forms of detail stepping and selective seeking of abstractions are also a central part of many everyday problem-solving situations and of intellectual inquiry ranging from historical analyses to detective-like thinking and to the noticing of relevant constancies, regularities, or invariants in scientific discovery.

Thought Box: *Generating Hunches: The Detail-Steeped Mind of the Detective*

A form of creative or generative reasoning, which philosophers some-times call "ampliative reasoning" or "abduction," involves a movement from a given set of observations to a new idea or a new construal of those observations.[9] The given set of observations is often puzzling, surpris-ing, or incongruous in some way. This type of thinking is closely linked to finely tuned sensory-perceptual awareness and has been described as a form of reasoning that detectives use, whether real or fictional; think of Sherlock Holmes.

Sir Henry Baskerville, newly arrived at a hotel in London, is sur-prised to find that one of his new boots has gone missing. Curiously, a short time later, the boot is returned, but one of his old boots dis-appears instead. Why would someone want and take a single boot rather than a pair? And why first take a new boot and then return for an old one? Ordinarily, a new boot would be preferred to an old one and a pair of matching boots would be much more valuable than a single boot.

What, though, if the stolen boots are not being used as footwear? But why come back for an old boot when you already had a new one? What can we say that is true of an old boot but not of a new one? They differ in their visual appearance, texture, and comfort, and . . . ah, yes, an old boot will be securely inhabited by the familiar odor of its longtime owner. What, then, if the boot has gone missing precisely for its smell? Why would that be important? Perhaps . . . perhaps a dog is being trained to use the scent to find Sir Henry? Perhaps, thinks Sherlock Holmes in *The Hound of the Baskervilles*, this is the key to the mystery?[10]

For a detective, facts are not simply assembled and then taken as given. Rather, some of the alleged facts appear odd, details or shadings of the purported facts seem out of sync with one another and with a broader or more abstract sense of what must have happened. To arrive at a solution the investigator attempts to suspend belief in one or more of these incongruous "would-be facts" by probing for what is "really there" in the gaps between the facts.

The detective's goal is to answer the question: What *really* hap-pened?—ingeniously piecing together the facts that he or she has available. The eventual insight into the most likely sequence of events is often arrived at when the detective does not simply accept the way events have been perceived, conceived, and communicated by others. The detective notices overlooked or miscategorized details and connects and reconfigures them into a new overarching and compelling account of the events.

Research Highlight: *The 62-Square Checkerboard Problem*

Researchers posed to participants an intriguing problem involving a checkerboard.[11] Participants in the experiment were presented with a standard 64-square black-and-white checkerboard *but* with two squares removed, one at each of two diagonal corners. The participants' goal was to cover the entire board using 31 dominoes, with each domino covering two horizontally adjacent or two vertically adjacent squares—or to determine that doing so was impossible. Diagonal placements were not permitted. Participants were asked to think out loud as they attempted to solve the problem.

It was found that the participants who solved the problem more quickly showed what the researchers called greater "flexibility in noticing." Those who solved the problem sooner noticed both more nonperceptual and more perceptual aspects of the problem. They noticed not only more things but also a wider variety of things.

In order to think more flexibly and creatively we should try to look and perceive more flexibly, noticing more about the problem space that we are in. To notice everything is simply impossible—and not really that helpful. The question is this: out of all the many often changing things and the many relations between things, what should we try to notice?

For the checkerboard task, noticing what remains the same or *invariant* across different attempts can direct attention to a key feature in the solution to the problem. At some point it may be noticed that the two squares that still remain uncovered at the end, after placing down all 31 dominoes, are always the same color, that is, the uncovered squares are either both black or both white. Because we know that each of the 31 dominoes must each cover two colors—that is, one white square and one black square—we know that the problem cannot be solved. The squares remaining on the board are not completely paired by color and so can never be completely covered by dominoes that must each cover one black and one white square.

In a large and complex realm of possible places to look when we are trying hard to gain a grip on a problem or a problematic situation, even a little guidance as to where we should be looking may be tremendously helpful. We should try to notice what *remains the same* in our various attempts to solve a problem. That is, what is *invariant* across different approaches whether it is a perceptual feature or something that is not perceptual.

As the researchers astutely observed: "The essence of discovery . . . is that you do *not* know beforehand where the solution may lie. If noticing invariants, and in particular perceptual invariants, provided even a little search constraint for the ill-defined task of discovery, then we have a cause for celebration."[12]

Abstract terms are powerful, but they can also be dangerous. Their power is that they enable us to travel across and capture our experiences in a highly compressed and efficient manner. Abstract concepts provide us with a potent mode of intellectual locomotion. Their danger lurks in exactly what makes them so powerful. If our thinking becomes too separated or overly distant from the concrete particulars that test and anchor them, we can become lost in speculations with outcomes that cannot be implemented or that, when implemented, lead to unanticipated detrimental side effects. Actually *acting* to realize our ideas, even if only in part, as in writing computer code or rapidly introducing prototypes, provides us with specific anchored feedback and harnesses the potential of the perception-action cycle to carry us beyond mere mental mullings and musings.

Excessive abstraction can also constrain the ideas that are accessible to us in our idea landscapes and narrow the possibility for breakthrough insights. We may miss richer, more fully embedded meanings that connect us to other people and their aspirations and to other objects through the world of the senses—how something looks, sounds, feels, tastes, and smells and the ways in which we interact with it. But without abstractions we may become mired in details, unable to see and move beyond the narrow confines of our current particular situation. Detail stepping—moving up and down and back again in our levels of abstraction and specificity—enables us to adaptively and creatively make the most of all of our mind's and brain's capabilities to encode and store and relate information from our experiences.

> The order in organizational life comes just as much from the subtle, the small, the relational, the oral, the particular, and the momentary as it does from the conspicuous, the large, the substantive, the written, the general, and the sustained.... To make sense is to connect the abstract with the concrete.[13]
>
> —*Organizational theorist and professor Karl E. Weick and colleagues*

PHYSICAL OBJECTS, PHYSICAL WORLDS

Ideas exist in physical forms. Physical instantiations or realizations of our ideas through sketches, diagrams, maquettes, mock-ups, prototypes—as well as snippets or snatches of written words, computer code, equations, or musical notation—provide essential ways of capturing, storing, and testing our evolving ideas. The physical support provided by prototypes, sketches, diagrams, or mock-ups can lighten the demands on our mental processing, relying on our **perception-action cycle** and the powerful interplay of brain and environment. External support frees up thinking resources, such as our short-term working memory, expanding our idea landscapes that can then be drawn upon for the revision and extension of our emerging thoughts. As we set aside or reencounter successive drafts or versions of our ideas, such physical records also empower us to repeatedly revisit and elaborate our ideas across times and spaces.

> Designers consistently used a combination of textual descriptions, pictures, graphs, and mathematical representations throughout the design process.... Our observations suggest that the mental representations that designers use are rich and multimodal in nature, and are organized at different levels of abstraction.[14]
>
> —*Computational and cognitive science expert Ashok Goel and colleagues*

One ready and robust tool to help us spur ideas is prototyping. In *prototyping* we make a physical embodiment or virtual instantiation of an idea or process in order to test the feasibility of our ideas. Prototypes also allow us to better communicate our ideas to others.

The prototypes we use may themselves be more or less precise, and we may want to quickly adopt a number of different partial or intermediate prototypes in a mode of rapid prototyping. Rapid or iterative prototypes "are intended to be inexpensive, easy to modify, and quickly made representations of ideas that can be tested against the actual use environment."[15] Prototypes may act analogously to what in computer programming is known as a "read-eval-print loop" in which the programmer can rapidly explore, iteratively test, and debug her code, receiving quick and concrete feedback.[16]

During the early stages of generating new ideas, it is important not to aim for perfection or polish in the drafts or prototypes that we work with. Our initial exploration and discovery may require intermediate levels of detail—partial drafts or low-fidelity prototypes that are only approximately correct and not highly precise. This may work best if undertaken with a moderate degree of purposeful cognitive control leaving adequate room for spontaneity and unanticipated directions. Quickly cycling through multiple unfinished and partial attempts has many benefits. This process gives us rapid feedback, opportunities for recalibration, and a sense of progress, leading us in promising directions.

Developing multiple ideas in tandem is another way in which we can productively harness detail stepping using our immediate environment. In *parallel prototyping* we concurrently pursue two or more possible ideas or prototypes rather than only a single one at a time. This parallel process may yield many helpful connections and point to potential difficulties as well as potential solutions early on and throughout our generative process. The concurrent generation of alternative prototypes may prompt us to notice fundamental similarities and subtle differences that would escape our attention if we successively step-by-step or serially attempted to refine a single idea.

Consider an experiment in which the participants were asked to create advertisements for a website under either one of two conditions.[17] In one condition, the participants were assigned to a *serial* prototyping process, in which they received feedback for their designs one at a time. Other participants instead were assigned to a *parallel* prototyping process, in which they received feedback for two or three designs at a time rather than one by one. Those who were assigned to a parallel rather than a serial prototyping process produced designs that were significantly more varied and effective. Experts rated the designs of those in the parallel prototyping condition as higher in creativity. These two different forms of prototyping, with their diverging outcomes, are schematically illustrated in Figure 2.5.

The creative process often involves multiple successive approximations toward a better understanding and realization of where our creative endeavor is going, should go, or might go. Particularly in the earlier phases of our creative process, the presence of multiple alternative prototypes can encourage our mental flexibility to recombine and appropriately redirect our

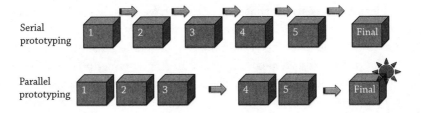

PARALLEL PROTOTYPING PROVIDES CREATIVE ADVANTAGES OVER SERIAL PROTOTYPING.	THE BENEFITS OF PARALLEL PROTOTYPING. Concurrently working on more than one idea or prototype at one time and then receiving feedback on those ideas was found to elicit more creative and effective solutions than was observed for a step-by-step serial process, with feedback given after each generated prototype.[18]

Figure 2.5

thinking. Parallel prototyping prompts us to capitalize on our natural abilities to better learn and perceive through comparison and contrast. We form useful differentiations and distinctions through juxtaposing—next to one another in space and time—objects or processes that share commonalities but also differences laden with possibilities.[19]

The recognition that we have alternative possible directions has an additional benefit. It may help us to avoid excessive investment of *emotions and resources* in any single idea, encouraging our ongoing openness to new as yet undiscovered possibilities. Ongoing openness and nondefensiveness then become part of a positive cycle of fluid, receptive, responsive interplay of ideas. We respond more positively and attentively to critiques and suggestions for improvement. Our emotional and intellectual investments then become and remain dedicated to the overarching creative process rather than to any one particular idea, approach, or instantiation.[20]

Despite the many potential aids and inspirations to creative thought that are offered by our immediately experienced surroundings or physical and social environments, we also need to be aware of the converse potential. As potent shapers of our idea landscapes, our environments can also lead us astray. Sometimes our environments, rather than helping us, may miscue us or unhelpfully hamper our efforts at novel exploration. What we encounter in our environments may unwittingly pull us and our thinking toward the conventional or toward the already familiar.

The ideas or suggestions that we or others have already produced can cue repetitive or habitual thinking, leading to an overly restrictive conception of what is possible. Such detrimental cuing effects are sometimes referred to as **design fixation**. Repeatedly encountering commonplace or familiar examples—as opposed to also experiencing unusual, less frequent, or atypical instances—can confine creative thinking even without our awareness.[21]

Unintentional reliance on prior examples is very powerful and can be difficult to notice. In a number of experiments it has been found that even when participants are explicitly told not to rely on specific examples, they continue to do so without realizing it. Suppose you are asked to design a measuring cup that might be used by a person who is visually impaired. Senior mechanical engineering students who were given an example page with a diagram of a potential design that deliberately included two obvious design flaws more often generated designs that were similar to the example—despite its flaws—as compared with students who were not provided with an example.[22]

Professional designers, too, either may be unaware of their inadvertent copying or mistakenly believe that the effects of example illustrations on their design thinking are positive. When presented with sample illustrations, professional designers, just like novices, generated fewer ideas and tended to imitatively incorporate features of those examples.[23]

Our own creative processes also leave a trail of examples. We need to ask whether our *self-generated* examples are helping to foster or hinder our creative ideas and approaches. We also need to consider the ways in which we use examples and prototypes across time. Perhaps paradoxically, an important way to counteract the potentially undermining effects of one or a few examples may be to generate varied and multiple ideas rather than just one single idea. As we have seen with rapid and parallel prototyping, a chorus of examples may be better than a lone one. Changing the way in which examples are provided or encountered, such as through using analogies or rerepresenting the problem through alternative categories, may also help us to reduce habitual thinking or the potential detrimental effects of examples.[24]

Our physical and virtual environments enter into and influence our creative processes in many often indirect ways. We should think carefully about how to structure and arrange our working and thinking environments to best encourage our ability to reach and hold on to promising ideas. Arranging our thinking and working environments so that the appropriate materials or tools are ready to hand can help us avoid branching off or detouring into distracting subtasks—preventing unnecessary clutter in our idea landscapes and in our short-term working memory. We also need ready access to supplies and materials with which to try out ideas, together with cleared and ample workspaces in which to experiment. Are there objects and images nearby that provoke your imagination? Can you easily reconfigure chairs and thinking/working spaces to allow the ready communication and expression of emerging thoughts between different individuals or teams? Does your making-and-finding environment allow sufficient privacy and autonomy, without undue or premature scrutiny, such that you and your team can fully and freely explore, iteratively test, and experiment? Do you "prototype your space" just as you do your creative projects, iteratively adapting and modifying your environment as you learn what most ignites and sustains your thinking?[25]

A creativity-friendly environment can maximize our access to promising ideas, feelings, and sensations that are incipient in our awareness. Environments that are friendly to our creative process can prevent us from losing preliminary fragments of ideas before they are no longer consciously accessible, also allowing us to integrate emotional premonitions or emergent tentative patterns. These and other ways in which our environments enter into our idea landscapes are abstractly summarized in Figure 2.6.

Although there is not a single ideal physical or virtual working-thinking space for everyone, paying closer attention to our own creative processes can help us to identify when objects in our environment are helping or hurting our ability to generate, pursue, and elaborate ideas. Do you find yourself frequently being reminded of irrelevant obligations or projects? If so, are there objects or notes or digital devices that you might place elsewhere or put away to help maintain your focus on the current project? If an idea emerges, can you capture it quickly and effectively with the materials and tools at hand? Are there things in your environment that you find productively stimulating and that fully engage your senses? Does your environment allow you to naturally move between periods of intense concentration and more diffusely but still focused attention? Do your collaborative physical spaces allow everyone to see each other and to readily make eye contact with one another? If you are having a discussion is everyone able to hear clearly? Is there sufficient room to walk around and to freely gesture?

> Looking at someone's office, kitchen pantry, bedroom, or even computer monitor, what one sees is an entire structure of cognitive and volitional scaffolding, a system that this person uses in order to accomplish (with varying degrees of success) routine tasks.... People who are good at environmental manipulation try to organize their affairs in such a way as to make certain activities easier and others harder.[26]
> —*Philosophy professors and social theorists Joseph Heath and Joel Anderson*

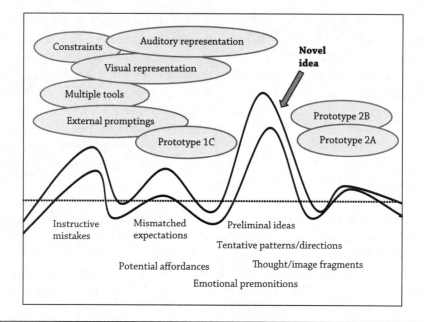

OUR ENVIRONMENTS ENTER INTO OUR THINKING PROCESSES IN MULTIPLE WAYS.	THE INTERPLAY OF OUR ENVIRONMENTS WITH OUR IDEA LANDSCAPES. Our ability to notice, capture, and creatively work through ideas is sculpted and shaped by our environments, including the opportunities the environment provides for the ready exploration of newly emergent ideas and their comparison and contrast. The dotted horizontal line represents our conscious awareness threshold.

Figure 2.6

Using our native aptitudes for perceptual grouping and pattern recognition to help us classify and arrange information, including symbolic information, can greatly ease the demands on our short-term working memory, freeing up room in our idea landscape for other relations and ideas. Think, for example, of how you name your digital or other files. Is the most important information included in the name of the file or its associated tags? Where, precisely, is that information in the name; does your eye naturally and effortlessly go to that information, or do you have to attend closely and search to find it? Are there ways in which you could use UPPERCASE or other__visual separators__to highlight the information you **need first** or *most often* in your work and thinking? If you are using a table to summarize data, might using a diagram or graph help you to better compare and readily extract relations and patterns?[27] Could you use colors or a color-coded heat map to easily visualize patterns? Grouping similar objects or materials together near to one another in space can help us to move away from a more coarse-grained categorization, allowing us to notice increasingly subtle perceptual and other differences.[28]

 Thought Box: *Words Are Physical Objects Too!*

The physical forms of words—whether spoken, written, or signed—may cue other words similar in sound or sense, as in alliteration, rhyming, and assonance.[29]

Think about playing a traditional game of Scrabble, with its smooth wooden tiles each with its own black-printed letter and score and the elongated wooden letter trays that allow us to easily shift and rearrange the tiles. Why does moving the letters around physically to a new arrangement on the tray often prompt new possible words that did not come to mind before we rearranged the letter tiles?

One reason is that we are able to transfer some of the mental demands for imaginatively recombining letters into possible words through the external physical support offered by the tiles themselves. But it may be more than this.

The constraints and pushes and pulls that bring to mind possible words in our *internal* idea landscape differ from the constraints that exist in the *external* world of the tiles. Beyond our ability to physically move and lodge the letter tiles, there are few limits in the external world on what we can place next to next. Physically any letter can go next to any other letter on the tray. In contrast, our ability to place letters next to next in our own minds is guided—wittingly or not—by what we know and have experienced in how letters make up words (lexical possibilities) or permitted sounds or sound sequences (phonology). Because our starting points and the "rules" for moving are different, our trajectories through mental versus physical spaces will be different.

In the language of one type of computer model of human thinking: "Mental rearrangements follow least energy paths in a lexical or phonological landscape, while physical rearrangement is sensitive to how easy or hard it is to move the [Scrabble] tiles. The state spaces [possible options] are different and hence the trajectories through those spaces will be different."[30]

In our mental landscape, we will also be guided by our goals to find words that could fit with others already on the Scrabble board and by strategies for optimizing our scores. These constraints do not directly apply to our physical movements of the letters. Our physical juxtaposing of the letters will generate many possibilities that simply are not feasible, but it may also uncover nonobvious options that we otherwise would have missed.

Moving the letter tiles about would not be beneficial if we ignored the changed options that come to mind or failed to spend time letting possibilities emerge. We need receptivity and dialogue or "back talk" with the materials at hand.[31] Placing words on a page or on a whiteboard, grouping them, subgrouping them, sketching connections with arrows, eliminating or erasing and questioning—all provide opportunities for such dialogue. Working with different types of materials may require different types of questioning and different expectations of making and finding or of intended and emergent outcomes.

Physical drafts and mock-ups are also communicative objects. Ready to hand can be ready to mind within not only our own creative thinking but also that of others on our team. Physical models and sketches can rapidly bring everyone together to the current situation and allow individuals to physically point or gesture as they seek to articulate their emerging ideas. As we saw in the electronic whiteboard example discussed in Part 1, such communal sharing of and access to ideas among a team can be especially important early in the idea-formation process and can improve design team performance on multiple dimensions.[32] Drafts, models, and mock-ups provide "living" specifications or constraints that can be up-to-date indicators of a project's evolving progress, tangibly scaffolding our mental access to ideas and the carrying forward of creativity and change.[33]

ENACTING KNOWLEDGE

Let's pause for a moment and vividly imagine that you are asked to complete the following three tasks in your mind:

1. Breaking a small birthday candle into three even-sized segments
2. Poking a "smiley-face" or "smiley" into a 3-inch square of thin paper using a toothpick
3. Tying a pair of shoelaces (without shoes) into a double knot

As you imagine each of these activities, what thoughts come to mind? What do you notice as you mentally simulate each activity in your mind's eye? Do you experience any surprises, stumblings, or unexpected discoveries as you imaginatively break the candle? What happens as you poke an imagined toothpick through the paper?

Now suppose that instead of *mentally simulating* the three activities you *actually perform* them with physical objects. Or, if you have any of these materials on hand, find them and work through the activities. What new information or insights do you gain or might you expect to gain from your direct and tangible interaction with the objects?

Informal classroom and group explorations that we have undertaken using these three activities showed a number of differences between the imagined mental simulations compared with actual physical enactments. Pairs of students or group members were asked to "think aloud" as they performed each of the tasks either exclusively in their minds or using pro-vided objects. Their think-aloud responses and retrospective observations revealed that there were unique benefits—but also pitfalls—to both the mentally simulated and the physical enactments.

Enactments with the actual materials evoked descriptions and obser-vations that were closely linked to the objects at hand and were in some respects highly literal. The color of the paper was noted as "blue" for the phys-ical enactment of the paper-based task, but its color was never mentioned for the **mental simulation/perceptual simulation**. In contrast, some mental enactments were accompanied by more schematic or generalized ideas, by analogical thinking, or by autobiographical memories or emotions. One stu-dent in her mental simulation saw an analogy between the broken candle and a leg fracture; another student, while attempting to mentally simulate forming a double knot, recalled a particular occasion of tying his ice skates.

Physical enactments tended to be accompanied by greater awareness of perceptual-motor difficulty. Poking small and regularly spaced holes through a piece of paper with a tiny implement, for example, required considerably more coordination and dexterity than was expected, as people discovered that the paper needed to be both firmly stretched and punctured at the same time. When asked to break the candle into three equal segments, many students in the imagined task made no reference to the wick. In contrast, physical enactments invariably elicited references to this hidden internal and central aspect of the candle. Students expressed surprise at finding that the candlewick resolutely resisted breaking and that the wax crumbled into multiple pieces around the wick.

Both physical enactments and mental simulations provide us with increased potential for innovative relational thinking. In mental simulations we imaginatively work through an interaction with an object or process, such as imagining ourselves walking through a revolving door or through a turnstile. Mental simulations can alter our ease of access to even very well known information, making it easier or harder to draw on related experiential knowledge. If we are asked to think of a watermelon, we may imagine its hefty weight and oval shape. If, though, we are asked to think of half a watermelon, we may bring to mind, instead, the light inner rind contrasting with the darker fruit and the nestled watermelon seeds.[34]

Suppose you were asked to imagine that "You are driving a car" or, instead, "You are washing a car," and then asked to answer questions such as "Can you touch the headlights?" and "Can you touch the wheels?" If research participants imagined themselves driving the car, they answered the questions more quickly when asked about the steering wheel or gas pedal than if they were asked about the car's trunk or tires. The opposite was true if the participants had imagined themselves washing the car; they then verified exterior features of the automobile more quickly than interior ones.[35]

These changes in the mental accessibility of relevant information occurred largely automatically as a consequence or by-product of mental simulation. Our mental simulations and our imagined spatial situatedness in our simulations directly influence the readiness with which we can gain access to long-term knowledge about how objects and object parts are spatially and functionally related. Deliberately varying our simulated physical perspectives and situations may enable us to connect and cross-connect a wider set of features of an emerging creative product or scientific endeavor.[36]

The type and degree of imagined and actual physical support we can best use in our creative endeavors depends on many factors. The complexity or multidimensionality of the ideas or processes that we are attempting to anticipate is important, as is the likelihood that we may overlook subtle or emerging features. Physical objects, too, differ in their degree of support. Sketches and diagrams provide valuable scaffolding for our thinking but, given their two-dimensional nature, also require additional imaginative reconstruction to be translated into three-dimensional space. As schematically shown in Figure 2.7, external representations differ in their degree of detail and physicality. The further explicitness and concreteness of three-dimensional over two-dimensional representations may prove valuable because the additional dimensionality reduces the demands on our imaginative reconstruction, freeing up our mental resources for other aspects of the creative process.

Comparing design teams who used two-dimensional as opposed to three-dimensional materials during a complex design project, one research study found that teams using three-dimensional materials produced designs that, across an extended series of design attempts, performed

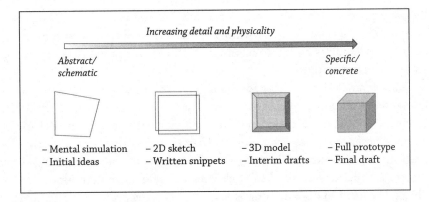

| CHANGING THE LEVEL OF DETAIL AND THE PHYSICALITY OF THE REPRESENTATIONS THAT WE ARE USING IN OUR THINKING PROCESSES MAY REVEAL NEW POTENTIAL PROBLEMS AND NOVEL POSSIBILITIES. | VARYING THE ABSTRACTNESS OF OUR REPRESENTATIONS TO SUPPORT CREATIVITY. During the formation and revision of our ideas, we can productively rely on multiple levels of abstraction and environmental support. The mental and physical representations of our ideas span a wide range from mental simulation through sketches, models, and prototypes, and from initial vague ideas through to a final written draft or full prototype. |

Figure 2.7

better, and showed reduced design fixation, than if only two-dimensional materials were used. Architects and landscape architects, for example, deliberately use many types of sketches, models, and mock-ups. Each representational format captures alternative levels of abstraction and schematically focuses on different aspects of the building or site, in turn revealing new potential problems and possibilities. Adopting—and flexibly alternating between—various external representations can enable us to see novel and unanticipated directions. Choosing multiple external representations supports deeper understanding and rich articulation of how objects and events truly unfold in time and space.[37]

Actually handling an object, moving it around, and interacting with it may provide insight into both how it actually works and how it might be used in alternative or novel ways. If we are thinking of a spoon as a scoop, it may not be too difficult to see that it could be used to smooth or level something. It may, though, be more difficult to see that it might also be used to pierce something, because this latter use likely requires holding the spoon by the cupped bowl rather than the handle. Functions are themselves complex, with actions embedded within actions, as where the spoon is gripped, so piercing requires a larger reconfiguration of our current idea landscape than does smoothing.[38]

Using an analogy, the current scooping use of the spoon is like a magnetic "attractor" that pulls or holds attention near to our current way of thinking. Using an object for one function ("preutilization") may block our noticing of alternative possibilities, even possibilities that we otherwise, without the preutilization, could readily recognize. If an object is already being used for a certain function, we tend to stick with or "glue" that function onto the object. We need to distance ourselves from the categorization of the object to see alternatives. Even identifying a single novel use for an object may stand in the way of identifying yet other novel uses, thus preempting further flexible formulations.[39]

Our more abstract schematic understanding of the usual functional purposes of objects may impede us from imaginatively seeing other uses beyond the typical or conventionally intended usage. This tendency for automatically categorizing objects based on their perceived intended function (known as *functional fixedness*) develops early in childhood and persists throughout our lives. Quite young children, of about five years of age or younger may, though, show *greater* flexibility or fluidity in how they think about objects and their functions.

When seven-year-old children were asked to suggest possible novel uses for a brick, they tended to provide variants on the standard function of the object. For example, they might begin with "to build a house" and follow that by "to build a wall," "to build a castle," "to build a school," and so on. In contrast, when still younger five-year-olds were asked the same question, they were more likely to include other plausible uses beyond those of the usual function, such as "to stop a door from blowing shut in the wind." For the youngest children, what an object looks like or how heavy it is and whether it is porous or could hold a liquid of any kind are just as important as the object's abstract conventional function.[40]

What happens when we engage more fully and vividly in the imaginative and exploratory activity of thinking of as many different uses as possible for a common object such as a blanket, brick, or paper clip? In generating possible uses we tend to begin by relying on our memories for how we and others have used such objects in the past. After we exhaust this initial search of our memories, we may begin to expand our range of thinking by perceptually simulating what bricks look and feel like (sensory-perceptual simulation). We may also begin thinking about more general purposes that people have (for example, transportation or communication) and whether the brick then could be imaginatively adapted to meet those purposes or goals (abstract conceptual exploration).[41]

Through our sensory-perceptual simulation of a brick, we might generate the idea of using a brick as an abrasive to smooth a surface or as a writing tool to compose a prominent greeting (or directions) in the sand on a beach. Using the abstract conceptual approach, we might arrive at the idea of using the brick to attach a written note to be thrown over a high wall in order to communicate with someone on the other side (a combination of both communication and transportation). Movements up and down within these levels of representational specificity help to spark novelty and creativity.

Research indicates that engaging in a combination of interleaved movements between more concrete and more abstract modes of thought may facilitate our subsequent efforts at insightful and flexible thinking. As we saw in Part 1, simply asking people to think about different ways to use a familiar object, such as a paper clip or a chair, for only 10 minutes improved their ability to solve insight problems and other novel reasoning tasks. The participants who thought of novel uses for objects outperformed others who were asked to generate the first words that came to mind during a word-association task. The participants asked to generate novel uses for familiar objects also were more insightful and more flexible problem solvers than were those who didn't perform any earlier task.[42]

Detail stepping in our creative process is sometimes prompted by the automatic noticing of unexpected potentialities or affordances in our environment that will meet our pending goals or subgoals. As we have seen, **affordances** are the possibilities for action and interaction that objects—or their representations—offer us, such as, for physical objects, opportunities for grasping, pulling, lifting, or supporting. Affordances are typically thought of in relation to our own ability to act, as when a particular object may be seen to "afford" sitting for a small and slight child but not for a larger and heavier adult. Affordances may also be construed for objects in relation to other objects. Think, for example, of how a chair or box might "afford" stacking with other chairs or boxes.[43]

Being attuned to and incorporating such object-to-object affordances as well as person-to-object affordances can creatively inspire the design process. So, too, for *representational affordances*. How we perceptually or physically represent (re-present) our ideas may make it easier or more difficult for us to see our way through to our creative goals and subgoals. Just like physical objects, representations may themselves make some cognitive actions easier to perform than others. Think of trying to perform division or multiplication using Roman numerals. Or imagine evaluating route and route times for an extended hike without the benefit of a topographical map or

GPS, or constructing a contemporary building without access to plan, elevation, and section diagrams.[44]

Noticing affordances often occurs intuitively but may be facilitated by expressing our goals at a midlevel of abstraction. Contrast, for example, "What is wanted here is a raised surface that could provide stable support for my body weight" with "I need a stepladder." As we saw in Part 1, during complex design, individuals often move between different levels of detail as the problem they are working on offers new ideas. These changes in a thinker's level of abstraction frequently coincide with unexpected affordances, presented by the problem situation, for moving forward in solving a problem, such as specifying necessary constraints on the possible solution.[45]

These affordances in the environment may be associatively cued largely automatically without deliberate top-down thinking, and following them may momentarily reduce the need for higher and more demanding degrees of mental control. Acting on a given affordance may itself reveal additional affordances as our creative and thinking processes unfold over time.

As one contemporary sculptor explained an important discovery in how she might approach her materials:

I didn't have enough money to make big bronze sculpture to fill this exhibition, and I was going for a walk every evening, and a swim on the beach. And that was when the fisherman were bringing in their nets. And I started looking at those forms on the beach, and I thought, "Well, there's another approach to volumetric form, without weight." And I could ship [the nets] around; they'd fold up, and they could be extended. And I'm still working with those ideas.[46]

Beyond affordances, another way in which our bodies may enter into our own and other's thinking processes and detail stepping is through gesture. Gesturing with our hands as we speak and think may support the development and expression of our ideas. Gestures become active participants in our idea landscapes and can even precede our awareness of ideas or signal incipient ideas. Gestures, in themselves, are quite concrete (physical tangible actions) but may refer to, or substitute for, highly abstract ideas. Sometimes when we are thinking we may gesture to indicate a balancing of viewpoints, as in "on the one hand, on the other hand." Or we may gesticulate to indicate that "this equals that," or trace an arc to physically suggest a continuous movement through space or time. Our gestures often help us to organize and group our thoughts. Just like physical objects, gestures can open up room in our idea landscapes for us to devote to evolving creative ideas and relations.[47]

Gestures provide opportunities for mapping (perceptually indexing) between our mental representations and the external world, as when we might show the thought of balancing using a similar movement here and then a similar movement there. Gesturing helps us to selectively single out relevant information such as the objects, spaces, and actions to which our spoken words or symbols refer, providing contextual support for our thinking. Gesturing can make clear the affordances—possibilities for action and interaction—that objects offer.

As continuous movements in space, gestures can also themselves perform representational "work" for us, as when rotational gestures help us to better think through and mentally simulate a particular mechanical problem. Gestures enable us to package information into tangible perceptual-motor segments that we can then use to further scaffold our problem-solving and creative thinking.[48]

There are many advantages to both abstract and specific (including physically expressed) modes of thinking and processing information. Ideally, in our creative endeavors and efforts to promote positive change, we neglect neither and discover ways to build on both. We next explore a parallel point but now within the "metarealm" of our thinking about our thinking.

THINKING ABOUT THINKING

We can find ourselves at different conceptual distances and levels of detail in the content of our thoughts, or what our thinking is about. This applies not only to thoughts about objects and events outside of ourselves but also to how we are thinking about our own thinking. Our thoughts and creative processes may themselves be the topic of our thinking. We may wonder if we are taking a wrong turn in our creative path, if we should perhaps change the way we are approaching a problem, or if we should reinvigorate or recast our aims.

One way in which we may introduce freshness and necessary distance into our thinking is through drawing on analogy or metaphor. Analogies offer us a way of thinking about the similarities of the relations or likenesses between things or processes. Analogies help to isolate a relevant relation. If we say "cub is to bear as kitten is to cat," we focus our attention on a shared developmental commonality. If we characterize our thinking as "a stream of thought," we single out its continuity, fluidity, and directedness. Or, in the words of the philosopher and psychologist William James, "Consciousness, then, does not appear to itself chopped up in bits. . . . It is nothing jointed; it flows. A 'river' or a 'stream' are the metaphors by which it is most naturally described."[49]

Analogies provide an important mode of thinking that can be harnessed to empower us to think about or rethink a current problem, project, or process in relation to its similarities and differences with our earlier experiences. Some analogies or examples that we generate may be comparatively close to our current situation. Other analogies that we or our teams propose may be quite distant or remote from the current situation. Still other productive analogies may occupy an intermediate conceptual distance from the problem at hand. Combining two or more analogies or metaphors similarly may spark surprising ideas.[50]

What if, for example, you were asked to develop a new "baton" for the Commonwealth Games baton relay—where some 5,000 runners traversing over 60,000 miles will successively exchange the baton before the start of the games?

A team of designers challenged with this task drew upon knowledge from an apparently unrelated former project involving a digital antenna. The antenna was shaped like a long stick with a broader middle portion, which allowed for a lighted display depicting the strength and activity of the radio signals received. In the newly designed relay baton made of a conductive material, the broader middle portion featured a large blue LED display that pulsated up the baton in time with the baton holder's heartbeat. The baton then became a novel and dynamically embodied biophysical rhythmic message to the spectators along the relay route.[51]

This extension of the team's prior experience exemplifies a middle-distance form of analogical transfer. Like many instances of creativity, it also involves an inventive recombination, connecting previously unconnected ideas in a new form.

The use of analogies and examples may help us to move about in our idea landscape in terms of distance, range, and depth, allowing new possibilities to come to awareness. Examples that are nearer or closer to the problem at hand or are relatively commonplace may bring to mind numerous but somewhat less novel ideas, but these are likely to be more immediately feasible. Comparatively remote or far afield analogies and less common examples may lead to more novel idea generation, but the quality of the ideas produced may also be more highly variable, encompassing especially low- as well as especially high-quality ideas.[52]

Analogical relations are pervasive in our thinking. Speaking of "remote" and "near" analogies itself involves mapping distances of conceptual similarity to distances in physical space. Similarly, construing commonplace

examples as "attractors" that constrain our creative search involves analo-
gizing our thoughts to physical objects such as the field of a magnet attracting nearby objects that contain nickel or iron. These ideas are themselves
analogically captured in Figure 2.8.

Analogies are clearly important in the generation of ideas, but they can
also serve several other functions in fostering positive creative change.
Analogies enable us to use what we already know in order to better understand or grasp something that is novel or less familiar. In one study of projects aimed at developing new products, 6 of 16 people interviewed explicitly
noted that analogies helped to promote *communication* among team members,
designers, and engineers. Two of the interviewees even stated that enhanced
communication was the most important aspect of the analogy in the given
project. The communicative and explanatory functions of analogies may

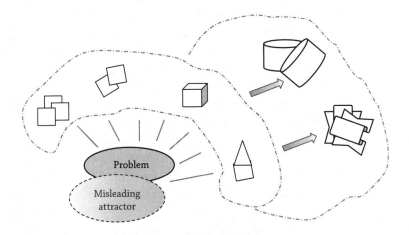

EXPOSURE TO DISTANT OR UNCOMMON EXAMPLES OR ANALOGIES MAY OPEN UP NEW CREATIVE POSSIBILITIES.	ANALOGIES CAN HELP US REACH NEAR OR FAR CONCEPTUAL SPACES. With a misleadingly narrow problem interpretation removed, our similarity space broadens and more options become available in our idea landscape. The consideration of far-field and less common exemplars compared with near-field and common exemplars may have a similar effect of increasing novelty and variability. However, far-field examples need to come to mind in the first place, and discovering their relevance may be challeng-ing. Intermediate levels of distance may also prove beneficial.

Figure 2.8

prove especially pivotal in bridging the gap between teams and individuals with quite disparate backgrounds, task priorities, and thought processes. Equally important, analogies can also help to articulate and clarify the distinctive or core goals of a design or engineering project.[53]

Analogies are, in part, abstractions, but they are so only in part. Like physical prototypes or models, they carry beneficial concreteness and details along with them that serve to anchor and reality-test creativity by helping us to think of the relations and interrelations between the various aspects of a process or product.

But how do analogies and useful recategorizations and reconceptualizations of our experiences arise? Analogies can be deliberately encouraged and solicited as part of a creative design process. They may also arise spontaneously, naturally, and regularly during thought and problem-solving situations requiring change, creativity, and adaptive agility. All but one of the 16 team members interviewed in the new product development study retrospectively reported that the spontaneous—unstructured and unplanned—use of analogies was a pervasive and frequent aspect of their thinking and creative process. Direct observations of science research lab meetings and teams have also documented that science teams frequently generate and rely on analogies.[54]

Professional engineers and masters' level engineering students who were asked to think aloud while working on a design problem demonstrated many spontaneous analogies. Abstract (schema-driven) and specific (case-driven) analogies were freely produced. The professional engineers, on average, generated over 50 schema-driven analogies and more than 10 case-driven analogies per hour. Stated differently, the engineers, during their design thinking, generated more than one analogy a minute. The engineering students, in contrast, spontaneously mentioned about 16 schema-driven analogies per hour and nearly double that many case-driven analogies, or about one analogy every 90 seconds. These results stand in marked contrast to findings from less naturalistic lab-based research studies, where participants have often seemed to fail to use analogies even when they had recently experienced events that were relevant to the analogies.[55]

Analogies may also be deliberately sought out. Consider the case of a ski manufacturer faced with the issue that the skis they produced would start to excessively vibrate when skiers exceeded a certain speed, making the skier's control difficult. The R&D team recognized that a solution might be found by searching for known solutions in other fields or industries that used dampening or cushioning to reduce unwanted vibrations. However, this deliberate search yielded far too many possible directions.

A viable solution emerged only when one of the team members stepped down in detail and decided to restrict the search to vibration frequencies over 1,800 Hz—the frequency at which the skis typically began to vibrate. With this additional specific constraint, the team found an analogous problem in the world of musical instruments—where bowed instruments such as violins and cellos sometimes also develop undesirable vibrational frequencies. Drawing on the experience of an expert in bowed instruments, the team incorporated an extra material layer in the ski, similar to the grid structure used in bowed musical instruments but tailored to the novel context. This analogy-derived approach eventually solved the vibration problem.[56]

Distributing problem information widely—to a diverse community of potential problem solvers concurrently or in parallel—may provide openings for new approaches by introducing the problem to individuals with expertise that is farther afield. Sharing intermediate or early results of problem-solving progress outside a team—an open exposure of evolving ideas—may promote the concentration of effort in promising solution approaches but also limit the wider range of ideas being explored. Removing barriers to entry for nonobvious individuals on the "outer circle" and inviting the participation of individuals and teams beyond the typically recognized expert community may be especially valuable in situations involving highly uncertain innovation problems for which predicting the solution direction or required expertise is also uncertain.[57] (We discuss the importance and role of innovation contests in Part 5.)

Biologically inspired design is one example of drawing on analogies from one field, in this case that of biology, to problems faced in other fields—such as engineering, materials science, architecture, or computer science—to foster new and surprising insights. This analogical approach (sometimes referred to as biomimesis or biomimicry) involves the "crossover" of ideas from biology to challenging problems in apparently unrelated fields at the level of materials, structures, functions, principles, or systems.[58]

Reflect for a moment on the highly unpredictable demands placed on the Internet servers that we—and millions of others—use to access the Web and "cloud-based" resources on a minute-to-minute and hour-to-hour basis. Each time we seek to access a webpage or to use "the cloud," we are placing a specific request to a remote server. But the pattern of our collective requests is characterized by huge surges and lulls, with our demands on the servers volatile, and only partially predictable. It is crucial to efficiently allocate and prioritize server resources to minimize queuing or waiting and switching times.

How could expertise in the foraging behavior of nectar-seeking honeybees help us here? A honeybee colony, of up to as many as 50,000 bees, orchestrates its allocation of forager bees to dispersed patches of flowers with varying nectar yields. The yields fluctuate in time from abundance to scarcity, with the amount of nectar available changing from one day to the next by as much as a factor of 100 to 1. There are a surprising number of parallels between the honeybee colony and the Internet server scenario, such as the need for self-organization using decentralized mechanisms, the necessity for dynamic updating, and a call for a ready adaptability to changing circumstances. Recognition of these parallels led to the development of novel algorithmic approaches to Internet server allocations.[59] Variations on the honeybee algorithm have been extended to a wide array of other contexts, ranging from coordinating the supply of fuel and raw materials in manufacturing, to planning vehicle routing, to the scheduling of nursing shifts in hospitals.[60]

Now let's consider another example of biomimicry—that additionally illustrates the myriad ways in which the environment and the affordances it offers can guide intelligent action. Colonies of mound-building termites can build complex structures that are orders of magnitude their own size. They construct these intricate structures with each termite acting independently—each reacting to the local situation in which it finds itself, without any centralized decision making or planning. Could the natural principles of this form of self-organization (known as "stigmergy") guiding the behavior of mound-building termites be adapted to create independent, limited-capability robots—robots that would, like the termites, construct structures larger than themselves? If so, ultimately, such robot-produced structures might be used in situations where it is not feasible or safe for humans to build.

Inspired by the abilities of social insects to self-organize, engineers and computer scientists developed small mechanical robots, each with limited capabilities that follow simple rules, with all robots (like the termites) following the same rules.[61] Each robot can perform such simple actions as moving forward, moving back, and turning in place using wheel legs or "whegs." Each robot can pick up and place solid square "bricks" at their own level using local sensors that allow them to perceive only bricks and other robots immediately nearby. Each robot has a static representation of the target structure to be made but acts using the simple rules based on sensed brick configurations. The robots cannot communicate with one another: "all communication is implicit via the joint manipulation of a shared environment."[62] The robots, following low-level "traffic rules" and only reacting and sensing to their local situation in an autonomous, decentralized way, were able to achieve specific human design goals such as creating a stepped pyramid and complex structures with internal courtyards.

Successful search and identification of analogies relevant to a problem may itself involve detail stepping. If, for example, we are searching for novel approaches that allow an organism or system to stay cool, we may want to move up in our abstraction level to the broader, more encompassing concept of "thermoregulation." We might also attempt stepping down in our level of abstraction, attempting to identify specific "champion adaptors" who successfully tackle the problem of keeping cool, perhaps in especially harsh conditions such as an animal or a plant living in intense heat or a hot desert climate. In other situations, we may use detail stepping in our analogy search by changing the number or particular combinations of the constraints that we impose.[63]

Our search for useful analogies may itself require us to be flexibly creative in our modes of approach. We might query experts we know from various fields or query databases using terms and synonyms and near-synonyms or antonyms at differing levels of abstraction for actions, processes, and descriptors of each of these. Actions, for instance, are themselves frequently modified by descriptive adverbs that may help to narrow our search. Searches using verbs rather than nouns may yield more options, in part because they capture the notion of functions at a more abstract level.[64] These approaches, together with more structured efforts to facilitate analogical search—such as through knowledge-based computer-aided design—may help to prevent us from settling too quickly on a particular analogy and encourage more systematically varied search reaching far past our initial ideas or associations.[65]

Beyond analogies, changes in the level of abstraction in our thinking (and our thinking about thinking) also arise through changes in our situatedness in space or time relative to a given endeavor or problem. Sometimes we may be quite close to an endeavor or situation because it is very near to us in time or space. We may have been immersed in a creative situation for several hours or days. Or the important occasion of actually testing or realizing our ideas may be imminent and nearly upon us, as in the moments before the opening of an art exhibition, the opening night of a play, or a new-product launch. At other times, though, we may be more distant from our creative endeavor. Perhaps we have been traveling and are geographically removed from our project. Or we may have been engaged in other concerns for a number of hours, days, or weeks.

We may also change our distance from a creative endeavor through imaginative changes or *mental time travel* forward or backward in time.[66] Although an important event, such as a forthcoming theater production, may still be several months away, to more fully prepare and anticipate events we may imaginatively walk through precisely how we might reconfigure the stage set for the second half of the play.

In most situations, we tend to gravitate toward a somewhat abstract position, higher on the detail steps. We typically prefer to focus on the general meaning or gist of events, activities, and objects. However, a greater physical distance in space and distance in time may encourage us to adopt an even more abstract, general, or summary-based mode of thinking. When we are temporally or spatially removed from a project, we tend to see the forest and give less notice to the individual trees. We tend to be more rule-guided than guided by instances or cases. In contrast, when we are closer in time and space to a project or event, our thinking tends to be more concrete, specific, and contextually guided. Here we are likely to notice the individual trees and to be less focused on the forest.[67]

Placing ourselves forward in time, in the future, may increase the level of abstractness of our thinking, bringing with it both benefits and risks. Yet future thinking is not always abstract. Future thinking, too, can vary in levels of abstraction and—because this influences what we can readily bring or keep in mind—it, in turn, has implications for our ability to think creatively and solve problems.[68]

There are many parallels between how we typically travel backward in time to the past, and how we imaginatively seek to envision likely future scenarios or possibilities. Both involve pervasive detail stepping in our mind's eyes, ears, and other senses. We can step up in our level of abstraction to broader life phases or periods of time in our lives or to our long-term goals and overarching aims. From this abstract meta-view, we can also partially step down in our level of abstraction to memories that are generalized across many similar occasions. Or we can detail step even farther down, to particular episodes, with all their unique sensory and emotional experiences.

These varied degrees of abstraction in our imaginative projections forward or backward in time are visualized in Figure 2.9.

Just as we can recall and access events from our past in more general and gist-like, as opposed to more specific and detailed ways, we can imaginatively construct possible futures that are more schematic versus more richly concrete. Successfully simulating a future event often requires us to flexibly recombine *both* temporally and contextually specific information together with more abstract aspects into an integrated and coherent whole.[69]

Abstract conceptual memory may be particularly crucial in the generation of highly novel future events, providing necessary coherence and structure for less schematic information. Retrieving detailed unique memories may be especially beneficial during our open-ended flexible problem-solving efforts that require accessing a wide range of options. Details can then furnish us with concrete mental inroads to more diverse and grounded possibilities. When we fail to access such particularized and individuated memories of our experiences, we become "stuck" at an overly high level of abstraction. For example, during chronic worry we often rehearse concerns repeatedly

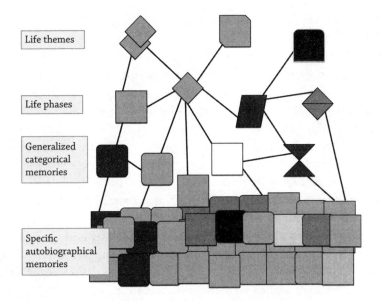

| Life themes |
| Life phases |
| Generalized categorical memories |
| Specific autobiographical memories |

| IMAGINING FUTURE POSSIBILITIES DRAWS ON OUR GENERAL AND SPECIFIC MEMORIES AT VARYING LEVELS OF DETAIL. | DETAIL STEPPING MOVING FORWARD AND BACKWARD IN TIME. Our autobiographical memories—whether individual, group, or organizational—form central parts of our idea landscapes and are stored at different levels of abstraction in relation to our ongoing goals and plans. We dynamically draw on the rich particularity of our past experiences not only in remembering but also in imagining and projecting forward into the future.[70] |

Figure 2.9

but in a very abstract manner without any practical or specific ideas of how to address the problem and move forward.[71]

We can also use detail stepping with regard to our goals and actions. Suppose we ask "What are you doing right now?" One answer you may provide is that you are seeing and reading words, with your eyes scanning across the page. Another answer, likely also true, is that you are trying to understand how detail stepping promotes creativity. At the same time you may have the goal of arriving at new insights into the many factors that support or undermine innovation and positive change. Although all of these (or some subset of these) characterizations of your current actions and goals may be true, which ones are most prominent to you and why?

Movements in the level of abstraction of our goals and actions often involve changes in our focus on *why* we hold certain aspirations (the reasons for or implications of our goals) versus *how* we might set about achieving our aims (the means to our goals). Repeatedly asking ourselves why we have a given goal or are choosing a given action can move us toward increasingly abstract thinking. Conversely, asking how we will accomplish a goal can move our thoughts in increasingly more concrete and specific directions. At lower levels of detail, we often focus on the feasibility or ease of attaining our goals and the specific implementations or concrete steps needed to achieve them. At higher levels of detail, we tend, instead, to dwell more on the desirability, prioritization, or function of our aims.[72] (We further discuss detail stepping in our goals in Part 6.)

Zooming out may allow us to bring to mind a wider and more inclusive array of possibilities and connections. Zooming in, too, though can be important, in alerting us to potentially pivotal details that can provide clues to new affordances and causal relations. Table 2.1 and Table 2.2 spell out these differing advantages—and risks.

Zooming out may also enable us to consider if, and how, our particular project or product would interplay coherently within a larger system-level context. Fully understanding a project's creative potential includes appreciating the more encompassing contexts in which an intended user of a new product or service might be brought into play, including how the "core" product or service might be better supported by supplementary services or accessories.

Table 2.1 ADVANTAGES OF DIFFERENT LEVELS OF SPECIFICITY

Abstract	Concrete
• Can be more readily extended and applied to novel situations	• Can be easier to remember and to access from long-term memory
• Emphasizes the most important aspects and downplays irrelevant details	• Some concrete details can informatively guide reasoning and inferences
• May encourage symbolic, context-free thinking and facilitate relational thinking	• May be easier to work and think through, with more tangible immediate feedback
• Enables flexible use of potent formal and symbolic representations	• Can capitalize on our sensory-perceptual pattern recognition and action capabilities

Both abstract and concrete modes of thinking and representing information offer distinctive benefits.[73]

Table 2.2 BENEFITS AND RISKS IN DETAIL STEPPING

	May promote	**May lead to**
More abstract or "stepping up"	• Rule-guided thinking • Big-picture view • Longer-term aims • Across-situation transfer or consistency	• Rigidity • Disconnectedness from actual contexts • Emotional distance • Remoteness
More concrete or "stepping down"	• Sensory attunement • Contextually sensitive variation • Connections to prior experiences	• Distractibility • Capture by examples • Inconsistency • Side tracking

Both moving up to more abstract and down to more concrete levels of abstraction offer accompanying benefits and risks.

> The total user need includes both a system-level solution and a detail-oriented focus.[74]
> —*Innovation experts and professors Marc H. Meyer and Tucker Marion*

> Some system properties can only be treated adequately in their entirety, taking into account all facets relating the social to the technical aspects ... These system properties derive from the relationships among the parts of the system: how the parts interact and fit together.[75]
> —*Systems expert and aerospace engineer, professor Nancy G. Leveson*

At a broader level, in teams, organizations, and complex processes of all kinds, zooming out may be crucial to identifying and learning from the sources of failures, accidents, or recurrent problems in larger systems involving many interacting parts or units. As we will see in Part 5, when we discuss "second-order problem solving," stepping up to a higher level of abstraction can allow us to perceive recurring issues or obstacles and to identify *why* something may be happening. Zooming out may also require changes in how individuals and members of a team think about possible sources of failures or problems. By zooming out we can often counteract a tendency to attribute missteps to individuals "individually" erring or to a unique and unfortunate co-occurrence of specific factors. Higher levels of abstraction help us to recognize, instead, how complex human systems have *emergent* practices. These emergent practices may support—or undermine—our longer-term goals and ideals.[76]

A capsule description of some of the complementary advantages of abstraction and specificity that we have discussed so far was provided earlier in Table 2.1.

Several of the advantages as well as the disadvantages of moving up and down in our detail steps were also earlier highlighted in Table 2.2. Maximizing our creativity and insight may require both ascending and descending in our level of abstraction at different times.

REPRESENTING MEANING IN THE BRAIN

In Part 1 we introduced the idea that all of our thinking and creating involves repeated cycles between what we see and perceive in our environment (what is open for us to notice and observe in the world outside of ourselves) and our actions (how we operate on the world and work with each other). Our perceptions of the external environment guide our actions, and our actions themselves lead to consequences that we can then again perceive and act upon, in an ongoing series of ***perception-action cycles***.[77]

In broad terms, the frontal regions of the brain are especially involved in representing and coordinating our actions and goals. More posterior areas in the back half of the brain are involved in representing sensory-perceptual information. But this broad division of labor in our brains is only one part of the story. Frontal and posterior regions of the brain speak extensively and incessantly to one another. There is pervasive large-scale connectivity—networks of interconnected neural fibers or white matter tracts—between frontal and posterior brain regions mutually associating sensation with action. Sensory information is processed partially in a "bottom-up" manner but is also greatly influenced by our prior knowledge and concepts, in a "top-down" fashion. When, for example, we first encounter an image where the figure and ground reverse, such as the duck-rabbit figure or an image forming either a vase or two faces in profile looking toward one another, it may be difficult to see that both alternatives are possible. Yet, once we have singled out both the duck and the rabbit or the faces and the vase it can be difficult to fully return to our initial perceptual naivete, as our "top-down" knowledge guides our "bottom-up" perception.

Sensory-perceptual and motor information based on our previous experiences in the world is a foundational part of our mental representations. Sensory-perceptual, motor, and physiological-emotional information is central to our understanding of concrete objects (e.g., bicycles) and actions (e.g., bicycling) and emotions and internal states (e.g., exuberantly racing along with the wind). Our understanding of more abstract ideas and relational concepts, though partially word-based, is also indirectly rooted in more concrete perceptual and action-based experience through metaphorical, figurative, and analogical modes of thinking.[78]

Understanding what something is and what it might potentially connect to and with is itself fundamentally anchored in detail stepping. Fully accessing and creatively forming new meaningful concepts, entities, and processes requires that we take into account both more concrete *and* more abstracted and cross-situational concepts and relations.

Let's reflect, for example, on our abstract notions of fairness or of impartiality. We may think of fairness in terms of "balancing" or evenhandedly "weighing" sides or perspectives—notions rooted in our experiences of action. Similarly, we may think of impartiality in terms of looking clearly, without obstructions or impediments to vision, at a given scene or situation. Alternatively, we might bring to mind the image of justice as blindfolded, suggesting neutrality and distance.

Now take a moment to try to vividly imagine or recall everything you can about a pear. What comes to mind? Did you think about the fruit's probable weight in your hand, its gentle curved shape and delicate color, its fragrant scent? How does your brain recreate these sensory-perceptual experiences without any direct support from your immediate environment?

The richness and vividness with which you can, in your imagination or memory, bring to mind a particular pear at this moment largely depends on how closely you have, in the past, attended to the look, feel, weight, texture, and scent of actual pears. Imaginatively bringing to mind objects, places, or people who are outside of our current situation induces activity in many of the same visual processing regions as when we were actually seeing and interacting with them. Similarly, remembering hearing a particular sound that we have often heard in the past, such as the sound of a foghorn or the song of a particular type of bird, leads to activity in brain regions near those that were active when we actually heard the sounds. There is also, though, activity in brain regions that may more abstractly combine or conjoin information from our different senses, including those regions that process and integrate language.[79]

Take, for example, thinking about a cat. If we are thinking of a hissing cat, this may activate regions of the brain related to the processing of auditory information or sounds. If, though, we are thinking of a purely jet black cat, this may activate cortical regions involved in processing visual information, particularly color. If we think of a cat having "nine lives," this might activate more abstract processing cortical regions involved in understanding linguistic expressions or idioms. If we are thinking about stroking a cat, we might activate regions in action-related cortical processing regions; but if we are thinking about watching a cat leap from a ledge, we might activate motion-related processing cortical areas. Our understanding of what a cat is and does is not isolated to one area of our brains but invokes multiple processing regions at different levels of abstraction. As Figure 2.10 shows, in a simplified form, multiple regions of the brain are called upon as we process the color, sound, or motion of things around us.

Our brains support and accomplish adaptive flexibility in our thinking by encoding information at varied levels of abstraction. As we saw in Part 1, there are graded sequences (continua or gradients) of abstraction throughout the brain supporting mental representations for different types of content. As schematically depicted in Figure 2.11, within the frontal cortex, the predominant regions that represent the ongoing requirements for our actions and goals change depending on the level of detail or abstraction of our goals. As we move increasingly further forward (in the anterior direction) within the frontal cortex, the representations of our actions and goals become increasingly abstract. Toward the back of the frontal cortex (in the

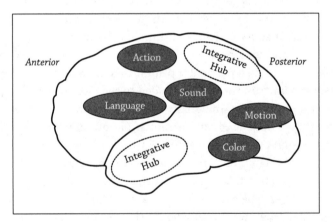

Figure 2.10 UNDERSTANDING CONCEPTS INVOKES MULTIPLE REGIONS OF THE BRAIN. When we think about or imagine ideas, multiple areas of the brain are activated. Bringing to mind sensory-perceptual features such as motion or color activates posterior regions of the cortex. Imagining actions or abstract language-related expressions activates anterior regions of the cortex. We may also activate cortical regions that integrate information across different modalities. There are a number of such integrative hubs in different areas of the brain, two of which are shown here in this simplified diagram, one in anterior temporal cortex (depicted in the lower part of the diagram) and one in parietal cortex (the angular gyrus, shown in the upper portion of the figure).[80]

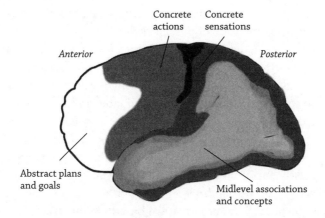

Concrete actions
Concrete sensations
Anterior
Posterior
Abstract plans and goals
Midlevel associations and concepts

THROUGHOUT THE CORTEX, THERE ARE BROAD GRADED SEQUENCES OF ABSTRACTION, WITH THE NEURAL REPRESENTATIONS OF PERCEPTION, ACTIONS, AND GOALS DIFFERING IN THEIR LEVELS OF SPECIFICITY.	GRADIENTS OF ABSTRACTION IN PERCEPTUAL, ACTION, AND GOAL REPRESENTATIONS IN THE BRAIN. White or lighter gray shading indicates brain regions in the cortex involved in more abstract processing (e.g., the prefrontal cortex). Darker shading indicates cortical regions that represent and process either comparatively more concrete sensory-perceptual information related to vision, touch, and hearing (in posterior regions) or comparatively more concrete action-related information (in anterior regions). Intermediate shading indicates cortical regions that represent relatively more abstract conceptual and associative knowledge that integrate information across different types of perceptual content (e.g., across vision, touch, and hearing) and across broader experiences of time and space.[81]

Figure 2.11

posterior direction, near to the central sulcus that divides the frontal cortex from the posterior parietal cortex), representations encode information about our concrete actions and goals.[82]

Noticing novel relations between situations or processes, or seeing "relations of relations" is a form of abstraction that frequently underpins the generation of creative metaphors and analogies. Both the generation and recognition of analogies, as well as solving complex visuospatial puzzles that require the flexible identification of novel patterns of relations (e.g., series), have been found to involve anterior regions of the prefrontal cortex (the frontal polar cortex). These regions may be important to enabling relational integration or the generation of possible rules.[83]

At an even broader level, the specificity of representations may differ in the right or left cerebral hemispheres of our brains. Although both the right and left hemispheres substantially contribute to object recognition, there may be some specialization for individuated and specific processing of objects compared with categorical object processing. For instance, representations of everyday objects in the posterior perceptual processing regions of the right posterior visual cortex may be somewhat more global or holistic, especially tightly encoding the particular instances of the objects we have encountered. The corresponding regions in the left posterior visual cortex may be comparatively more feature-based and abstract. These regions may be relatively specialized in representing the classes or kinds of objects we have encountered, with less detailed information about the particular instances.[84]

In the case of language, again, although both hemispheres are significantly involved in the representation of the meaning of concepts (semantics), concepts may be represented in a relatively focal way in the left cerebral hemisphere but more coarsely represented in the right cerebral hemisphere. A coarser representation may facilitate the noticing of comparatively remote associations between ideas because the representations tend to show greater overlap and so share more interconnections. Comparatively coarse representations can enable us to comprehend novel metaphorical and nonliteral expressions and to notice less direct associations between words or concepts. A coarse representation of "sourness" might overlap in the right hemisphere with the semantic fields for "lemon" and "sweet," whereas these might not overlap for the relatively narrow and fine-grained semantic fields in the left hemisphere.[85] (Recall our discussion in Part 1 of the pattern of associations that might be evoked in our minds upon overhearing someone say the word "green.")

The level of abstraction at which we attend to, encode, and later retrieve (bring to mind) information has crucial implications for how we create and innovate. The availability of both specific and abstract gist-like representations enables us to remember and use information in different and new ways. Somewhat abstract or gist-like representations that are not too closely tied to our initial experiences enable us to extend our experiences to novel situations that only resemble our earlier encounters in some ways while differing in others.

Note the intimate intertwining of the particular with broader meanings in this recollection of the poet, artist, and singer-song writer Patti Smith, walking, as a very young child, alongside a river with her mother:

I saw upon its surface a singular miracle. A long curving neck rose from a dress of white plumage. *Swan*, my mother said, sensing my excitement. It pattered the bright water, flapping its great wings, and lifted into the sky.[86]

Repeating the word to herself, "swan," Smith is not entirely content. She feels a yearning for something more, something that could capture the full richness and emotional power and immense movingness of what she has just witnessed. In this moment, a lifelong recurrent theme is born and recognized: to meaningfully say more than simply "swan," conveying and freely releasing sense and sound and sight.

On the one hand, abstraction can help to increase the flexible generalization of our experiences to new situations. On the other hand, if our level of abstraction shifts to an overly abstract level, or if we remain at a highly abstract level for a prolonged period, we may not be able to bring to mind the rich and vivid details of past experiences that can themselves also provide new directions for our thinking and creativity.[87]

Excessive abstraction may also impede our ability to draw on past learning to imaginatively project into the future. If, though, we become immersed in too concrete a level, we may find ourselves trapped in overly literal or narrow approaches that do not afford us options if something differs from the expected and planned.[88]

The art and science of creativity and innovation lies in our deft and dynamic detail stepping, whether up, down, or across in our levels of abstraction, within the ever-changing intersections of mind, brain, and environment.

~~~~~~

 Creativity Cross Checks and Queries

Questions to encourage reflection and connections to your own work and practice:

⇒ In how many different ways have you, or your team, tried detail stepping?
  - Have you tried detail stepping in your search for promising analogies, expressing your problem at a higher level of abstraction—or moving down in your abstraction level, trying to identify and forage for exemplars that are "champion adaptors"?
  - Have you tried to identify near-, middle-, and far-distant analogous cases or systems to the creative challenge that you are facing? Have

you deliberately searched for examples that had to meet not just one but two or more of the convergent constraints that you are currently facing?

- Have you sought external sources of information from experts and databases in various different fields?
- Are there computer-generated cases or synonyms or near synonyms that might fruitfully help you to broaden or hone the search space you are in? Are you searching using verbs as well as nouns?
- When is something the same and when is something new and different? Are the examples that you are exploring genuinely multiple prototypes, instances, or ideas?

⇒ As you think about your current creative engagements, do you step up and down in your perceptual noticing and sensing? Here is how the video and sound installation artist Bill Viola encountered something both new and very ancient through detail stepping:

> The Anasazi ruins in particular captivated us. Approaching them on foot from afar was like a gradual zooming in, a continuous magnification that unfolded layers of detail. One day, arriving right at the walls after a long hike, we looked closely between the mud bricks at the mortar, and realized that we could see thumbprints there of the people who made them. Stepping back, we saw that other rows had thumbprints too. There were hundreds of individual imprints.[89]

- What are the "thumbprints" in your creative worlds?
- What new vantage points would enable you or others to better notice or uncover as yet unseen or unforeseen details?
- Is it best for you to ascend or descend in your level of abstraction in a relatively smooth and continuous manner, as if on a ramp, or in more discrete and distinct steps, as if on a stairway?

⇒ Where, how, and when do ideas meet one another in your creative process and that of your colleagues and contributors?

- In what ways do you capture and share ideas? At what point do you and others see—and touch and play with—emerging ideas?
- How do you translate your creative direction to others? Are there analogies or figurative or symbolic ways of conveying key ideas that would help to propel and sustain creative momentum?
- Observe your own use of gestures, and the gestures of others. What "thinking work" are the gestures doing? How could you extend your use of gestures to better help others and yourself express your ideas and carry them forward?

⇒ How are you using mental simulation and mental time travel to change your own and your team's idea landscapes?

- What time frame are you thinking in, and have you tried changing it?
- How near at hand in space are you imagining a new product or process? Have you imagined other people far away and very different from you interacting with it or observing the process or system? If you imagine that you are giving the final presentation or unveiling a performance in a few hours, what new aspects come to mind?
- Have you tried moving from a mental simulation to an actual simulation, or the reverse? Are there hidden and overlooked "candle-wicks" in the creative scenario that you are facing?
- By closing our eyes we may be able to more fully immerse or reimmerse ourselves in a past or future situation; this may also provide us with more detailed information to envision (and hear). When you are generating new ideas, do you sometimes close your eyes?
- How do you access the deep pools of accumulated event-specific memories and experiences that you and each of your team members uniquely possess, as well as those that you share in common? Do you approach creative and future-oriented search through different time windows? Do you try midlevel generalized categorical memories alongside specific cue combinations to prompt unexpected new directions?

⇒ Consider the following perspective on international economic development:

> Reform discussions focus on the need to get away from "one-size-fits-all" strategies and on context-specific solutions. The emphasis is on the need for humility, for policy diversity, for selective and modest reforms, and for experimentation.[90]

- How might the broader viewpoint and sentiments expressed here apply to change efforts in your organization and group?
- To what extent are you closely evaluating the context in which you are attempting to instigate changes or new policies?

⇒ Are your analogies focusing your attention on the most relevant aspect of your situation?

- Consider a case recently argued before the US Supreme Court. The government argued that police officers have the right to search all of the data on a cell phone belonging to someone they had just arrested because the cell phone is, like a wallet or purse, an object that people often carry with them. Police can legally search property on or near a person who has been arrested. Is a cell phone, then, like a wallet or a purse? Why or why not?

By shifting its level of abstraction the Supreme Court came to realize how a cell phone is relevantly different from a wallet or purse in both a "quantitative and a qualitative sense," capable as it is of aggregating in one place an exceptionally wide range and amount of personal information. As the Court explained:

> The [Government] asserts that a search of all data stored on a cell phone is "materially indistinguishable" from searches of these sorts of physical items. That is like saying a ride on horseback is materially indistinguishable from a flight to the moon. Both are ways of getting from point A to point B, but little else justifies lumping them together. Modern cell phones, as a category, implicate privacy concerns far beyond those implicated by the search of a cigarette pack, a wallet, or a purse.[91]

Are there instances where you are confusing a ride on horseback with a flight to the moon? Are you "lumping" where you should be "splitting"?

⇒ How are you shaping and preparing your thinking and making environment?

Consider this observation:

> In flower arranging it is customary to leave around discarded by-products, such as twigs and ferns, on the off-chance that they will prove useful in striking on a felicitous design. Pieces that seem most likely to be helpful are kept closer. Spatial layout partitions by-products into categories of possible use.[92]

- Do you use your physical environment to make certain thoughts or plans more accessible to you, and in the right order, at the right time?
- As you think through a creative problem, do you help your environment do some of the representational work for you?
- Do you strategically hide distracting affordances and uncover helpful prompting affordances in the environment, to automatically guide your attention to pertinent and promising opportunities?
- Do you selectively "seed" your environment with "scraps and remnants," idea fragments, phrases, or images that may later happen to be just right for your creative purpose?

Part 3

Staying the Course *and* Letting Go: Varying Our Degrees of Mental Control

Thinking prompts

- Why should we develop both relaxed *and* stringent modes of cognitive control?
- What are "thinking scaffoldings"? How can we use them to modulate our mental control?
- What are "times in between" and how do they change our idea landscapes?
- How can we attune and flex our attention to discover newness?
- How might we best proactively structure our creative task environments?

It may seem that a high degree of mental control would be uniformly help-ful in enabling us to be persistent, systematic, and analytical, avoiding dis-tractions and consistently pursuing our goals. But is it? Are there costs to deliberate cognitive control? Can we have too much control? Does control sometimes stand in the way of creativity but at other times help? How does our degree of cognitive control shape our idea landscapes? Think of the type of person who can never let go, always needing to know exactly what is com-ing next that day and in the next five minutes, and all of the steps to be taken to get there. Are there benefits from sometimes relaxing our mental control, or might it be useful to be at one degree of control at one time and at a different degree of control at another? How can we modulate our control or "control our control" to be flexibly adaptive and innovative?

There are many settings on what we will call our cognitive control dial, a metaphorical dial that we ourselves can turn toward greater or lesser degrees of cognitive control or that may be shifted by our circumstances at one time toward deliberateness, at other times toward spontaneity. A dial is something that can be turned in a single sweep, moved through gradual increments, or held at a particular setting.

If we are, so to speak, "dialed higher" in our **control dialing**, we are in a more deliberate, focused, and purposeful mode of thinking. This mode relies on comparatively top-down attention and planning processes in the brain in response to our current physical, social, and symbolic environments.

In contrast, if we are "dialed lower" on our control dial, we are in a more spontaneous, diffusely receptive mode of thinking. This mode relies predominantly on bottom-up processes in the brain that are largely associative or automatically cued and prompted by our environments.

No one setting on the continuum of mental control is always ideal for creativity. The best setting depends on what we are trying to accomplish and where we are in our making/thinking process. Creative processes involve incrementing, decrementing, or holding steady our degree of cognitive control across time, within not only our concepts and categories, but also our emotions, our perceptions, and our motivations/goals. Our degrees of control form a continuum.[1] We need *both* flexibility and persistence to maximize our creativity and resilience.[2]

When we are mentally agile, we fine-tune and contextually adjust our degree of mental control. Across time, we increase or decrease our mental control and, at any one moment of time, we may be at differing degrees of control in each of the four interrelated constituents of our thinking (concepts, emotions, motivations, and perceptions). These possible variations in our degree of mental control across time and at any one moment of time are schematically illustrated in Figures 3.1 and 3.2.

Research in the cognitive and brain sciences has shown that when we are adaptively flexible we adjust our degree of cognitive control on a moment by moment basis, responsively altering the intensity and direction of our control as we meet with obstacles or success. One recent neuroscience account suggests that the level of cognitive control that we are exerting at any given moment is based on two factors. One factor is a "control signal" that our brain is currently receiving about the optimal level of control that we should expend. The second factor is our ability to actually carry out that level of

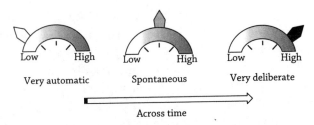

Very automatic　　　Spontaneous　　　Very deliberate

Across time

Figure 3.1 FLEXIBLY ALTERING OUR DEGREE OF COGNITIVE CONTROL ACROSS TIME. To be optimally agile and creative across time and situations, we need to flexibly increase and decrease our degree of cognitive control, sometimes dialing toward greater deliberateness and sometimes dialing toward comparatively automatic responding. At certain points, greater control may be called for; at other points, a higher level of spontaneity may best provide new insights and clarity.

control. In this "expected value of control" account, a region deep within our brain (the anterior cingulate) integrates information about our current state, about what we are trying to achieve and how likely we are to succeed, together with how much effort is needed and how "expensive" that effort would be for us to exert.[3]

Control brings clear benefits but also potential risks.[4] Exercising a high degree of mental control is essential for persistent goal pursuit and for achieving our longer-term aims, including fully realizing our creative projects.[5] Yet deliberate mental control may also lead to detrimental effects—particularly if our efforts at control are prolonged over long time periods or are too incessantly maintained without intermixed phases of more spontaneous and receptive thinking.[6]

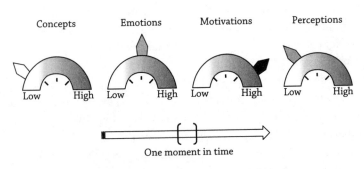

One moment in time

Figure 3.2 OUR DEGREE OF COGNITIVE CONTROL AT A SINGLE MOMENT IN TIME. At any moment of our creative and problem-solving process our degree of control may differ within each of the four interrelated constituents of our thinking (concepts, emotions, motivations/goals, and perceptions).

Excessively high control may reduce our flexibility by creating unnecessary bottlenecks as we process and respond to information. When trying too hard, we may proceed in a more serial step-by-step manner than is actually required by the task, thus losing the benefits of more concurrent and automatic modes of cognitive processing.[7] Exerting less control can sometimes, in the right circumstances, be more effective. "Less can sometimes be more (in terms of cognitive control), especially if the environment provides sufficient information for the cognitive system to behave on autopilot based on automatic processes alone."[8]

One well-recognized path to the emergence of creative ideas involves diffusing or defocusing our attention. This allows a spreading of neural activation across a wide range of idea associations, including loosely or tangentially connected thoughts and concepts.[9] Nonfocused attention may enable wider and deeper intuitive access to associations that are only remotely associated with the problem at hand or with what is at the forefront of our awareness.

Such defocused thinking often involves concrete visual or sensory content, sensitivity to subliminal stimuli or feelings, and perhaps also spontaneous analogical insights.[10] Ideas may occur to us, suddenly and unsought, in moments of nonfocused attention or reverie. These moments of unlooked for emergence of ideas or meaning-related knowledge surfacing into awareness have been evocatively described as *mind popping*.[11]

However, such diffuse or defocused attentional states on their own are rarely sufficient for the complete formation, realization, and articulation of creative insights. Intentional goal-directed thinking processes are nearly always necessary.[12] Initial insightful ideas often gain much in novelty, profundity, and feasibility through additional systematic search and experimentation, planning and reasoning, and careful recombination, revision, refinement, and evaluation. Successful entrepreneurs, for instance, reported using a *balance* of intuitive along with analytical thinking processes, with neither approach predominating.[13]

In our larger creative projects and undertakings, we may benefit from cycling through multiple successive phases of comparatively undirected imaginative search alongside more directed thinking. Throughout such creative and other endeavors, our goals and subgoals may also change and move up and down within our conscious awareness.[14] Rather than simply being better at defocused attention, evidence suggests that creative individuals may show *a wider range of modulation* in their degrees of mental control. Individuals who are highly creative may be able to dive more deeply into either defocused attentional states or focused controlled attentional states depending on context.

> Creative people are better at adjusting their focus of attention depending on task demands . . . in essence, creative people exhibit *differential* [attention—flexibly changing their levels of attention] rather than reduced focusing of attention.[15]
>
> —*Creativity researchers Oshin Vartanian, Colin Martindale, and*
> *Jonna Kwiatkowski*

> The attentional style of highly creative people may be a double edged-sword: while initially defocused attention may switch quickly, cognitive control may take longer to switch. Nonetheless, both edges of this sword have potential benefits for creativity.[16]
>
> —*Cognitive neuroscientists and creativity researchers Darya Zabelina and*
> *Mark Beeman*

Often, as we will learn throughout this book, while working creatively we move between what has been characterized as phases of "see, move, see," or cycles of perception, action, and renewed perception.[17] A key aspect of gaining creative expertise involves learning to use what we will call "thinking scaffoldings" to help alternate between deliberate proddings of our thinking and a more spontaneous intuitive noticing of patterns and possibilities. There are also intermediate forms of control. Sometimes we begin intentionally thinking about a creative problem and our mind continues to work through the problem in the background of our awareness.

In this Part we will encounter various ways we can creatively benefit from aptly modifying our degree of cognitive control. We first look at control dialing in situations that invoke or involve less directed thinking. Next, we progressively move through combinations of control and spontaneity, to practice and habit, and then highly deliberate top-down attention. We close with a discussion of some of the brain correlates of cognitive control.

INSIGHT, OPEN GOALS, AND UNDIRECTED THINKING

Recall the timekeeping example we explored in Part 1, in which engineering students were asked to generate novel ways to measure short units of time using an assortment of standard household objects. Information distantly related to the timekeeping task was substantially helpful in fostering insights and ideas only if individuals had already begun working on the task for awhile and so had the *open goal* of creatively producing new ideas that met the task constraints. Ongoing or open goals prompted the spontaneous noticing of otherwise remote, seemingly irrelevant possibilities by attuning the attention of the students to new and promising associations, principles, and connections.

Frequently there are subcomponents of the creative tasks or change initiatives we are pursuing that cannot be immediately fulfilled. We may need to await the arrival of appropriate circumstances, such as finding the right materials or having the opportunity to confer with a particular person or group. We might then form the intention to be on the lookout for moments when we might arrange to work with that particular person or group or to be on the alert for the required visual image, phrase, or access to equipment. By deliberately setting an open goal we allow ourselves later to be more receptively attuned to potentially relevant information and to more *automatically* and effortlessly notice opportunities to move toward fulfilling our intentions.

Creative thinking and action often rely on our ability to notice that an opportunity to fulfill an open goal is at hand. When we set an open goal it may be especially beneficial to explicitly bring to mind specific aspects or features that would, in the future, provide a good opportunity to realize (or resume pursuit of) that goal. Bringing to mind particular possible future scenarios that could permit acting on our postponed goals may reduce the need to "remember to remember" and make way for more spontaneous, reflexive reminding.

Implementation intentions are "if-then" rules that support less effortful future remembering.[18] We might think to ourselves, for example, "if I am in the drawing archives, then I should look again at that piece by Ellsworth Kelly," or "the next time I work with my vocal coach, we should talk about new warm-up exercises for next month's performance." In a group or team setting, the team likewise may choose to adopt a proactive "if-then" strategy to improve their decision making. A team might agree, for instance, that once they reach a decision about what they think they most prefer, they will carefully again review the advantages and disadvantages of the top three alternatives. Recurring phases of "if-then" thinking can prompt us to systematically spell out the "who, when, what, and where" of our hoped-for outcomes—demonstrably improving the likelihood of realizing our individual and team plans.[19]

Deliberate intention setting also can be a way of offloading demands from our short-term working memory onto the external environment and so unclutter our thinking space. At the time of forming an intention we rely on conscious and planful thinking using a high degree of effortful control, but then we may relinquish much of that control, permitting environmental cues to later associatively spontaneously prompt our remembering of our intentions. Deliberately and specifically imagining possible future contexts that could allow us to more spontaneously meet our temporarily postponed aims is a form of future-related or prospective memory. Such explicit strategic anticipation of future circumstances, or "strategic automatization," allows us to consciously act at one moment in a way that will later enable us to act automatically with little effort once we encounter the circumstances that we have earlier imagined.[20]

Our use of "if-then" implementation intentions may be strengthened through a process of what is known as **mental contrasting**, whereby we first fully envision a future outcome or goal that we believe is possible for us to achieve. But then we also explicitly bring to mind potential *obstacles* to our outcome or goal.[21] For example, we may anticipate being pressed for time when we next visit the drawing archives and so explicitly plan to look at the Ellsworth Kelly drawing as soon as we arrive. By first vividly imagining a desired probable outcome and then also conjuring up possible real impediments to that outcome, we form an associative connection so that, when we think of the outcome, we may also automatically relate it to the potential barriers that may stand in our way. This associative pairing of an achievable future goal with a present and tangible obstacle helps to prepare us in dealing with intervening setbacks and significantly enhances our likelihood of success. We will return to the advantageous process of mental contrasting in Parts 5 and 6.

We often, too, may have brief periods of time when goals that we were not actively pursuing reemerge into our thoughts and we newly reassess and reprioritize them, to accommodate our current circumstances and aims. Such **times in between**—as when we are taking a brief break, snacking on a piece of fruit, or momentarily gazing out of the window to check the weather—offer us opportunities to notice newly emerging ideas and connections between ideas relating to our creative goals and projects. During such times our attention is often only partially occupied with the immediate and perhaps more habitual or automatic activities at hand, permitting ongoing subconscious or preconscious progress toward our creative aims. They are opportune moments for the sudden emergence of ideas into awareness where the idea was not intentionally sought.[22] When we are in a situation that does not call upon our full attention, new associations to ongoing or recent aims may spontaneously come to awareness.[23]

Times in between change what is accessible in our idea landscapes in several ways. They provide altered environmental input. The changed external circumstances may be fortuitously relevant to our creative goals, as in happy reminders or in serendipitous finds. Or our changed environment may subtly shift our thinking in new directions that are not directly related to our creative endeavor but which initiate new promising perspectives. Times in between also provide a temporal space for fluctuations in our idea landscapes.

With time, ideas—and the associative connections between ideas—that were in our peak awareness may recede or dissolve and new ideas or associations formerly in peripheral awareness or beneath awareness may emerge. We all have had the experience of knowing that we know something—such as a person's name, a fact, or a phrase—but that we cannot, just at that moment, seem to bring to mind. It is, as we say, on the "tip of the tongue" and we even may be able to say what the first letters are or the number of syllables, but the actual word eludes us. Yet, with the lapse of time and sometimes a change of context, the elusive name or fact may spring into awareness.[24]

One of the benefits of lower degrees of cognitive control may be that less salient but potentially relevant information enters our awareness, and enables us to think about a problem in a new way. Times of relaxed control may allow new ideas to emerge or to become strong enough to supplant unhelpful ideas that continue to occur. Additionally, lower degrees of cognitive control may be associated with a less strict or restricting/constricting focus of attention. This might be particularly beneficial if our attention has become "caught on" misleading or incorrect information.

We might even attempt to use different times of day to alter the degree of control that we bring to a creative endeavor. Our cognitive performance at different times of the day has been found to fluctuate and different individuals often tend to prefer working in the mornings, or instead, in late afternoons or evenings. At our preferred time of day, we may more readily and easily inhibit distractions, and this can help us to approach novel, difficult, and demanding tasks that require focused attention.[25] Unlike many other types of tasks where performance is best when they are undertaken at a preferred time of day (in line with our circadian rhythms), performance on insight-type problems may be enhanced when we are *out of sync* with our preferred time of day. On insight-type problems that require more diffuse or remote associative, conceptual or meaning-related connections, increased distractibility may prove beneficial.[26]

Times in between, when we engage in briefer necessary routine activities, may facilitate the formation and emergence of ideas in another way. The routine tasks we perform (simple actions of personal hygiene such as showering, brushing one's teeth, tidying or cleaning up around the house, or rearranging items at the office) are familiar and well structured, so that we receive clear immediate *feedback* on our progress.[27] Such feedback, or "progress signals," may be accompanied by mild positive emotion.[28] As we saw in Part 1, mild positive affect may enhance the flexibility and inclusiveness of our thinking. Mildly positive emotion may also prompt the insightful noticing of appropriate associations that are only remotely linked to one another, as in successfully finding the connecting word in the word triples or remote associates task.[29]

Times in between are related to the idea of incubation but are broader and more varied. **Incubation**, as we noted in Part 1, is a phase in which we maintain a problem in thought, subconsciously "brooding" on it. Incubation is typically understood as occurring after we have reached an impasse in our deliberate and prolonged top-down efforts to solve a problem and refers to the process of subconsciously recombining ideas when we have moved away from deliberately working on the problem.[30] Time away from an ongoing problem, including during a night's sleep or an afternoon nap, may enable us to insightfully reconfigure it. The reactivation of memory representations during sleep can allow for the neural reorganization of memories. Sleep may help to isolate the most valuable or invariant aspects of a problem and enhance our ability to generalize these patterns to new situations.[31]

Beyond incubation, times in between occur in a wide range of contexts. Even momentary times in between, such as those needed to switch between using one tool and using another, may open us up to the intimations of new creative directions when we did not yet know consciously that a new direction was needed.

In-depth observations of composers of electroacoustic music uncovered multiple instances where movements between work areas or from one computer application to another led to insightful bursts of creativity. As characterized by the researchers:

> One composer got out of his computer chair to pick up a metal tube nearby, recorded the sound of the hit tube into the computer and then continued to work on the computer. Even though the time spent away from the computer was less than five minutes, it became evident from the procedural protocol of the observation that in the following 15 minutes the composer went on to create the most "significant" (in his own judgment) sound structure of the whole seven-hour composition day.[32]

Apart from times when we deliberately take a break or change tasks, our attention and thoughts may happen to drift to something other than what we are currently doing. Spontaneously generated task-unrelated thoughts may distract us from what we are doing and may sometimes be harmful in separating us from the here and now[33] but—depending on context and content—they may at times be beneficial.[34]

When people are asked what they were thinking about during such moments of **mind wandering/task-unrelated thinking**, relatively often they report they were anticipating future activities or working through current or upcoming goal-related opportunities. They might, for example, report that they were wondering where they should take their visiting out-of-town friend for dinner. Such goal-guided but often involuntary exploratory thinking may offset the possible costs of less than full attention to our current task. It may allow us to approach an upcoming situation with greater mental flexibility, a wider range of options in mind, and more tangible preparation.[35]

SCAFFOLDING OUR CREATIVE THINKING

Just as our environments provide extensive support for our thinking, there are structures within thinking, or what we call thinking scaffoldings, that can help us to explore, extend, change, and vary the direction of our creative problem solving and action. **Thinking scaffoldings** are a way of productively guiding our perception-action cycles. They are intentional queryings and quarryings of our idea landscapes that are intended to help bootstrap (that is, "scaffold") our idea-generation processes.

Thinking scaffoldings are ways of deliberately invoking and putting to work our perception-action cycle, assisting us to transition and keep moving across ideas, prodding us to recategorize and shake up or unsettle creative objects or their configurations. They are ways to encourage our insights that are neither highly general nor highly specific but are of midlevel abstraction and related to action. Thinking scaffoldings help us to see things we could try or attempt without an assurance that what we are trying will work. They prompt us to test and revise, look and revise, and test again.

~~~~~~

 Thought Box: _The Many Spaces_
of Reading and Thinking

How do we think of reading a story or an extended narrative? Perhaps we tend to think of such explorations as involving a linear progression through a story line or a temporal trajectory. But story, thinking, and reading may be approached and experienced as _volumetric_. Story, thinking, and reading may be volumetric in space and time and in the ways in which they allow navigation within the intermingling thinking constituents of concepts, motivations, perceptions, and emotions.

From such a "volumetric perspective," how do we approach what we read, and why? Consider how the writer Alice Munro "goes into" a story written by someone else:

> I can start reading them anywhere; from beginning to end, from end to beginning, from any point in between in either direction. So obviously I don't take up a story and follow it as if it were a road, taking me somewhere, with views and neat diversions along the way. I go into it, and move back and forth and settle here and there, and stay in it for a while. It's more like a house. Everybody knows what a house does, how it encloses space and makes connections between one enclosed space and another and presents what is outside in a new way.[36]

We might construe this metaphor of a story as a house as itself a thinking scaffold: by intentionally picturing our story reading (or story writing) as moving about inside a house, we are released from a too insistent press in a single direction; we're given a mental model that effortlessly incorporates multiple vantage points and activities. Although, as we will see, there are many formal methods of scaffolding our thinking, we can also develop our own or tailor methods to our own ways of working.

Scaffolding suggests a structuring and a supporting rather than free-floatingness. It also suggests goal guidedness within constraints and a degree of effortfulness. Think of how a scaffolding structure surrounds a building that is being renovated. The scaffolds offer sets of stable supports that help individuals and teams safely and steadily reach and work in new spaces. After they have served their purpose, scaffolds are then dismantled to later be reused and newly configured for different projects. Thinking scaffoldings likewise are ways for us to first deliberately intervene and then (for a time) "let go" of our thinking.

Let's consider two concrete examples of thinking scaffoldings in action.

Suppose that you were asked to take on the role of a product designer. Your project for today is to sketch new and creative salt-and-pepper shakers. The salt-and-pepper shaker sets should rely on one or a combination of seven basic three-dimensional geometric forms, including sphere, cone, cube, cylinder, pyramid, box, or a prism shape. Although they should complement each other, the shakers should not simply repeat the same geometric form. Try to take into account how the two shakers will actually work, including how they will be filled and cleaned; if you like you can also specify the material and color of the shakers.

You are given a design brief with images of the seven basic geometric shapes and are explicitly charged to create concepts that are highly creative and imaginative. The ideas that you propose should be novel but also pleasingly fitting for their intended purpose. Next you are given eight standard 8.5- by 11-inch sheets of paper. You are asked to sketch a different design on each page, using the space around the sketches to jot down any accompanying explanatory comments or details.

Imagine that you are given only these guidelines and a total of 40 minutes to generate as many creative design sketches for salt-and-pepper shakers as you can. How would you go about this task? What approaches might you take? How might you use control dialing to help you to generate promising ideas? Are there ways that you could cycle between periods of more deliberate and intentional strategies and phases of more spontaneous discovering?

Would it help if you were prompted to think about ways of *nesting* one geometric form in another or of *merging* two or more of the forms together? What if you were asked to think about one of the forms as being *enlarged* or *miniaturized*? Would these explicit and deliberate prompts help you to spontaneously notice and recombine the seven basic geometric shapes in novel ways?

The design activity we just asked you to consider engaging in is closely based on one that 120 first-year university students were asked to undertake in an experimental setting.[37] One of the main purposes of the experiment was to test the effectiveness of explicit instructions to use a form of thinking scaffolding involving design heuristics such as trying to *merge, nest,* or *rescale* one or more components or objects in a creative design challenge.

Design heuristics are intentional strategies that introduce systematic variation into the problem space of the design. They "serve as a way to 'jump' to a new subspace of possible design solutions, or even to expand the original space of possible designs."[38] As illustrated in Figure 3.3, design heuristics relate to particular features of a design problem, providing new ways in which to look at those features, and they can be applied in appropriate circumstances to a wide range of situations in order to generate new ideas.

The students in the salt-and-pepper shaker experiment were selected because they were novices and not experienced or trained designers; thus they would not have been formally introduced to design heuristics. Six design heuristics were provided to them with a brief description of each. They were *changing configuration, merging, nesting, repeating, rescaling,* and *substituting.* These particular heuristics were chosen because they were frequently and effectively used by a professional designer that the researchers had earlier studied intensively and because each heuristic could be used independently.[39]

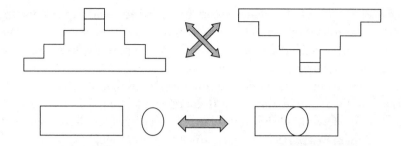

| ONE WAY TO EXPAND OUR CREATIVE THINKING SPACES IS TO DRAW ON THINKING SCAFFOLDINGS OR DESIGN HEURISTICS, SUCH AS "FLIPPING," "MERGING," OR "NESTING." | INTENTIONAL PROMPTINGS CAN STIMULATE SPONTANEOUS CREATIVE DISCOVERY. Powerful aids to expanding and transforming our creative problem spaces are focused queries that are posed at a midlevel of abstraction, such as "What if I flipped this?" or "What would happen if we merged this or subtracted that?" These questions help us to move productively across deliberate and less deliberate degrees of cognitive control. |

Figure 3.3

All of the students were first given general guidelines for the design task and were explicitly instructed to produce designs that were novel, imaginative, and functional. The students then were randomly assigned to one of four groups. For one group, all six heuristics were provided together and the students were asked to choose the heuristics they wished to use in generating their sketched designs. For two additional groups, the heuristics were provided one at a time, at timed intervals, and the students were asked to use the current heuristic in their design to produce a set of six sequential designs using each of the heuristics in turn. To decouple the possible effects of any one particular sequencing of the heuristics from sequential ordering in general, one of these groups received the heuristics in the order of *merge, change configuration, substitute, rescale, repeat,* and *nest;* the other group received them in a different order: *merge, repeat, change configuration, substitute, nest,* and *rescale.* The fourth group was a baseline control group in which the students were not provided with any design heuristics at all.

Three judges, who were not told the purpose or hypotheses of the study, evaluated the creativity of each student's set of sketches. Approximately 40 percent of the sketches were awarded a score of 5 or higher on a 7-point creativity scale by at least one of the judges. These more highly creative sketches were then shuffled and intermixed with one another, and all of the judges were now asked to make a more fine-grained creativity evaluation of the sketches by sorting them into one of seven piles of increasing creativity. This procedure enabled the judges to readily compare the sketches within each creativity category.

Which of the four groups do you think produced the most highly creative designs and why? Take a moment to imagine that you were in each of the four groups. How would the requirement to use any of the design heuristics, or to use them in a particular order, affect how you thought?

Students who were provided with the six heuristics and then were also offered a free choice of which heuristics to use and in what order generated the most successful, highly creative, top-scoring designs. Next were the two groups of students who were sequentially walked through each of the six design heuristics. The control group, who were not provided with any heuristics, produced the fewest highly creative designs.

Comparisons of the highly creative sketches showed that, relative to the control group, the groups that were explicitly provided with design heuristics generated sketches that were more visually detailed, with more extensive notations as to how the salt-and-pepper shakers would specifically function. Overall, the students in the control group tended to rely more narrowly on their own personal knowledge through analogy and association and rarely supplemented these with more form-related heuristics such as nesting or rescaling.[40]

An often asked question is "Can creativity be learned or trained?" Based on the outcomes of the salt-and-pepper shaker experiment, we can see that even simple instructions and strategies substantially bolstered the creativity of novices, leading to the generation of more imaginative and novel designs that were more varied in visual form. Deliberate consideration of possible strategies may have prompted students to more effectively engage in a perception-action cycle or a "see-move-see" interchange[41] where changing degrees of control allows us to freshly discover new perceptual insights and explore positive unintended consequences. (We will encounter further examples and applications of the expansive possibilities offered through understanding the "see-move-see" process in Part 4, "Making, Finding, and Improvising.")

Such deliberate variations in our degree of cognitive control may also attune us to varying levels of specificity in our creative problem space, effectively traversing and expanding our idea landscapes. An important aspect of expertise may involve learning to intermix and combine thinking scaffoldings throughout one's creative process.

In-depth study of the hundreds of design sketches that were created by an expert industrial designer for a particular project over the course of approximately two years showed that, from one sketch to the next, he used differing combinations and types of design heuristics. As schematically diagrammed in Figure 3.4, some sketches involved many different heuristics (more than a dozen) and others as few as two.[42]

The number of design heuristics used in novel problem solving increases with experience and training. When asked to design an inexpensive portable solar cooker that could easily be set up and used by individual families, engineering students and practitioners relied on a wide range of heuristics. Across the 36 participants, a total of 62 design heuristics were identified in their sketches and think-aloud protocols. Although everyone used multiple heuristics, on average less experienced students used 12 different design heuristics while more experienced students and practitioners employed significantly more, bringing into play an average of 17 different heuristics.[43]

The salt-and-pepper shaker and the solar cooker design experiments involved product design, but thinking scaffoldings can help us in all creative realms. In writing a poem or in composing music, we might ask ourselves "What if I ended here instead or what if I invert or flip this?" "What

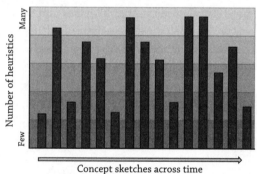

Concept sketches across time

VARYING OUR DEGREES OF COGNITIVE CONTROL USING THINKING SCAFFOLDINGS CAN PROMPT NOVEL INSIGHTS.	CHANGING DEGREES OF CONTROL DURING CREATIVE DESIGN. Across time, new ideas emerge from varying our degrees of control by the deliberate and spontaneous application of varying numbers and types of design heuristics or thinking scaffoldings. This figure is schematically adapted from the case study of an expert designer's two-year design process.[44]

Figure 3.4

if I folded this in?" "Is there a way of decoupling or separating the parts?" "Could I condense and capture opposing senses or meanings here?" In the sciences and the social sciences too,[45] we can prompt and expand our exploratory and creative thinking by deliberately asking ourselves questions such as "What if I changed the context of this phenomenon?" "Is this really only one effect, or are there two or more things going on here?"

   This process of questioning the direction of our work may at first be difficult and unsettling. It may seem to undermine our creative progress. Yet with time and practice, the questioning may itself become a natural part of our creative working process. In the words of contemporary singer-songwriter and musician John Fullbright:

> For years, even well into my career, I couldn't edit or re-write a song. But now I'm finally at a place where I can and it's fantastic. . . . You can have a great idea and hold onto it for a long time until you get what you actually need out of it, instead of throwing out a bunch of great ideas because you can't go back and change anything. I can edit now and I do, often.[46]

After a time we may begin to use thinking scaffoldings or generative heuristics or other questionings in a more effortless and seamless way, sometimes without even realizing that we are using them. Then they may become integral parts of our ways of working and acting and exploring—part of our procedural know-how and know-to.

> A designer sees, moves and sees again. . . . At local and global levels, and in many different ways, designing is an interaction of making and seeing, doing and discovering.[47]
> —Design experts Donald Schon and Glenn Wiggins

PRACTICE, REPETITION, AND STRUCTURING OUR IDEA SEARCH

You and your friend regularly enjoy afternoon coffee together. Today, your friend offers you a cup of coffee in a new, attractive mug. You begin to take a sip and are startled to find that the cup is decidedly heavier than you had anticipated, at least twice as heavy. How might the unusual weightiness of the mug influence your thinking compared with if you were drinking from a typical coffee mug?

Would you expect that encountering the heavy mug would change your degree of cognitive control or your level of abstraction? Would it change how you thought about what you were doing?

Although you might most often characterize your afternoon coffee routine in rather abstract terms—as time spent relaxing, conversing, and sharing ideas—your encounter with the unexpectedly heavy mug might instead lead you to think more concretely. Now you might attend to how—exactly—you were lifting, tipping, and drinking from the mug, finding yourself thinking about swallowing, avoiding spilling, and placing the mug on the table with extra care. These many fine-grained and separate subcomponents of the activity of drinking coffee are usually subsumed under your more abstract or "higher-level" way of framing your actions and goal of sharing time together. They quickly emerge, though, into the foreground of your awareness when your actions meet with unexpected difficulty or unanticipated change.

This example, based on research findings, is an illustration of a change in what is known as our level of *action or goal identification*.[48] We typically prefer a somewhat higher level of abstraction in how we identify our actions or goals. We think of ourselves as engaging in actions such as "driving home," "visiting a friend," or "making breakfast" with little attention to the many connected steps and substeps needed to achieve these goals. Often this way of thinking about what we are doing or trying to accomplish is all that is necessary for many of our routine and highly practiced activities.

When we encounter unforeseen obstacles or difficulties in performing an action it can dramatically shift our thinking about even highly practiced actions. Upon meeting with difficulties in performing a routine activity we tend to step down in our level of action or goal identification, now focusing our attention and effort on evaluating and adjusting our behavior for the subcomponents of the activity. Upon encountering a sudden downpour of rain, instead of just "driving home," we might find ourselves focusing on where we were in the lane, how well the windshield wipers were working, and carefully slowing down to adjust the distance from the cars ahead of us.

One of the benefits of extensive practice in a creative activity—such as playing a musical instrument, drawing, or writing computer code—is that it allows us to form and effectively carry out our goals and actions at higher levels of abstraction. We can then focus our attention and effort on other aspects of our experience and expression. Deliberate practice involves focusing on and progressively honing and refining our partially acquired skills, making them increasingly effortless and allowing us to combine and recombine them in novel configurations.[49] This form of practice involves patient and persistent edging forward in our level of mastery by continually attending to particular subcomponents of a skill, absorbing feedback on consistent gains and progress. As we edge forward, we continually set and reset our creative goals.

Extensive experience and practice also can allow very rapid decision making even under severe constraints of time and information by enabling what is known as *recognition-primed decision making*.[50] If we reach a high level of expertise based on extensive practice we can exceedingly rapidly classify a situation, responding to the situation with little deliberate thought or systematic evaluation of alternative options. Based on their deep prior experience experts may simply "see" what they can and need to do; they then make rapid online adjustments to suit the current situation instead of deliberately and extensively weighing their options.

Research Highlight: *Varying Degrees of Control in the Operating Room*

Systematic observations of surgeons revealed that they engaged in several different ways of "slowing down" at different points during surgery. This slowing down was not necessarily physically slowing down in their movements but often involved deepening their attentional focus and regrouping their mental efforts. Based on first-hand observation of surgeons and in-depth interviews, researchers identified six distinguishable types of adjustments that surgeons frequently showed in their degrees of cognitive control.[51]

In *stopping*, surgeons actually stopped a procedure to seek further information, such as reviewing x-rays or other images or consulting a patient's file. Stopping sometimes occurred in response to the evolving emergent situation. At other times stopping took place in a prearranged proactively planned way. Here, the surgeons might make sure that all necessary resources were at hand, and that team members were ready; they might then pause to engage in mental rehearsals to focus themselves and to focus the team to the impending task. Stopping often took place at critical junctures. Following a critical juncture, once the first step was initiated, the subsequent steps would follow in a rapidly unfolding cascade of required events.

By *removing distractions* such as conversations and teaching instructions, either by verbal or nonverbal cues to the rest of the surgical team, surgeons would make additional cognitive and attentional resources available to themselves to devote to a potentially critical part of the procedure.

A somewhat more subtle modulation of control involved *focusing more intently*. Surgeons would confine their attention more narrowly to the immediate procedure, screening from awareness the incidental remarks of team members or other environmental distractions.

Fine tuning occurred very often during surgery at many points of minor transition during which the surgeons subtly increased their ongoing attention and responded on a moment-by-moment basis to emergent cues, constantly monitoring the changing situation.

When such continual fine tuning and monitoring did not occur and surgeons moved closer to highly automatic responding, an undesirable form of *drifting* could emerge. During drifting, which tended to arise during very routine and familiar procedures, the reduction in situation awareness posed the risk of leading to mishaps and mistakes.

Changes in these degrees of control could occur abruptly, without proceeding through a strict series of stages. Based on their observations, the researchers proposed that, as they developed increasingly skilled and automatic responding in one aspect of a procedure, the surgeons would "reinvest" the additional cognitive and attentional resources they gained into a *metacognitive or metaperceptual monitoring* of the broader situation, providing ongoing self-corrective feedback.

"On the basis of what we observed in the operating room, we propose that being in an automatic mode is not an 'all or none' phenomenon; rather, it can be further characterized by *how much attention* is being reinvested into monitoring activities during the [surgery]."[52]

Practice is not just about practice itself but also about the effects it may have further afield. Practice, and a prepared mind, may help us to develop and master skills and competencies that set the conditions for what have been characterized as *flow states*. When we are in a flow state we have a high level of concentration without any feeling of effortfulness. Developing the subjective experience of flow depends on two preconditions: a close match between what we are trying to do and our skills for doing it, and clear indications of our progress. In the first of these preconditions, we face "Perceived challenges, or opportunities for action, that stretch (neither overmatching nor underutilizing) existing skills; a sense that [we are] engaging challenges at a level appropriate to [our] capacities." In the second, we have "Clear proximal goals and immediate feedback about the progress that is being made."[53]

During flow states we are able to effortlessly immerse ourselves in creative or other challenging activity with intense attention to an unfolding task. We enjoy the experience for itself. There is an intimate merging of our action and awareness with a deep sense of control and intrinsic involvement because of the close fit between our skill level and the challenges at hand.[54]

A crucial determinant of whether flow states will emerge in our experience is the compatibility between our skill level and the level of demands and complexity of our current activity. States of flow may often be associated with the simultaneous presence of the capability to *see or anticipate difficulty* together with a capability for *mastering difficulty*.[55] Flow states may be an important contributor to motivation and expression in creative performances in, for example, dance, music, or drama.[56]

We know from a study of professional classical pianists that flow states involve "effortless attention," an apparently paradoxical state of a high degree of attentional control combined with positive emotion. Detailed physiological measures of the pianists' depth and rate of breathing, heart rate, and blood pressure suggested that flow was accompanied by a distinctive physiological state.[57] In a flow state as in other states of creativity or in certain forms of meditation, there may be highly interactive cooperative dovetailing of physiological subsystems enabling higher attention and performance. Flow states and other forms of absorptive attention involve complete immersive attention, drawing concurrently on all of our perceptual, motor, imaginative, and emotional capabilities.[58]

Incessant or unpredictable interruptions of our thinking process—due to demands on our attention such as incoming text messages, telephone calls, or unexpected visitors—decrease the chance that we will achieve or maintain a flow state. Rather than immersively and enjoyably engaging with the task at hand, we may find ourselves scattered and jolted from one demand on our attention to another. Attempting to simultaneously divide our attention across two or more different complex activities leaves both activities shortchanged.

When we try to work on several things at once, we are at risk of losing track of our progress and may experience insufficient immersion in those tasks. The quality of our work may also suffer. Even when they had ample time, participants in a lab-based study wrote essays of significantly lower quality when they had been interrupted several times during either the planning of the essay or its writing than in instances when they had not been interrupted.[59]

Yet not all forms of "task switching" are the same. We need to also take into account the *time scale* on which we are moving between tasks and how much choice we have in *if* and *when* we switch tasks. Different types of task switching may have different implications for our creative progress.[60] As we have seen in our discussion of times in between, disruptions or breaks in our working process can sometimes be helpful. They can rechannel the direction of our thinking—recall the burst of creativity that followed the brief interruption of the working process of the electroacoustic composer that we saw earlier in this Part.

Interleaving two or more tasks—beginning one, spending some time on it, then turning to another task for a period of time before returning to the first—can refresh our idea landscapes, with subconscious processes continuing to work toward our open goals in the background of our awareness.[61] The interleaving of different activities may also serve a preventative function—preventing us from reaching a point where we are feeling completely stuck, with the accompanying feelings of frustration only compounding the problem.[62]

When we sequence our actions in this way, we can devote ourselves to the task before us and also give ourselves the needed time to transition between each project. People differ, though, in their ability to effectively interleave creative tasks, and finding the conditions that work best for you may require some experimentation. Some people, for example, may find that they work and create best if they predominantly work on one project across an extended period of time, mostly completing one before advancing to the next. Others, however, may thrive by more frequently alternating across different creative projects.[63]

Are there other ways in which we can more readily and completely immerse ourselves in our creative projects? Our immersion may also be fostered through experience with mindfulness training or meditation, which can enhance our capacity for deliberate and prolonged attention or for more open and receptive attunement. During forms of meditation involving concentrated or directed attention, the meditator intently focuses on, for example, his or her breathing or intently and successively on different parts of the body. In contrast, in receptive or open-monitoring meditation, the meditator attends to the present moment without any effortful reining in of thoughts, emotions, motivations, or perceptions. Most meditation may involve aspects of both concentration and receptive openness.[64]

Mindfulness meditation aims to counter our excessive reliance on verbal or conceptual information and to reorient us to a fuller range of sensory-perceptual, emotional, and bodily experiences. Engaging in mindfulness exercises may enhance our ability to control our attention and help attune us to where we are on our control dial, giving us a wider range of adaptive control.[65] In practiced meditators, a brief period of open-monitoring meditation promoted flexible associative thinking and the fluent generation of creative ideas.[66] Even a short mindfulness training session using a 10-minute meditation video has been shown to enhance insight problem solving among undergraduate students.[67] By taking part in mindfulness exercises we may more readily overcome a too-ready automatic reliance on habitual responses, including responses that are highly commonplace. "Meditation may result in honing the general skill of refocusing attention on actions and cognitions that were previously habitual."[68]

Let's consider how habit and repetition may prevent us from noticing novel solutions to a problem and how forms of meditation may counteract cognitive rigidity. In the classic "water jar task," participants are asked to use three hypothetical jars to obtain a specific amount of water to fill a target container.[69] They might, for instance, be given jars that can hold 3 units, 21 units, and 127 units and be asked to fill the target container with 100 units of water. Using only addition and subtraction, they need to find the simplest and most efficient way to achieve a result of 100 while using only units of 3, 21, or 127. So, for this example, the problem might be solved through the sequence $127 - 21 - 3 - 3 = 100$.

If people are given a number of such problems, each of which can be solved using the same sequence of steps, they often continue to rely on the same practiced multistep sequence even when a shorter and simpler solution is available. However, individuals who had just completed a six-week training course of different types of mindfulness meditation were less prone to falling into this unthinking reliance on routine.[70]

In another study, participants took part in seven two-hour group sessions and a half-day retreat that introduced them to five different types of meditation. The first four types asked them to sit still with their eyes closed and focus on their breathing (breathing meditation); to follow instructions to successively focus attention on different parts of their bodies (body scan meditation); to remain receptively open to sensations of the present moment, such as sounds or smells (open awareness meditation); or to wish for release from suffering or distress for a person they cared about and a person they were in conflict with (compassion meditation). The fifth type involved walking meditation, wherein participants were asked to walk silently and slowly, noticing the varied aspects and sensations of their walking. Although in solving the water jar problems everyone relied on habit to some extent, the meditation group was significantly more likely to notice if a shorter, simpler solution was available than was a baseline control group that had not undertaken the meditation training.[71]

As we can see, from the water jar example, increasing experience or expertise is not uniformly beneficial for creativity or insight. Sometimes greater skilled action and the increasing abstractness of our goal and action identification may, paradoxically, stand in the way of our seeing and noticing. We may automatically and habitually substitute objects or features based on what we *expect* rather than paying attention to all that is actually there.

We may also overemphasize what we know well, unthinkingly falling back upon well-learned procedures. We may "overzealously" transfer what we know to an inappropriate context, failing to notice important differences or distinctions.[72]

Consider what happened when groups of first-year and senior-level mechanical engineering students were charged with developing next-generation breakthrough alarm clocks. One group (subdivided into first-year and senior-level subgroups) was asked to interact with two actual alarm clocks in a typical manner. A second group (also subdivided into first-year and senior-level subgroups) was asked to do so while wearing oven mitts, blindfolds, and both earplugs and earmuffs to perceptually *and* emotionally simulate limited dexterity, dark conditions, or deep sleep—circumstances we might face upon groggily hearing a clock's wake-up alarm early in the morning.[73]

The group faced with the challenging sensory limitations during their explorations of the clocks developed significantly more original and feasible designs. The sensory limitations *enhanced* the innovation of first-year students and senior-level students, but the first-year students under sensory constraints were judged to be significantly more innovative than were senior-level students under those conditions. The group with the imposed sensory challenges may have been encouraged to incorporate a wider range of ideas into their design thinking, beyond their habitual or readily mentally accessible concepts, emotions, perceptions, and goals.

Upon examining the sketches and drawings that the students had generated, it became clear that the senior-level students were using the skills they had acquired in their undergraduate courses. Yet they may have *overrelied* on those well-practiced and more routine skills; "they seemed to be more fixated on creating feasible designs with high levels of certainty, rather than exploring a variety of potential improvements and changes to existing designs." In addition, the senior students stepped down to a highly detailed level too soon, "Their drawings often included different projections of the concept and relatively high levels of detail on potential attachments between modules and other engineering details."[74] Although highly specific diagrams may often be appropriate, during the process of initially generating possible design constructs, less detailed and even somewhat ambiguous sketches might productively provoke diverse interpretations.[75]

Deliberately plunging designers into sensory, physical, or cognitively challenging situations during the design process is one aspect of the empathic design approach. In **empathic design**, designers intentionally adopt constraints and processes that help them empathize with potential users.[76]

Empathic design is one of a diverse and wide range of semistructured or structured approaches to guiding idea generation. What this panoply of

techniques has in common is that each technique seeks to guide and strategically modulate the degree of cognitive control that individuals and groups
are using in their creative or innovation processes. These many approaches
to idea generation differ in their level of structure and the extent to which
they rely on different forms of external visual or sensory support. They also
differ in the degree to which they explicitly involve successive expansions or
modifications of ideas over time and across different contributors.

Key dimensions on which semistructured or structured approaches to
idea generation techniques differ from one another include:

- The types of representations that are used (e.g., sketches, verbal
  annotations, sentences).
- Who shares with whom and when (e.g., whether there is an initial
  idea-generation phase for individuals and then a form of rotation or
  display of those ideas to additional individuals or groups).
- Which thinking processes are explicitly encouraged (e.g., comparison, elaboration, resolving contradictions or trade-offs).
- The explicit goals of the approach (e.g., quantity or quality of ideas,
  novelty or feasibility, and the explicitness of the problem or opportunity constraints).

A few of the more frequently used idea-generation approaches we outline
here include brainstorming, collaborative sketching or C-sketch, the 6-3-5
method and other forms of brainwriting, the gallery method, and TRIZ or
TIPS. We first introduce these methods and then discuss how and when they
work best and why.

Brainstorming, and its many variants, emphasizes the spontaneous and
intensive generation of numerous ideas to meet a given goal or set of constraints, with relatively minimal guidelines such as injunctions to bracket
criticism, build on others' ideas, and welcome all contributions.[77] Although
brainstorming is commonly thought of as verbally expressing ideas in
face-to-face group interactions, ideas may alternatively be expressed in written form (on paper or digitally) or in sketches.

In *brainwriting*, individuals silently write down their ideas on pieces of
paper and place each separate idea sheet in the center of a table. Individuals
in the group can then opt to select and review the idea sheets of others.
Alternatively, individuals may pass their idea sheets along. In the *6-3-5
method*, an alternative form of brainwriting, six people generate three ideas
individually and write them on a sheet of paper; they then circulate them
to each other, building on the ideas of others, until each sheet returns to its
originator.[78] A variant, called *C-Sketch* or collaborative sketching, involves

generating sketches and circulating them silently.[79] In the *gallery method*, individuals each separately sketch concepts and then display the sketches for group viewing and discussion; then they cycle through the process again.[80] In *electronic brainstorming*, different approaches may be taken, but all rely on the basic idea that individuals develop their own ideas independently before sharing them through a computer network.[81] All of these methods tend to rely on relatively more spontaneous and less controlled modes of thinking.

A comparatively more systematic and deliberate approach to creative and innovative design decomposition and analysis is *design by analogy*. Recall that we explored earlier, in Part 2, design by analogy and biomimetic concept generation; recollect the vibrating skis problem that was solved by calling upon comparisons to cellos and violins, or the development of internet server algorithms based on honeybee foraging. Another systematic approach, intended to help reveal new interrelationships or configurations of a problem, is *TRIZ* (from the Russian, *teoriya resheniya izobretatelskikh zadatch*) or as translated into English *TIPS* (the theory of inventive problem solving).[82] This design decomposition and analysis method explicitly recognizes the frequent trade-offs that regularly occur in mechanical and product design, such as the opposing demands for material strength versus weight or of speed versus efficiency. It treats these trade-offs as promising opportunities for innovation through a systematic or structured exploration process. TRIZ provides an abstracted problem matrix developed from data on tens of thousands of patents. As a stimulus to thinking through the current problem the method provides a "design contradiction matrix" that identifies design contradictions and then allows the user to map to successful solution principles used in the past.

In considering the possible benefits and drawbacks of any method for generating ideas we can try to think about how the method will shape and sculpt the idea landscapes of individuals, subgroups, or the entire group or team. The different techniques are ways to attempt to beneficially enter another's idea landscape without disrupting the creative/associative processes that are already emerging. For any given technique we should ask ourselves the following questions:

- Does the technique potentially disrupt or truncate the flow of thinking of each person? Are all good ideas being captured or are some being submerged because they are competing with others?
- Does the technique introduce new perspectives at the right time(s)?
- Does the technique encourage and allow time and space for elaboration of ideas and making connections among ideas?

- Does the technique promote a truly wide and inclusive diversity of ideas and "takes" on a problem? How large and varied is the group?
- Are the goals of the idea generation process clear and clearly communicated? Is the predominant aim of the exercise to generate as many novel ideas as possible or to elaborate ideas by building on successive ideas?
- At the most general level, does the technique capitalize on the benefits of our mind's exquisite sensitivity to "associative cuing" from our environments and from each other? Or does the technique leave us vulnerable to thought prompts that are poorly timed or distracting?

We need to take into account several factors in selecting and modifying an idea-generation method for a particular project or purpose. One important factor is **associative cuing**. As we saw in Part 1 with the example of our chancing to overhear the word "green," encountering an idea associatively cues other thoughts related to that idea.[83] Such cuing can be beneficial, as it introduces multiple perspectives and expertise into a shared dynamic thinking space. But sometimes associative cuing can detrimentally channel thoughts into an overly uniform or narrow direction, limiting novel associative possibilities. We need to be on the lookout for poorly timed associative cuing. Equally important, though, we can make associative cuing do creative work for us through what we do *before* we meet. By discussing the nature of the problem at hand and by providing background information or reading we can trigger beneficial associative cuing prior to the idea-generation session.[84]

Another significant factor is *output interference*. We can retain only a limited number of ideas in focal awareness at any given time, and ideas that are now being expressed ("output") by ourselves or others may interfere with or limit our ability to access other ideas that are still forming or are not yet expressed. Ideas compete with one another for emergence in our awareness and sometimes can be lost if we do not rapidly capture them by "outputting" them into spoken, written, or other forms. A typical instance of output interference can occur in a group ideation or verbal face-to-face brainstorming session when someone must delay expressing an idea but then finds it has been lost in the interim while he or she was waiting to speak. Output interference combined with associative cuing may also impede the incipient development of ideas by attracting or pulling our ideas in an alternative direction before they have the opportunity to be fully formed, articulated, or expressed.

Output interference and detrimental associative cuing are two fundamental reasons why simpler forms of face-to-face group brainstorming have not proven to be effective. Despite the popularity of verbal group brainstorming, many studies have shown that interacting face-to-face groups produce *fewer* unique (nonredundant) ideas and ideas that are of *lower average quality* than do an equal number of individuals generating ideas separately on their own.[85] Verbally expressing our ideas to the group too soon may lead to a single shared idea landscape without the beneficial input of each individual's contributions and successive reworkings. Variations on simpler face-to-face group brainstorming are attempts to avoid the drawbacks of jumping into a single idea space too soon.

The possible "productivity costs" of brainstorming—the frequently observed finding that individuals working alone produce a larger number of novel ideas than do interacting groups—can be counteracted by individuals capturing ideas on their own *before* they share them with others, as in electronic brainstorming or the 6-3-5 method. There may also be detrimental productivity costs if we share ideas with the entire team all at once. For this reason it may be best to share ideas in pairs and then pairs of pairs so as to maintain the greatest diversity of ideas until the very end of the process. We should ask ourselves how soon the idea landscapes of individuals or subgroups should be meshed or intercombined. Might the timeline of the idea generation process be extended, with everyone given several days to reflect on and develop their ideas? Would it be beneficial to allow multiple communication modes, both online and offline? Is integrating idea landscapes across individuals and teams itself a priority?[86]

Rotational viewing, or the sharing of ideas with others in a sequence rather than open full-group gallery viewing, may allow more people to maintain and "grow" good ideas semi-independently of one another, with enough input to spark new ideas and connections but not so much as to swamp or sweep everyone up in the same direction. The same may be true for sharing ideas digitally. Some forms of electronic brainstorming may similarly balance the need for allowing time to individually develop our ideas with the need for opportunities to encounter others' suggestions in order to re-ignite our own thinking through associative cuing. Sparking promising ideas off of those of others in electronic brainstorming may be especially likely in larger groups of more than eight participants[87] or when participants are exposed to comparatively larger numbers of ideas (say about 100 ideas rather than about 25).[88] Many of the idea-generation techniques or aspects of the techniques can be beneficially used in combination, and the boundaries between them in terms of degree of cognitive control are not sharp.[89]

A third important factor is the availability and explicitness of external representations of ideas. What external representations are available to the group and produced by it? How do these externalizations of ideas facilitate the perception-action cycles or see-move-see of the individuals or group? How open are the representations to alternative interpretations?

Approximate sketches or jottings can help to both articulate and sculpt ambiguous or not fully formed ideas and may evoke productive associations in ourselves and others.[90] As we have seen, in empathic design methods, the use of sensory constraints deepens our consideration of sensory-perceptual and motor interplay in using an object or process. Introducing sensory challenges can provide us with a way of moving away from our habitual action patterns and promote novel ways of noticing.[91]

A final consideration that we should take into account in selecting and modifying an idea-generation method for a particular project is the extent to which the idea-generation technique or techniques make room for variations in degrees of control. Restructuring our environments or external representations can be a deliberate action (as in structured search for analogies or using a TRIZ or TIPS matrix), but then the outcome of that action may provide the impetus for *spontaneous* pattern recognition and perceptual and conceptual comparison and contrast processes.

All idea-generation techniques, like the creative process itself, involve trade-offs between the benefits of continuing exploration versus the need to constrain thinking within particular time or other requirements. Trade-offs in idea generation often include dedicating time and effort to developing new options (generation or discovery) versus revisiting, extending, and revising ideas (elaboration and evaluation). Yet both are necessary. Indeed, two of the common ground rules for brainstorming—participants are exhorted to welcome unusual or wild ideas ("freewheeling"/generation) and to combine and improve ideas ("building-on"/elaboration)—may themselves encourage undesirable trade-offs between generation and elaboration. In any idea-generation technique, we may want to decide whether generation or elaboration is most important at a given time and to tailor our process and stated goals accordingly.[92]

EFFORTFUL PLANNING AND DOING

We have now reached a consideration of those points on the control dial where we are most effortful, deliberate, and planful. In our endeavors to foster creativity and change, effortful planning and doing are prominent in the processes of choosing and meeting problem constraints and in evaluating our creative attempts and our creative processes. Equally, effortful top-down deliberate control is essential in enabling us to maintain our focus and persistence despite setbacks or obstacles and in prioritizing and reprioritizing our innovative and creative directions. All of these take place over the longer term, in working/playing environments that we deliberately and actively structure and restructure.

The constraints or requirements that define and form our creative and change spaces are in part selected or chosen by us, and in part imposed or necessitated by external considerations. Constraints vary in kind, from time constraints, to material or resource constraints, to client requirements and beyond. Some initial basic constraints are usually explicitly specified in a design brief or project specifications. In addition, the creative and innovative process itself frequently requires further and iterative deliberate interpretation and the application of additional requirements, either inherent to the problem or introduced through the acquisition of new information. The constraints may be based on our individual experience or expertise or deduced, based on our analysis of the problem or of already defined constraints.[93] Rather than creative leaps, the creative process often involves the building of successive temporary and emergent bridges between problem spaces and solution spaces—or subproblems and subsolution spaces—by identifying a key idea.[94]

> It seems that creative design is not a matter of first [identifying] the problem and then searching for a satisfactory solution concept. Creative design seems more to be a matter of developing and refining together both the formulation of a problem and ideas for a solution, with constant iteration of analysis, synthesis and evaluation processes between the two notional design "spaces"—problem space and solution space.[95]
>
> —*Design researchers and educators Kees Dorst and Nigel Cross*

In Part 4, which follows, we further explore the key roles of constraints, including both those that we choose and those that are imposed, in the context of the continual iteration of making and finding.

Closely related to this process of iteratively moving between our problem spaces and solution spaces is the similar interchange or taking turns between *generating* ideas and *evaluating* ideas and plans.[96] When asked to think aloud while drawing, artists with extensive experience in drawing and nonartists with little drawing experience similarly made evaluative comments between 15 and 25 percent of the time as they drew. But the artists more often made positive evaluations whereas nonartists more often made negative evaluations. Throughout their drawing processes, besides describing their drawings, both artists and nonartists made explicit references to their plans and their goals.[97]

Artists made twice as many references to goals and nearly twice as frequently commented on the ongoing progress of their *entire drawing*, making more global assessments. They spent significantly more total time on both preparing for and carrying out their drawings, and their drawings were independently rated as much more creative, demonstrating higher quality, originality, and skill. In addition to greater initial expertise and investment of time, higher creativity depended on deliberate control, as shown in more planning, more attention to goals, and more careful assessment of the overall project.[98]

Given that these various forms of deliberate control can be so valuable, how might we selectively and strategically introduce more control into our creative process?

One especially effective approach involves **reflective verbalization**. For complex and extended activities, we can explicitly describe, explain, evaluate, and justify our attempted design or creative solutions to someone else; this may help us to identify gaps, promising next steps, or the need to reprioritize. We do need to be careful, though, in verbally characterizing our impressions, so that we do not allow our verbal descriptions to enter too completely or overshadow more elusive sensory-perceptual experiences.[99]

Suppose you were asked to sketch designs for a new outdoor garden grill. The grill should have an easily removable and stable cooking grid and coal pan, with a grid that could be adjusted and secured at distances from 2 to 10 inches from the coals. After you had completed your designs, suppose further that you were asked to answer questions by someone unfamiliar with your design and the project itself. For each of the components and functions of the grill, you might be asked questions, such as "How does this work?" "Why did you do it like this?" "What advantages and disadvantages does this solution have?" "What could a better solution look like?"[100] Having responded to your questioner, imagine you were then given an opportunity to return to your original design and make revisions or changes. How and why might your question-answer exchange influence your ultimate design?

When students without any formal engineering or design background were asked to design such a grill and then either answered reflective questions or completed an unrelated questionnaire (that is, the baseline control group), the question-based reflective verbalization led to the generation of significantly more alternative design modifications and corrections. These modifications resulted in higher-quality designs that more completely met the design specifications.[101]

Why might the reflective verbalization process have produced, in the end, better design outcomes?

Interspersing our creative process with phases in which we explicitly attempt to explain our thought and action processes to one another encourages us to step up and down in our levels of abstraction (e.g., asking both how and why). It also requires us to move between modalities (e.g., visually sketching and verbally describing) and prompts us to notice and more thoroughly consider the interrelations among components and features. Explicitly explaining our thinking and actions to someone else may also encourage us to gain a wider perspective on our creative or change project, allowing increased separation or distance from our prior thinking patterns and solutions, thus extending our idea landscapes.

> Through the practice of talking about your work, you say things you didn't know you were aware of ... talking out loud is another way of thinking, and ... new thoughts come out through that process.[102]
> —*Design professor Chris Bertoni*

An important benefit of working in pairs or in teams may be the opportunity to take turns in articulating and conveying ideas both through actions (e.g., sketching, configuring objects, gesturing) and words (e.g., verbal or written descriptions, explanations, or questions), in dynamic interaction with our external environments. Such turn taking may help us to see broader, more abstract options and opportunities, including new ways of representing and approaching our problem or project.[103] More generally, reflective verbalization, including to ourselves, may provide an impetus to probe our thinking, including our thinking about the interrelated aspects of a project, beyond what might be prompted by a checklist or a template.[104]

There are other powerful direct and deliberate ways of becoming aware of our noticing and of introducing novelty into our creative and other actions. We can deliberately or mindfully pay attention to nuanced distinctions in an otherwise well-practiced routine activity. Or we can deliberately change—and reward—our varying responses.

In working with the creative processes of dancers, the dancer and choreographer Gill Clarke observed how encouraging the dancers to focus on their full kinesthetic and sensory experiences opened new possibilities. Clark noted, however, the importance of inviting this intentional noticing as a form of novel experiential *sensing* or "tasting" of their internal bodily proprioceptive sensations during the movements rather than the dancers' familiar emphasis on more externally forming movements. As she explained of the dancers: "I was impressed by their capacity to turn attention and curiosity to noticing small changes and proprioceptive feedback from their own moving, just so long as the task invited responses motivated by 'tasting' sensation rather than the forming of movement, and was therefore able to be apprehended as an unfamiliar territory dissociated from their habitual dancing."[105] We will look at these and other approaches to learning to vary in Part 4.

Higher degrees of cognitive control are also crucial in enabling us to maintain focus and to persevere in our creative and change endeavors despite setbacks, both on shorter time scales on the order of minutes or hours and on longer ones comprising days, weeks, or years. Our performance of even brief creative ideation tasks (e.g., generating alternative uses for a common object such as a penny or a paper clip) is initially supported by more automatic processes (e.g., based on memory retrieval). With continued time and engagement in the task, however, we increasingly draw upon our more effortfully persistent attempts at analysis and structured exploration.[106]

We may need to exercise focused deliberate control in order to overcome our tendencies to take the "path of least resistance,"[107] persisting past our ready-to-mind thoughts to find novel combinations and possibilities. The *dual pathway to creativity model* proposes that, beyond cognitive flexibility, we often need persistence or perseverance to realize our creative directions.[108]

Higher degrees of cognitive control may also be positively related to our ability to actively hold information in mind, including goals and branching into subgoals, thus allowing greater integration of ideas and their interrelations. Keeping multiple ideas in mind may facilitate improvisation. Experienced cellists who were able to actively mentally retain and work with high amounts of information (that is, those with a relatively higher short-term working memory capacity), when asked to improvise, were judged to be more creative and original across a series of short improvisations.[109]

In the longer term, individuals who show a propensity for comparatively higher levels of deliberate self-control, such as self-regulation or resistance to immediate temptation, demonstrate many advantages, such as higher grade point averages, better relationships, and enhanced interpersonal skills.[110] Delay of gratification in preschool children—as measured by a child's willingness to postpone eating a cookie or a marshmallow immediately in order to receive two such treats at a later time—was significantly positively related to their degree of cognitive control on a difficult laboratory-based inhibition task 10 years later.[111]

The many and clear benefits of a highly controlled, future-oriented, comparatively abstract perspective may, however, lead us to adopt such a perspective too uniformly or continuously. We may relentlessly emphasize future goals and plans in an abstracted manner that leaves us overly removed from the present. Such abstraction, as shown by daily mood reports from experimental participants, may be linked to a diminished awareness or expression of both positive and negative emotions. It may also be associated with reduced awareness of embodied or physiological aspects of our experience that, in turn, enable empathy, self-understanding, and spontaneity. Adaptively changing our degree of control and our temporal perspective, intermingling perspectives of the past, present, and future, may counter potential costs of excessive abstraction and control.[112]

Exerting cognitive and self-regulatory control at a high level and over a long time also raises the possibility that we will stretch our mental, emotional, and physical resources too thin, which could leave us vulnerable to relying on mundane, commonplace, or habitual responding. Continued pursuit of a given effortful activity is often associated with both fatigue and changing opportunity costs as we continue to forgo other, potentially more rewarding, activities that we might engage in instead of the one at hand. We need to pay attention to the *informational signal* provided by the subjective experience of fatigue, as this can help us to adjudicate between our many goals and promote our longer-term adaptive flexibility. As we saw earlier, one recent neuroscience account suggests that there is an integrative hub in our brain (in a subregion of the anterior cingulate cortex, further described in the next section on the brain bases of cognitive control and spontaneity) that continuously computes the possible costs and possible benefits of exerting cognitive control. This hub is proposed to guide us toward an appropriate level of control, including how much and where to invest cognitive control, in line with current incentives, goals, and our broader motivational state.[113]

If we stretch our control too long and too relentlessly, we may be more likely to default into a less deliberate mode of processing even when—from a broader more overarching perspective—this is not what we would otherwise choose. Both in the longer and the shorter term it is important for us to flexibly and creatively develop ways in which to counter and prevent such overextensions. By doing so, we continue to have maximal choice and capabilities for when and how successfully we do exert deliberate control.

One option involves taking breaks or giving ourselves shorter or longer phases of "time away" when it is contextually appropriate to do so. This approach not only helps to directly reduce a continual demand on our deliberate control but also provides an avenue for comparatively automatic and spontaneous thinking to come to our aid in our endeavors. Breaks that offer us immersion in natural settings such as walking among trees in a park or alongside water may be especially mentally rejuvenating and restorative of our ability to exert deliberate attentional control.[114]

Another related approach involves changing how we ourselves think of our creative endeavors and goals. We can ask if there are ways in which we could think of our goals that make goal pursuit and goal effort less demanding and more naturally unified with our inclinations. A key contributor here involves considering how we view our goals. Do we see our goals as our own, as something that we (and our teams) actively endorse, and that meaningfully fit within a bigger picture? Or do we see (or feel) that our goals are imposed, that they are not endorsed by us, and that we lack a clear sense of why we are pursuing them?[115] Questions about goals and also of prioritizing and reprioritizing our innovative and creative directions, are explored in Part 6.

Actively structuring and restructuring our working/playing environments is yet another way in which we can exercise deliberate control in our creative pursuits and also reduce demands on our control.

Imagine that you are asked to take part in a hypothetical medical diagnosis experiment. You have no medical training and no medical training is required. You are given some information and are asked to make diagnoses about patients, but you are asked to order as few lab tests as possible (to reduce costs). You are provided with materials to take notes.

Would you use these materials to take notes, and what kind of notes might you take? How could you structure your environment to help you navigate this novel task?

In this situation, a comparison of undergraduate and graduate students, both without medical training, showed clear differences in the environmental structure they created for themselves.[116] Undergraduates immediately moved into the diagnoses without taking notes, but graduate students made extensive lists, matrices, and decision-tree diagrams. Creating these diagrams initially slowed down the graduate students considerably, although they were just as accurate in their diagnoses as the undergraduates. The diagrams gave them a significant advantage—the graduate students succeeded in their goal of pinpointing just the right lab tests to request. When faced with novel cases, the matrix or decision-tree diagrams that they had earlier made also enhanced their efficiency in arriving at a decision.

This form of proactive or *prospective adaptation* of the environment is an example of deliberately and methodically creating a representational tool that can outperform habit and routine. Prospective adaptation refers to how we initially set up a working or thinking space for a challenging problem, including particularly how we represent the problem in words, symbols, charts, or diagrams. "A good representation can greatly improve problem solving ... and introducing a representation can help with a class of related instances, even if they are not fully known beforehand."[117] Importantly, with experience or training, the decision to structure information in effort-reducing external representational forms may itself become habitual.

There are myriad ways in which we can repurpose our environments to make them more friendly or congenial to our current goals and needs.[118] We should take time to purposefully structure our external environments. By restructuring our creative environments we can often enhance our actual working and playing spaces, improve the tools we have to hand, expand the options that our spaces and technologies offer for different modes of thinking and working, and better integrate emotion and perception with our goal pursuits.

Especially promising temporal windows in which to intentionally restructure our thinking/working/making environments and establish new desirable habits are provided during times in which those environments are changing for other reasons. We can take advantage of the temporary abeyance of our usual habits that arises when we change our place of residence, embark on a new course of study, or launch a new project or business venture. At such times, research demonstrates that both our environments and our habits are especially malleable and open to change. The fresh environment has not yet accumulated strong associative cuing prompts for us, and so gives us greater degrees of freedom and offers us relative ease in establishing new positive habits.[119]

We offer a capsule summary of several of the advantages and disadvantages of dialing up and dialing down in our degree of mental control in Table 3.1.

Table 3.2 outlines some of the ways in which we can typically adjust our degree of cognitive control to maximize flexibility and variation.

Table 3.1 ADVANTAGES OF DIFFERENT DEGREES OF COGNITIVE CONTROL

Higher control	**Lower control**
May promote	*May promote*
• Long-term perspective	• Context sensitivity
• Systematic and analytical thinking	• Pattern recognition
• Persistence	• Exploration
• Objectivity and emotional neutrality	• Receptivity and empathy

Both higher *and* lower degrees of cognitive control offer distinctive benefits in our thinking and creativity.

Table 3.2 MODIFYING OUR COGNITIVE CONTROL

To increase control	To decrease control
• Consider the long term	• Attend to the here and now
• Focus on the abstract/general	• Focus on the concrete/specific
• Keep alertness high	• Relax
• Remove distractions	• Receptively explore

We can increase or decrease our degree of cognitive control in various direct and indirect ways.

BRAIN BASES OF COGNITIVE CONTROL AND SPONTANEITY

The different components of our creative processes—involving variation in the degree and mode of cognitive control—may call upon different networks and subnetworks of our brains. Although particular forms of sensory information, such as sounds, or colors, or motion, are each processed in relatively localized and spatially contiguous cortical regions, complex forms of cognition depend on widely separated and interconnected networks. These widespread networks themselves connect and interconnect many local networks, integrating information both across different modalities and with our prior learning. These large-scale networks—spanning the right and left cerebral hemispheres as well as the anterior and posterior regions of the brain—flexibly couple and decouple with one another across time. They are configured and reconfigured as we alternate between more open-ended and receptive phases devoted to the formation and generation of ideas and phases of more closely focused controlled attention, planning, and creative evaluation.

One such neural network is the **executive control network**. It is designated as "executive control" for its highly consistent role in a range of activities that require cognitive coordination and control, such as focusing or shifting our attention, planning, and monitoring our goal progress.[120] As schematically shown in Figure 3.5, key brain regions in the executive control network are the right and left dorsolateral prefrontal cortex (important in holding goals in mind and short-term working memory), anterior cingulate cortex (important in error monitoring and evaluating our progress), together with the right and left posterior parietal cortex (important in guiding attentional control and attention switching). Increased brain activity in regions of this executive control network has been observed in a wide array of creative generative tasks calling upon different skills and techniques, from musical improvisation to graphic design.

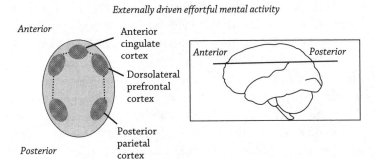

Executive control network

Externally driven effortful mental activity

Figure 3.5 A BRAIN NETWORK IMPORTANT IN EFFORTFUL CONTROL.
A simplified diagram illustrating key brain regions within the executive control
network. The right panel shows the brain in profile; the horizontal line indicates
the thin layer, section, or "slice" of the brain that is schematically shown in the left
panel. The left panel schematically depicts the slice as if we were looking down from
above, onto the top of the brain.

Activity of the executive control network has been identified during creative story generation,[121] piano improvisation,[122] problem solving through
insight,[123] the formation of novel analogies,[124] and visual art design.[125]
Remarking on their findings that dorsolateral prefrontal cortex was called
upon during musical improvisation, researchers emphasized how this quint-
essential executive control brain region contributed to "the creative aspects
of a complex and ecologically relevant behavior, where the free selection of
responses is adapted to an overall goal of producing an aesthetically satisfactory end-result."[126] Collectively, these research outcomes underscore the
often underrecognized contribution of deliberate attentional and evaluative
processes to our creative endeavors.

Three other neural networks have been shown to significantly contribute
to the imaginative, receptive, and emotional aspects of creative thinking,
either working in tandem or staggered in time, with the executive control
network. One network, initially discovered to be most active when experimental participants during brain scanning were taking breaks or pausing
from perceptual-cognitive tasks, is referred to as the default-mode network.
This distributed collection of brain regions tends to become more active
when the activities that we are engaging in are not especially demanding of
our top-down attention or mental effort.

The **default-mode network** is called upon in a diverse set of complex imaginative and reconstructive mental activities, such as our anticipations and
plannings for future events, and empathically imagining the thoughts and
feelings of other people. Comprising multiple subnetworks that span the left

and right hemispheres and both anterior and posterior brain regions, the default-mode network functions "to facilitate flexible self-relevant mental explorations—simulations—that provide a means to anticipate and evaluate upcoming events before they happen."[127] As shown in Figure 3.6, key brain regions in the default-mode network are the ventromedial prefrontal cortex (important in processing self-related and emotional information), the posterior cingulate cortex (important in mental imagery and autobiographical reexperiencing), and the right and left posterior parietal cortex (important in guiding attentional control and attention switching).

During creative endeavors, two other brain networks—one that may itself sometimes couple with the default-mode network and one that may help to switch between the executive and default modes—are, respectively, the mediotemporal network (not shown here) and the salience network. The mediotemporal network, including the hippocampal and parahippocampal regions, is fundamental to enabling retrieval from memory and for encoding novel combinations.

The salience network is important in integrating and detecting incoming and internal information that has significance (that is, "salience") for us. The **salience network** is often activated during the processing of emotional (affective) information. This network, including especially the anterior insula cortex, is important in integrating highly interpreted sensory information with other internal information about how we feel, its significance to us, and our

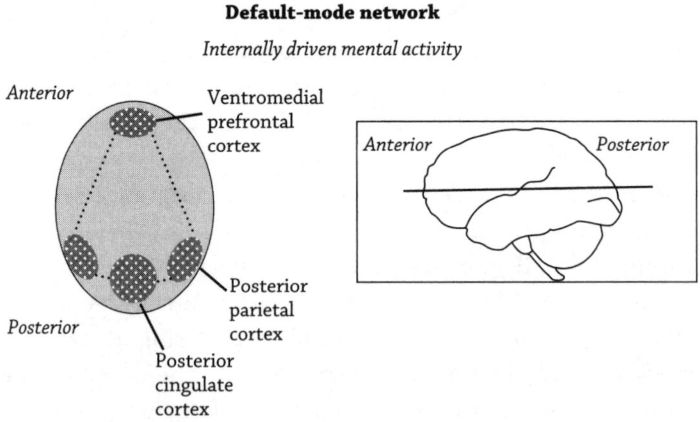

Default-mode network

Internally driven mental activity

Figure 3.6 A BRAIN NETWORK IMPORTANT IN INTERNALLY DRIVEN SPONTANEOUS AND IMAGINATIVE THINKING. A simplified diagram illustrating key brain regions within the default-mode network. The right panel shows the brain in profile; the horizontal line indicates the thin layer, section, or "slice" of the brain that is schematically shown in the left panel. The left panel schematically depicts the slice as if we were looking down from above, onto the top of the brain.

physiological responses (visceral, autonomic, and hedonic).[128] We further elaborate on the functional role of the anterior insula cortex later in this section. As schematically depicted in Figure 3.7, the left and right anterior insulae and anterior cingulate cortex (important in monitoring and evaluating our progress) are key regions in the salience network.

Analyses of the precise timing and direction of changes in brain activity has revealed that activity in the salience network may "generate the signals to trigger hierarchical control"[129] and to modulate cognitive systems.[130] These findings suggest that these brain regions may enable us to adaptively switch between the executive control network and the default-mode network.

The proposed role of the salience network in dynamically switching between the executive control and default-mode networks is schematically depicted in Figure 3.8.

Engagement in endeavors that place high demands on creatively adaptive thinking, such as forming new analogies, creating novel artistic designs, and imaginatively planning one's future goal-related pursuits has been found to lead to couplings of brain networks that are more frequently found to work in opposition to one another.[131] Typically, increasing activity in the executive network is accompanied by decreasing activity in the default-mode network and vice versa. But this oppositional relation is not found in all cases.

In a recent brain imaging study, visual arts students designed various book covers in response to brief written book descriptions while they were in a functional magnetic resonance imaging scanner. The students were

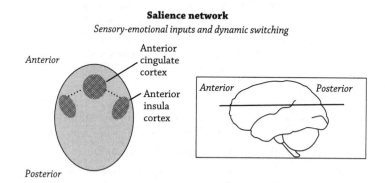

Figure 3.7 A BRAIN NETWORK IMPORTANT IN INTEGRATING SIGNIFICANT (SALIENT) EMOTIONAL, MOTIVATIONAL, AND SENSORY INFORMATION.
A simplified diagram illustrating key brain regions within the salience network. The right panel shows the brain in profile; the horizontal line indicates the thin layer, section, or "slice" of the brain that is schematically shown in the left panel. The left panel schematically depicts the slice as if we were looking down from above, onto the top of the brain.

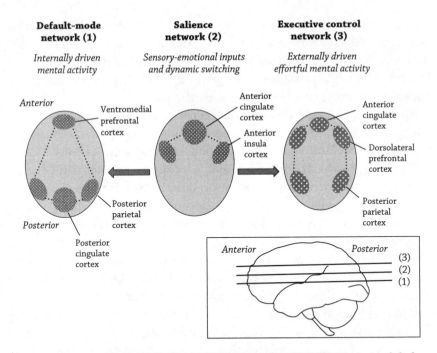

Figure 3.8 DYNAMIC SWITCHING BETWEEN BRAIN NETWORKS. A simplified diagram illustrating the proposed role of the salience network in adaptively signaling or initiating changes in our degree of cognitive control (suggested by the horizontal arrows). The salience network might prompt the default-mode network to relax our cognitive control or introduce spontaneity. At another time, the salience network might signal the executive control network to heighten our level of attention and degree of deliberate control. Each network is made up of several nodes that extensively communicate with each other. Some of the major nodes are pictured here. The lower panel shows the brain in profile; the horizontal lines indicate the thin layers, sections, or "slices" of the brain that correspond to those that are schematically shown in the upper panel.[132]

instructed (at particular points) to attempt to creatively *generate* a cover and at other points to creatively *evaluate* or simply *trace* what they had produced. The results pointed to the intermingled nature of both thinking and feeling, deliberation and spontaneity, in creative evaluation. The researchers concluded that creative evaluation may "allow for the combination and integration of both cognitive and affective as well as deliberate and spontaneous forms of evaluative thought" and that it may "be an extended form of analytic processing that combines processes that do not ordinarily act in tandem in order to produce optimal thinking conditions for creativity."[133]

So far we have emphasized that, throughout the brain, there are large-scale widely distributed neural networks that tend to be relatively stable in how they intercommunicate. It is important to note, however, that in addition to these large-scale networks, there may also be smaller-scale "flexible, temporary, and opportunistic" couplings of small groups of brain regions that form "process-specific alliances"[134] as we attempt to meet dynamically changing unique demands on our thinking.

Returning to the salience network, let's focus on the anterior insula. Enfolded deep within the frontal cortex, the anterior insula represents and integrates diverse sorts of information about what is important to us. Different subregions within this complex brain structure progressively represent and integrate successively, "homeostatic, environmental, hedonic, motivational, social, and cognitive activity to produce a 'global emotional moment.'"[135]

Based on brain imaging and other evidence, it has been proposed that intuition may involve sensitive attunement to internal physiological and visceral states represented in the frontal anterior insula. Such intuitive decision making has been defined as "the rapid assessment of the probability of a favorable or unfavorable outcome of a planned behavior in a situation of uncertain outcomes, which is dependent on previous experiences rather than on serial processes of inductive and or deductive reasoning."[136] It has been suggested that the presence of a particular type of neuron with especially long-ranging connections—found predominantly in the frontoinsular region of the brain of humans and other mammals with complex social interactions (e.g., elephants, bottlenose dolphins, and great apes)—may be involved in such highly integrative modes of decision making. Intriguingly, this particular type of neuron has also been postulated to be important in neutrally representing our "selves" across time.[137]

From a broader perspective, our ability to exercise cognitive control is also modulated at many other levels beyond that of large-scale brain networks, including the levels and interactions of neurotransmitters. One such neurotransmitter is dopamine, with sometimes exquisitely fine-tuned dopaminergic levels needed to allow the "just right" balance between too much control and too little.[138] Neurotransmitter broadcast release mechanisms spread neuromodulators widely throughout the cortex and subcortical regions, exerting effects at the cellular level. They work in tandem with "topological reconfigurations" of brain regions and subnetworks, and with integrative converging informational hubs such as the anterior insula, to enable us to meet our changing goals in changing circumstances. Relatively momentary and transient states of cognitive control may make it easier or more difficult to switch from our current manner of thinking to alternative modes of responding. In the brain, too, there may be a trade-off between staying with a given task or task configuration (stability or persistence), and opting for a different task or configuration (flexibility).[139]

We revisit the role of dopamine at the close of Part 4. Next, though, we delve more fully into broader questions of the interplay between flexibility and stability throughout our making-and-finding endeavors.

Creativity Cross Checks and Queries

Questions to encourage reflection and connections to your own work and practice:

⇒ What range of settings have you been using on your mental control dial?
  • Have you been trying too hard and too directly for too long?
  • Are you overly deliberate and controlled in your approach—or not controlled enough?
  • Could some indirection help you move forward in your creative problem space?
  • What are your transition zones and how do you use your times in between? Could you reconfigure how you think and respond to some minor obligations or requirements on your time so that they become useful times in between rather than unwanted distractions?

⇒ Are you providing permissive pauses around your ideas and during your creative projects? Here is how contemporary photographer Ryan McGinley and the novelist and poet Michael Ondaatje, respectively, describe a part of their processes:

> Usually it's about three or four [candidate photographs] and I'll put them up on the wall, and just have them in my peripheral vision for about a few weeks. It really becomes evident which one is the most important image.[140]

> I never have a strict controlling governor present during the first draft of a book. I write as if it were a rehearsal, I attempt or try out everything, though of course a subliminal editing is taking place. But I'm not thinking of that. And I find I am always surprised later. A scene I might think is too casual when I am writing it will later, in context, have just the right tightness.[141]

⇒ When should you speed up and slow down in your creative processes?
  • Are there intermediate or midlevel degrees of attention and control that might help you move forward, so that you invest more attention selectively, allowing your know-how to have its own appropriate autonomy?
  • Do you formulate for yourself appropriate timelines, including intermediate and final deadlines that give you impetus but do not impose undue pressure? Do you understand the origins and rationale for the deadlines that you or your team are working toward?
  • Do you allow spontaneity through your chosen constraints, as anchored in your earlier deliberate practice?

- Singer/songwriter Gillian Welch observes: "A lot of the songs [we record] are done in one take . . . Maybe two."[142]
  And the photographer William Eggleston notes:

  > I work very quickly and that's part of it. I only ever take one picture of one thing. Literally. Never two. So then that picture is taken and then the next one is waiting somewhere else.[143]

Might these approaches help you in increasing the range of your control? As you think about this, consider also the artist Robert Rauschenberg's observation that:

> One gets as much information as a witness of activity from a fleeting glance, like a quick look, sometimes in motion, as one does staring at the subject.[144]

⇒ Do you deliberately prompt yourself with broad, open-ended queries?
  - Have you tried intentionally focusing on action/verb possibilities to move about in your creative problem space? Have you asked yourself, *"What if I substituted an element here?" "Or flipped or inverted part of this idea?" "What if I or we tried ".* . .
  - What are the thinking scaffolding questions or the midlevel prompting queries that work best for you?
  - Are you keeping track of these questions and do you return to them when you are creatively stymied or losing creative momentum?
⇒ What encourages you to "play" and imaginatively stretch your boundaries? Have you tried mildly exhausting yourself with a long walk or a long swim before you sit down to write, compose, or design? Or have you tried writing as soon as you wake up in the morning?
⇒ Many good ideas emerge for us during routine activities such as showering, tidying, or walking. Some important features of "shower times" are that they tend to be uninterrupted, with an approximately expected duration. There is a clear sense of progress or completion as the task at hand is well understood and not highly demanding. Such times also are typically pleasant and mildly relaxing; they involve multiple senses with accompanying sounds, movements, touch, and so on.
  - How are you using your shower times?
  - What is special about these times, and are you using them to best creative advantage?
  - Do you allow yourself enough idea-generation shower times or should you be finding or making new ones?
  - Can you generate or discover "mini-shower times" in your creative process: moments that permit background idea reconfigurings to

fully emerge and form? Here is how a user experience and product designer described his process: "I often generate a UI [user interface] design, iterate a little, and if I'm not getting good diverging ideas, sometimes I work on details, polishing it. I don't for a minute think that I've necessarily got the best design, but it's a low-demand activity that's kind of pleasant and keeps the problem in front of me."[145]

⇒ Have you structured what you know and represented it in the external environment in a way that maximizes your ability to work with it and to see interrelations and relations?

• Consider this writing advice on the crucial role of actual words on a page from the psycholinguist and cognitive scientist Steven Pinker:

> Too many things have to go right in a passage of writing for most mortals to get them all the first time. It's hard enough to formulate a thought that is interesting and true. Only after laying a semblance of it on the page can a writer free up the cognitive resources needed to make the sentence grammatical, graceful, and, most important, transparent to the reader.[146]

⇒ What are your beginnings—do you plunge into your ongoing projects or do you gently wade in?

• Do you often start with something that is comparatively easy and more automatic (for example, reviewing and revising the text of the day before, expanding and organizing point-form notes), slowly reinstating and returning to your earlier idea landscape? Or is it sometimes better for you to dive directly into new material and contexts—resisting the reentanglement of your earlier attempts?

• What works best for you in getting you started? Do you understand and make way for (anticipate) good starting places? Do you sometimes allow yourself to "sneak up" on getting started by beginning to work almost surreptitiously, without any explicit declaration to yourself that you're about to work?

• Do you give yourself and others open opportunities to say out loud what has been done and what the next intentions are? Do you ask such questions as "Why did we do it like this?" "How does this work?" "How does this fit with where we are going?" Are you taking turns listening and explaining?

• The opera singer Jessye Norman reveals, "Truly, one of the most joyous things that I do in preparing for a performance is the warming-up part."[147] How do you warm-up and why?

Part 4

Making, Finding, and Improvising

Thinking prompts

- How do constraints guide and sometimes misguide our creative endeavors?
- How do we learn to vary the ways in which we make and find newness?
- Why and when should we improvise?
- How often and why do we alternate between action and receptivity?
- Where does creativity begin—and begin again?

Creative thinking takes place in more than just our heads. Thinking occurs in our minds and brains, situated in our bodies, which are continually exploring our environments through both perception and action, in what we see and what we do, and what we see again as a result of what we have done. We sense and perceive our physical, social, and symbolic world but also act in it and then perceive once more how our actions have changed the world.

Earlier, in Parts 1 and 2 we referred to this ongoing, dynamic interplay of our goals and actions with our perception of how our actions shape the world as the "perception-action cycle," or as "see-move-see" in Part 3. As we seek to realize our goals, we repeatedly cycle between perceiving (sensing and making sense) and acting (moving). We see what our actions have accomplished and then adjust, revise, or change course accordingly. We both make and find. *Making* is based on our aims and what we hope to accomplish. *Finding* is what we perceive and sense in the world as we make moves to realize our aims.[1]

Alternating between making and finding (and finding and making) may also allow us to maintain forward impetus because we replenish as we go, interleaving moments of higher deliberate control with more spontaneous responding to what the world offers us. Then we can move repeatedly between moments of attentional focus on what we are trying to accomplish and moments of receptive "finding" that inspire alternative takes on our making.

This ongoing dynamic cycle of making and finding, call and response, or of our intended and emergent realizations is portrayed in Figure 4.1.

Let's begin by looking at the trajectory of the thinking activities of some senior undergraduate engineering students who were asked to design a neighborhood urban playground for about 12 children between the ages of 1 and 10.[2] Any playground equipment they designed would have to meet many constraints. It must remain outdoors throughout the year, must not be too costly, and could only be made from materials available at a local lumber yard or hardware store. The playground equipment must be safe for children, must comply with the Americans with Disabilities Act, and had to be ready within two months. Additionally, the playground would have to allow for at least three different types of play activities, and its design would have to be fully developed and explicit so that a third party could build it using the plans alone.

The engineering students were able to ask for additional written information throughout their design process and were given up to three hours to develop a complete solution. They were asked to "think aloud" as they worked their way through the process. Their design-related thoughts were

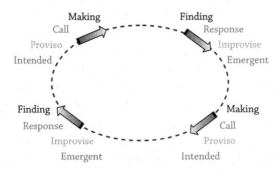

| OUR CREATIVE EFFORTS INVOLVE A CONTINUAL, INSTRUCTIVELY CONSTRUCTIVE CYCLE OF MAKING AND FINDING. | THE CONTINUING CYCLE OF MAKING AND FINDING. In our efforts to discover and create we alternate between making (guided by what we intend) and finding (responding to what emerges as a consequence of our intentions). |

Figure 4.1

recorded and classified into eight categories, such as identifying basic needs or purposes and describing how to tangibly realize an idea.

We'll focus on the final design plans of just two of the students. One student's design was rated as being of high quality. It met the many constraints and used appropriate materials while being unique and feasible. The design plan of the second student was rated as of substantially lower quality.

The trajectory of each student's thinking processes during the first hour, as they developed their playground plans, is shown in Figure 4.2.

What differences do you notice in how the two students thought through the design challenge over time? Which of the two thinking trajectories do you suppose resulted in the higher-quality design, and why?

These design trajectories are two examples taken from a larger study of 50 civil, industrial, and mechanical engineering students, all of whom were given the urban playground design challenge. A key difference between students who created higher-quality designs and those who developed designs judged to be of lower quality was the number of category shifts or *transitions* between design activities.

Students who generated higher-quality designs more frequently shifted among different design activities, such as identifying problems and exploring possible solutions. They made more transitions across the varied design activities of problem scoping, developing alternative solutions, and deciding and communicating how to realize their project plans. Design quality decreased when students spent an especially large portion of their overall time in any one part of the thinking process.

Looking once again at the first hour of the thinking trajectories of the two students shown in Figure 4.2, we can see that the student in the lower panel moved much more frequently across the eight broad types of design activities. No one of the types of design activity predominates in their thinking or is neglected. The design quality of the playground plan of the student displayed in the lower portion of Figure 4.2 was higher (it achieved an overall quality score of 63 percent) than that of the student shown in the upper portion (given an overall quality score of 38 percent).

By transitioning frequently between types of design activities, students were able to flexibly notice and uncover more opportunities to meet constraints, improving both the feasibility and uniqueness of their designs. Dwelling primarily on one aspect of the design challenge meant that the amount of information a student encountered was too narrow and not well integrated into the design plan. Or as one student who produced a high-quality design described it: "I think it's important to go back like that to problem definition. Once you get information you have to look and see how it pertains to what you defined. I went through with preliminary ideas.

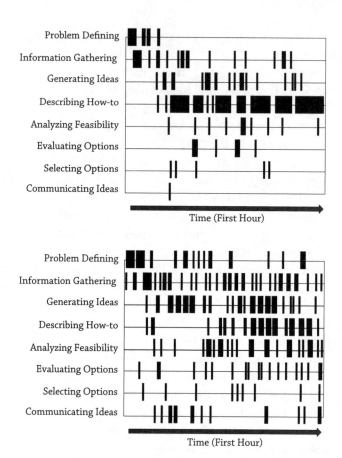

Figure 4.2 THINKING ALOUD DURING THE PLAYGROUND DESIGN PROBLEM. The comments of two senior engineering students as they worked through the first hour of the playground design problem as classified into eight categories: identifying basic needs or purposes (*Identifying Needs*); defining the problem, such as determining constraints or criteria (*Problem Defining*); gathering and searching for information (*Information Gathering*); generating ideas or alternatives (*Generating Ideas*); describing idea realization such as dimensions or measurements (*Describing How to*); feasibility analysis (*Analyzing Feasibility*); comparing and evaluating options (*Evaluating Options*); deciding on an idea or solution (*Selecting Options*); and communicating ideas or solutions to others (*Communicating Ideas*). The frequency and duration of thoughts in each category is schematically shown, with brief thoughts indicated by a narrower bar and longer considerations shown by increasingly elongated bars, with the length of the bar proportional to the amount of time spent.[3]

You go back and see what other information you need. You need to look at your problem again. It's totally iterative." [4]

In this Part, we continue to delve into the making-finding cycle with its deep and varied contributions to creativity, improvisation, and change. We begin by further exploring the nature of made and found constraints. We then broaden our vantage points to focus on, in turn, the roles of active experimentation and play, what things motivate us to explore and keep exploring, and the often overlooked contributions of deliberately learning to vary. In two final sections, we take up making and finding in teams and groups and touch upon how our brains both shape and are shaped by our making-finding explorations.

MADE AND FOUND CONSTRAINTS

> Materials that you think you drive could drive you.
> Or, you can take turns. [5]
> —*Digital media artist and design professor Kelly Dobson*

A significant source of information regarding where our efforts should be focused during creativity and problem solving are the "constraints" of the task that will guide our goal pursuit and thinking. Indeed, one definition of creativity itself is, "novel generation fitted to the constraints of a particular task." Discovering and defining the constraints of a creative or change project is an essential characteristic of the *coevolution* of a creative challenge and possible solutions. Rather than taking place in discrete phases, the processes of articulating the nature and limits of a challenge and its possible solutions work hand-over-hand in tandem. [6]

Constraints are both made and found. The constraints may be real and explicit—that is, actual requirements or specifications for the to-be-achieved product or process that are provided to us, or discovered by us. Or they may be implicitly assumed, sometimes correctly, but sometimes incorrectly. If incorrectly assumed, presumed constraints can unwittingly stand in the way of our wider explorations. As we will see, intentionally identifying and revisiting what we take to be our constraints, and clarifying their source, can prevent us from unnecessarily narrowing our creative options.

Constraints can be considered from many perspectives. Any one problem may have multiple concurrent constraints that channel, focus, or limit an individual's or group's explorations into particular subsets of their broader idea landscapes. Artists, for example, may deliberately choose constraints or combinations of constraints. To foster their creative seeking, they may deliberately eliminate or preclude a conventional way of working, in turn promoting novel approaches. Constraints simultaneously preclude and promote.[7]

Think of the painter Claude Monet. Early on he asked himself "How does light break up *on* things?" Monet's attempts to answer this self-imposed challenge in painting created a new series of works that evolved into yet a further quest: "How does light break up *between* things?" This rich inquiry into the effects of light surrounding an object, such as a grain stack or poplar tree, itself later merged into an even deeper and "deceptively simplified" constraint: "representing how light—by itself, not on things or between things—breaks up."[8] In pursuing this question, Monet's earlier particular ways of working with depth and finish, with focus and point of view, penetrate into still another world. In the words of one artist and psychologist:

In *Water Lilies, Reflections of Weeping Willows* (c. 1916), we no longer look from the shore but from above the pond and very close to its surface. We look at fragments: lily pads horizontally, summarily stroked in dark, saturated blue-greens, with magenta outlines that fall outside or over the blue-greens; and reflections presented by separated vertical strokes, darker greens and blacks for the willows, and lighter lavender for the sky. Things are not clearly separated. The lavender is under and on top of everything. It even falls inside the magenta outlines of the lily pads.[9]

In zooming out from this luminous example and thinking about all of our change or creative efforts, large or small, it can be helpful for us to group or classify the constraints we are facing. One widely applicable classification of constraints, particularly with regard to design, involves six possible dimensions relating to the *timing* of the constraints (initial to late); their *flexibility* (nonnegotiable to negotiable); their *importance* (from nice to have to must have); their *source* (e.g., user, client, task); their *domain* (e.g., internal, external, inherent); and their *purpose* (e.g., validity, nonfunctional, quality).[10] Constraints on design may also be broadly classified as deriving from four mutually interrelating origins, including (1) the *legal and regulatory context(s)*; (2) the *design problem, goal, or need*; (3) the *process* through which the solution is achieved; and (4) *constraints arising from the emerging solution itself*, as some decisions restrict options for future choices.[11]

I design and make. I can't separate those two.... Form and the material and process—they are beautifully intertwined—completely connected.[12]

—*Chief Design Officer at Apple Inc., Jonathan Ive*

An intensive case study of an engineering design company revealed that constraints might be present on some, several, or all of these dimensions at once.[13] At different points within a project, design teams might consider how truly fixed (rigid, inflexible) and necessary or real any of the believed/perceived constraints were. Meeting multiple constraints in a novel or highly parsimonious manner was sometimes viewed as grounds for evaluating a solution as especially creative. Such happy conjunctions of simultaneously meeting multiple aims may be a form of *goal synergy* and represents one aspect of the process of "goal tuning" that we explore in Part 6. Goal tuning also assumes an important place in helping to prioritize our constraints, with some constraints emerging as more definitive of the needed direction of a project than other more minor constraints.

The case study of the engineering design company revealed four broad ways of treating constraints. One approach was *blackboxing*, or treating some constraints as fixed and inflexible so as to allow for a focus on other more crucial requirements. Two other approaches were *removal*, or temporarily assuming that a particular constraint no longer applied, and the converse, an intentional *introduction* of a new constraint. Introduction involved internally or externally supplying a constraint that had not previously been specified, such as requiring that the product be environmentally friendly. These self-generated constraints were described as "kickstarters," as they often helped open up new avenues for exploration after a creative standstill. *Revision* of constraints was the fourth approach observed. The engineers revisited constraints to see whether some of them might be tweaked or shifted to give them additional flexibility. They also returned to constraints to assess if they were truly externally imposed rather than optionally adopted during the earlier idea-generating processes.

Observations of the engineering design teams in the early stages of their new projects showed that they referred to the outer limits of the project (project scope) as "inside" or "outside" the "corner flags" and to "moving the corner flags" to change the potential direction of the design. At later stages of the project, the term "frame" was used by the teams to describe more specific, formal, and concrete "absolutes" of the project. It was observed that sometimes product teams implicitly relied on tacit constraints that had subsequently been removed. One such tacitly accepted constraint concerned problems with a given material that had actually been solved earlier within the company. When explicitly brought to awareness through discussion, these beliefs could be appropriately updated, transforming the possible idea landscape for the project.

Explicitly and directly discussing what we understand to be the full set of current constraints on a project—both at the outset and at periodic phases throughout the process—can help us to identify constraints that we have mistakenly assumed to apply or to pinpoint constraints that are no longer necessary or relevant. Direct and recurring discussions of this sort can enable us to appropriately reprioritize and update constraints. For example, direct discussions may keep track of changes in the importance of a constraint, an altered time line, or the discovery of unrecognized interrelations among constraints.

We should also be alert to the level of abstraction at which our constraints are articulated and understood. Specifying a challenging constraint at the highest level of abstraction that is possible, while still faithfully capturing the aims of the constraint, permits us the largest number of degrees of freedom in creatively meeting the requirement. Think, again, here of the particular yet spaciously open-ended questions that Claude Monet posed to himself, such as "How does light break up *on* things?" and "How does light break up *between* things?" These questions were constraining while allowing for a remarkable range of motifs and themes.

 Thought Box: *Walking, Thinking, and Making Landscapes*

A firm of Swiss landscape architects was commissioned to help plan the site surrounding the Tate Modern, an art museum in London. In their preliminary thinking about the site, the architects deliberately changed their habits, as this would help them to *perceive* differently. As part of their initial scoping and interpreting of the project, the architects flew from Switzerland to London's Heathrow Airport and then took a train to a station that, intentionally, was a four-hour walk from the museum. Walking for several hours along the banks of the River Thames to get to the Tate rendered the scale and complexity of London more fully tangible and present to them.[14]

Emphasizing a walker's perspective as deeply informing their design processes, the architects explained that, "the rhythm of walking brings us into a frame of mind conducive to discussing ideas."[15] Although some landscape architects do not explicitly tap into street views as an essential part of their design process, these particular architects used model-based design, including photographs from eye level to promote more fully immersed human-scale viewing. They planned the height of elements based on local horizons and built in new local horizons at the scale of a walking pedestrian.

Its very place on the river is a defining feature of the site. From the Tate Modern there are stairs along the south bank leading to a "beach" on the Thames, where people can walk their dogs and "beachcomb." The ebb and flow of tidal waters twice a day uncovers and discovers new objects and fragments, including "horse bones, antique medicine bottles, pottery shards, Roman coins, and flint arrowheads."[16] To meld the ebb and flow of the tide into their conception of the landscape the architects included a terrace that is stepped down toward the river. Material of clay in the surrounding landscape is also generously incorporated. The original Bankside Power Station—the precursor building that later became the Tate Modern—is built of London bricks made of clay from near the site.

Making and finding for these landscape architects relied on constraints of multiple origins, including the spontaneous emergence of possibilities arrived at through their extensive exploratory ambulation. The architects also relied on varying levels of abstraction, of scale, and of the specificity of the site and its history, including its cultural situatedness, in their ongoing processes of making and finding.

The level of abstractness of our constraints may also involve whether the constraints specify only the *outcomes* to be achieved, or also the *method* or process to reach those outcomes. Do the constraints of our project specify only the ends or also the means we are to use?

For open-ended and collaborative activities, "The best statements of team purpose are those that clearly specify the *ends* a team is to achieve but that leave it to the team to decide about the *means* it uses in pursuing those ends."[17] Goals formulated at an appropriate level of abstraction promote our individual and collective ability to flexibly identify problems and appropriately adapt our work processes.[18] Focusing on ends may promote our resilience and flexibility, but focusing too early or too exclusively on means may leave us brittle in the face of change or the unexpected.

Another important type of constraint integral to change and creativity, particularly in situations requiring high levels of reliability and stability, may be the requirement to impose the *minimum amount of change* necessary to accomplish an aim.[19] Constraints for projects or products involving many complex and interrelated components—such as commercial jet aircraft, large computer programs, or renovating historically significant buildings—may cascade within and across components and at different levels of specificity. In cases involving many complexly interrelated components, some constraints need to be taken as nonnegotiable or be assumed to be so in order to proceed at all. In very large projects that take place over an extended period of time, some materials and ways of working can be changed only at great cost to what has already been accomplished. Sometimes, though, such costs are necessary.

It is not only the constraints themselves but also the origin and source of the constraints that matter. A constraint may be perceived as rigid or fixed when it should actually be more flexibly interpreted once we understand its source and purpose. In larger projects or multiperson projects, the "ownership" of constraints may be important in allowing us to evaluate when and if a constraint can be modified or ignored.

Without clarity on the source of a constraint or the expected procedures for modifying a given requirement, we may simply continue to follow it unnecessarily or unhelpfully. "Constraints without background, explanation and/or a clear owner could thereby be a strong barrier to creativity."[20] Implicitly assumed but mistaken or no longer relevant constraints can also impede creative change and may be actively countered through explicit exploration and updating of a project's status. A broader culture of openness to questioning and the inclusiveness of varying perspectives likewise are excellent antidotes.

A commonly experienced constraint is limited time. In an interview study of four R&D creative product teams in the corporate research lab of a large multinational corporation well known for innovation, each of the product teams frequently identified constraints relating to time pressure and deadlines. Overall, 84 percent of the team members mentioned time limitations as a key constraint.[21]

For the R&D teams, deadlines seemed to work best if they were not overly aggressive and were perceived as genuine, rather than merely fabricated to inject a sense of urgency. More generally, although deadlines have been proposed to undermine creativity by narrowing the team's and individuals' mental scope for exploration, research suggests that under the right circumstances deadlines, like other constraints, can be beneficial to creativity. When the deadlines are not excessively tight but a reasonable challenge, then, like other forms of constraints, they may spur creativity. As with other types of constraints, there may be a "sweet spot" for time pressure and timelines—a level of time pressure that is neither too unrealistic nor too permissive. When they successfully target such a sweet spot, deadlines motivate and guide teams without shutting out their openness to exploration, team autonomy, or intrinsic enjoyment.[22]

Other types of requirements, such as legal and safety regulations, may also prompt innovation. Constraints limit but also open possibility spaces. In the realm of the construction industry, new governmental building regulations or building codes for reducing adverse environmental impacts and increasing safety have been noted to spur new innovations. One study of a 55-year period in the Dutch construction industry found that nearly 40 percent of registered innovations in the industry in recent decades were related to the introduction of new regulatory requirements. In quite another realm, that of intellectual property, such as patents or copyright, imposed limits may paradoxically open the way for novel creative inspiration. Take the genesis of *Star Wars*, for example. "George Lucas crafted the plot for *Star Wars* only after he failed to get a license for a remake of *Flash Gordon*. Unable to use the precise creative universe he initially identified, he distilled particular visual and thematic aspects of that universe and used them to construct the now-familiar setting a long time ago in a galaxy far, far away."[23]

Constraints guide creative cognition in many ways. They are important, too, in improvisation. Although it is probably easiest for us to see the pervasive role of constraints in acts of deliberate creativity, constraints crucially guide how we generate and interpret spontaneously produced improvisational expressions. We can readily understand verbal expressions that we have never before encountered.

Think of such expressions as "octopus apartment," "elephant complaint," or "motorcycle blanket." Despite our unfamiliarity with these phrases, we can readily generate multiple plausible interpretations of these novel combinations. An elephant complaint, for instance, might be a very large complaint or a complaint that cannot be ignored.[24]

Given additional context we might narrow our interpretation of novel and ambiguous expressions to one or a few possibilities. For example, a "motorcycle blanket" overheard in the context of a sudden downpour may mean something different than it would in an indoor garage or in a young child's bedroom. Constraints in these situations derive from the possibilities for perceiving and acting that are present in the particular physical or social context. In a child's bedroom, a motorcycle blanket might be a small soft blanket patterned with images of motorcycles; in an indoor garage, it might be a vinyl protective dust cover for an actual motorcycle. Various physical and meaning-related constraints may be rapidly pulled together in our minds, meshing into a novel, coherent, and plausible interpretation of words we've never before encountered.[25]

Constraints of all sorts offer both guidance and goads. How we use, choose, or iteratively make and revise constraints profoundly propels the generation and refinement of innovative ideas.

We next turn to some of the surprising ways that we can foster open exploration and receptivity to making and finding newness in ourselves and in others.

MOTIVATING EXPLORATION AND LEARNING TO VARY

Imagine that you were asked to run your own virtual lemonade stand in a large town. In this computerized game scenario, you will choose the type of lemonade you will sell (its sweetness, lemon concentration, and color), where you will situate your stand, and the price of the lemonade. Imagine, too, that you are given some background information from the former manager of a similar virtual stand. In a "letter," he provides you with valuable and honest advice about a business strategy that worked well in a particular location he had experience in—selling expensive, low-sugar, high-lemon, green lemonade in the business district. Although he had experimented with different lemonade recipes in the town's business district, he had never located his stand in other locations, such as one near a school or a stadium.[26]

After choosing the attributes of your particular lemonade, where you will locate, and the price you will charge, you learn about your sales, profits, and customer feedback after each of 20 sales periods. You can use this information to change, if needed, the location of your lemonade stand and to modify aspects of your lemonade or its price.

Now suppose that your lemonade business will be based on one of three incentive schemes: (1) a fixed and reasonable wage per period; (2) pay for performance, where you will be paid 50 percent of the profits for all 20 periods; or (3) pay for performance, but where you will be paid 50 percent of the profits for the *last* 10 periods. What differences, if any, do you think these alternative reward arrangements might make in your approach to the lemonade stand challenge? Which of the three arrangements would most encourage *you* to explore and to find the best opportunities?

When 144 university students were randomly assigned to these three incentive options, a number of differences in their thinking and choices emerged. Those students who were given the third option, with their rewards dependent on their performance in only the second half of the 20 sales periods, much more often discovered a new, highly profitable location that also required altering the lemonade formula and price. These students experimented widely in the first 10 periods, finding new opportunities and making new choices that, in turn, later yielded the highest success (significantly greater average profit). They also voluntarily tracked their decisions throughout all 20 periods much more closely than did most individuals in either of the other two groups, providing themselves with more detailed and integrated information for their further explorations. Yet even within the fixed-wage condition, individuals differed widely in the degree to which they explored and kept track of their decisions, with people who explored more widely achieving significantly better results.

In a quite different domain involving biomedical and life sciences research, longer-term reward structures similarly appeared to encourage exploration, including embarking on new research directions and fostering deeper and higher-impact research discoveries. A study compared the research impact of two groups. One group comprised distinguished early career prizewinning scientists who received funding through shorter-term (typically three-year) project-focused grants that were difficult to renew. The second group of equally accomplished researchers was funded through relatively longer-term (typically five-year) investigator-focused rather than project-focused grants, with typically at least one five-year renewal and the first renewal emphasizing new projects embarked upon rather than completed work. The second group also received more frequent critiques, advice, and encouragement, with such feedback providing timely opportunities to hone or redirect their research questions or approaches.[27]

The group with longer-term support, rich feedback, and encouragement of intellectual experimentation published almost 40 percent more scientific articles. Compared with the group with shorter-term support, these research publications included nearly twice as many articles with extremely high citation rates, indicating that other scientists more often found the work valuable to build on. This research was also relied on by scientists from a wider range of specialities and disciplines. As with any attempt at innovative exploration, not every new direction was equally successful. The larger number of publications for the scientists with longer-term support included both very highly cited, high-impact research papers alongside some research papers (about one-third) that were much less influential.

The longer-term research directions of the two groups of scientists also differed. Tallies of the keywords classifying the topics of their articles indicated that the group with longer-term support tackled scientific topics that were more on the cutting edge. The classifications additionally revealed that the scientists with longer-term support pursued more varied research trajectories, reflecting a dynamic broadening of their research agendas. These differences between the groups emerged clearly only after a period of about four or five years.

Similar evidence of the importance of longer-term incentives to exploration and originality has been documented in other areas. In the realm of corporate R&D, longer-term reward structures for senior executives have been found to be associated with both more heavily cited patents and patents of greater originality.[28]

Explorations in science, industry, and medicine may be encouraged through multiple means. It may be that the most flexible and nuanced approach is offered through "innovation policy pluralism—with patents, prizes, grants, and tax incentives all playing a role in efforts to encourage research and development."[29]

The lemonade stand, the life sciences research, and the corporate R&D findings underscore several important distinctions with implications for creativity, innovation, and change. How we reward and motivate experimentation and exploration matters—as do the *time scale* of our incentives, the *feedback* we provide, and our *tolerance of failures*.

Experimentation and discovery themselves vary in kind. Some of our experiments or trials involve comparatively minor fine-grained testing within existing constraints. Other experimental ventures that we embark on are more ambitious, open-ended, wide-ranging, and potentially risky. Devoting time, energy, and resources to minor revisions and tweaks may more often lead to incremental innovation. Casting and searching in less well known directions may increase our chances of making more profound and radical discoveries, but these chances might be slim and the risks of failure higher. The trade-off between making minor but less risky tweaks as opposed to taking on novel ventures that may offer higher rewards but with greater risk is known as the *exploration vs. exploitation* trade-off.[30]

This trade-off occurs at multiple time scales and at individual, group, and organizational levels. Take, for instance, a theater that may need to balance keeping its loyal subscribers returning year after year to see its productions while also responding to the need to attract new audiences and offer alternative experimental programming. If the theater management and artistic direction simply pursue slight variations on existing approaches, this may preserve the status quo, but the theater may miss out on broader emerging opportunities, some of which may prove unsuccessful but others of which may yield essential longer-term benefits and promising organizational trajectories. (We return to this example in Part 5.)

Individuals and organizations may at differing times and in differing contexts, excel at both exploration *and* exploitation. They may show contextual versatility[31] or other productive ways of balancing to derive the most benefit from each form of discovery.[32]

In the lemonade stand experiment, we noted that even within the fixed-wage condition, some individuals explored and experimented much more widely than others, keeping closer track of the effects of their various actions and on average achieving a more favorable outcome for their virtual business. These individual differences illustrate that we cannot exclusively focus on external reward structures in understanding exploration and how willing we are to vary our behaviors and approach. External reward structures are often associated with extrinsic motivation, but intrinsic motivation likewise plays a central role in exploratory search. Equally important, as we will see in a moment, extrinsic motivation is not all of one kind. Extrinsic motivation itself assumes varied forms, with some forms closer to our long-term goals and identity than others.

Many of us tend to think of motivation as a single "engine" for action. Yet, instead, research has shown that **intrinsic motivation and forms of extrinsic motivation** are separate or *dual dimensions* that may interact and complement (or compete) with one another. We may be at a high level on one form of motivation (e.g., intrinsic) and low on the other (e.g., extrinsic), but each of the other combinations is equally possible. As diagrammed in Figure 4.3, individuals can be high on extrinsic but low on intrinsic motivation, low on both intrinsic and extrinsic motivation, or high on both.[33] Depending on context, each of us may show any or all of these combinations across time.

When we are intrinsically motivated we are driven by enjoyment, curiosity, and the inherent pleasure of engaging in an activity for its own sake. When we are extrinsically motivated we are most likely acting in order to obtain financial or other tangible incentives or consequences such as positive recognition or accolades from others.

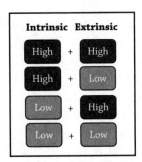

Figure 4.3 COMBINATIONS OF INTRINSIC AND EXTRINSIC MOTIVATION. At different times we may draw upon varying levels and types of motivation. Sometimes both our intrinsic and extrinsic motivation may be high; in other situations one or the other may predominate or we may be low on each.

But extrinsic motivation itself, as we suggested earlier, comes in degrees or gradations. At one extreme, extrinsic motivation feels very controlling and external to us and seems imposed on us as a type of external regulation. At the other extreme, extrinsic motivation is recognized and accepted by us as personally important, yet our actions are still undertaken as a means toward an end rather than for their own sake. Extrinsic motivation here is seen as involving more *autonomous control*, in which we value a particular activity given that it helps us to achieve a self-endorsed goal.

Think of readying our tools and materials, such as a painter cleaning her brushes or a photographer cleaning his lenses, or the members of a musical ensemble tuning and retuning their instruments. These activities may not be inherently enjoyable, but they may still be pursued as part of essential creative preparation and as a means toward a valued end. Likewise, a creative writer or research scientist may not greatly enjoy meticulously proofreading his or her manuscript, but recognize that it is an important step toward effectively communicating their ideas. These more autonomous instances of identified or *self-directed extrinsic motivation* are especially crucial when we engage in activities that are not themselves consistently intrinsically rewarding but that are necessary to successfully achieve our creative or change endeavors.[34]

Self-directed extrinsically motivated activity can also have the important function of carrying us across periods of low intrinsic momentum in our creative work. Engaging in a task such as organizing our notes and materials can set the preconditions for the emergence of intrinsic rewards by encouraging us, through the perception-action cycle, to become immersed in our task situation and environment. Not only intrinsic motivation but also self-directed extrinsic motivation is similarly important in large scale collaborative creative projects such as those involved in film production, symphony orchestra performances, or the design of a new aircraft.[35]

We typically pursue creative endeavors neither solely through intrinsic motivation nor solely through extrinsic motivation but by combining elements of each. Ideally, the two work in a complementary fashion. Intrinsic motivation helps us to concentrate our attention on the activity at hand, keeping us excited, absorbed, and energized. Extrinsic motivation, however, helps to keep us oriented toward the longer-term if needed and can carry us through less inherently fascinating but nonetheless essential phases of our projects. Because our creative enterprises take shape over time, our innovative goals may not be best realized through an exclusive reliance on intrinsic motivation.

For many of us, our peak creative moments emerge when our actions and thoughts are fueled jointly by both intrinsic and extrinsic motivation.[36]

This was found to be the case for undergraduate students who were asked to write a brief poem within highly specific constraints, to engage in a drawing task, and to find solutions to ambiguous mathematical problems. Trained raters evaluated the creativity of the students and the students also completed measures of intrinsic motivation. Creative performance was significantly predicted *both* by the student's intrinsic motivation and by more self-directed external motivation and their interaction.[37]

We can sometimes deliberately structure our extrinsic motivations. In an experiment with two groups of writers experiencing writer's block, a researcher asked one group to write at specific times each day and also to make a substantial donation to a cause they did not like if they failed to write on three consecutive days. The second group was encouraged to write only when they felt freely and spontaneously prompted to do so. The writing productivity and the self-evaluated creativity of the first group over a 10-week period markedly exceeded that of the second more exclusively intrinsically motivated group.[38]

External rewards are not always beneficial for creativity, nor are they always harmful. It depends. Sometimes external rewards and extrinsic motivation can undermine creativity and initiative, especially if they act to reduce our sense of autonomous choice or are focused on goals that we do not fully endorse or understand.[39] At other times external rewards may serve an important and synergistic *informative role*, conveying information that creativity is both valued and valuable.[40] Maybe it is not fully clear that creativity is a priority for a team or organization. Other values such as efficiency or standardization or avoiding risk may be perceived to have a higher priority. Explicit rewards for innovative actions may signal that creativity is prized and sought for, particularly if such rewards are combined with programs designed to extend creative competencies. Field- and lab-based investigations have underscored the potential synergistically positive effects on creativity of combining extrinsic rewards with techniques to boost creativity, as this combined approach also serves to reinforce intrinsic motivation.[41]

Beyond their effects on motivation itself, we also need to take into account the ways in which rewards relate to our learning of skills and the building of our competencies and confidence. Providing thinking scaffoldings for creativity, such as those discussed in Part 3, can also enhance intrinsic motivation—which in turn enhances creativity.[42]

As diagrammed in Figure 4.4, intrinsic motivation and engagement are themselves energized by our actions and the feedback our actions provide. Sometimes intrinsic motivation emerges through the process itself of engaging in our work. We don't need to passively wait for intrinsic motivation to kick in. The very act of working through ideas or with objects can ignite our

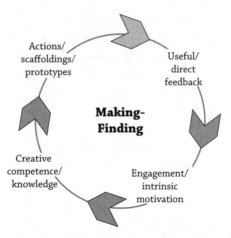

Figure 4.4 INTRINSIC MOTIVATION CAN EMERGE FROM ACTION. Taking tangible actions in pursuit of our creative goals (making) such as sketching or working on a draft or prototype can promote informative discovery (finding), in turn promoting both our engagement and our further competence.

absorption, initiating cascading benefits in our creative process of making and finding.

Given the crucial role of motivation and its many forms, an important question to ask ourselves is "What do we think we (and others) are being rewarded for?" Although creativity and innovative thinking are valuable and valued, other aspects of thinking are also important, and it may not be clear in any one case whether creativity trumps such other values as efficiency or consistency. If the conditions that need to be met to receive rewards are left vague or underspecified, we may default to assuming that what is to be rewarded is conventional, efficient, or habitual action. It is crucial, however, to reward *useful variability* if innovation is desired.[43]

Research conducted with children suggests that we may inadvertently reward each other for uncreative and conventional behaviors. Praising their intelligence or ability when children had shown high levels of performance on a challenging task encouraged them to focus mainly on how well they had performed, rather than on how well they were learning or mastering the task. Praise for intelligence may have implicitly promoted an interpretation of intelligence as something that is a fixed and unchanging internal entity. In contrast, praising their efforts or hard work led children to focus on the more malleable and situationally varied motivational aspects of intelligence.[44]

Praise concerning children's efforts increased the likelihood that they would later choose challenging problems that provided opportunities to increase their learning and skills, rather than "safe" problems that they could more easily answer correctly. Praise for effort rather than ability also changed the type of information children most often requested. If given a choice between learning about how others had performed on the task or instead learning about strategies that could help them to improve their own performance, children praised for their ability more often chose to learn about how other children had scored on the task. In contrast, children praised for their efforts were more likely to choose to be given strategy information that could help expand their own mastery of the task. Additionally, in the face of failure, children earlier praised for their "fixed" or "trait-like" intelligence showed lower levels of persistence and effort, more negative emotion, decreases in task enjoyment, and decreased performance compared with children earlier praised for their efforts. Viewing our level of intelligence or more generally our personality predispositions as "fixed"—rather than something that is amenable to change and improvement through our efforts and experiences—may render us less resilient in the face of setbacks than we would be if we viewed these as qualities that can and do develop.[45]

Rewards can lead us to develop both adaptive (and nonadaptive) habitual, conventional, or repetitive behaviors. Less well known, however, is that the types of behaviors or outcomes that are rewarded may powerfully shape the *opposite* of predictable behavior. We can reward highly variable, nonrepetitive, constantly changing, and innovatively creative actions. We can be rewarded and reward ourselves not only for repeating but also for *not* repeating. That is, we can be rewarded for *learning to vary* as well as for learning to repeat. Rewarding variability, whether in ourselves or in others, has been found to lead us to explore more often and more persistently.[46]

Deliberately varying our actions helps to bring different sets of thoughts and procedures close together in time and space within our individual and group idea landscapes. This, in turn, allows us to combine and reconfigure aspects of ideas and ways of doing things to make novel combinations. The likelihood and ease of such cross-fertilization of different ideas is increased if a number of different approaches have been used recently and so are relatively accessible in our idea landscapes and in our action repertoires. It is not always an entirely new approach that is needed. Sometimes "repeating with a difference" frees us to see new options.

Greater spontaneous variation and flexibility in using different strategies may provide grounding for our subsequent learning. Using a variety of strategies—such as different explanations or alternative arguments and gestures as well as speech in domains ranging from mathematical problem solving to mechanical reasoning problems—has been found to be linked with (positively correlate with) later mastery, generalization, and effective transfer of knowledge and skills to novel settings.[47]

Procedural flexibility—knowing and appropriately applying or adapting multiple possible approaches for problem solving—may help to enhance individual and team performance. Under some conditions, even beginners solving problems may gain flexibility by being introduced to alternative methods. Introducing alternative methods may itself support our further explorations and variations—including encouraging us to ask ourselves which procedure is best suited for the particular task at hand.[48]

 Research Highlight: *Acting to Learn*

In a long-term study of the relations between the motor actions of infants at only five months of age and their much later academic achievement as adolescents, it was found that infants who had explored more actively, extensively, and effectively at only five months showed higher academic performance as 14-year-old teenagers. This was so even after taking into account such factors as their social competence, verbal intelligence, gender, the quality of caregiving, and the home environment.[49]

Why might this be?

The ways in which an infant, less than half a year old, can physically interact with his or her immediate environment shapes and sculpts many surrounding events and learning opportunities. Being able to act on objects, such as grasping them or mouthing them, provides important information about the infant's ability to control events and the consequences of particular actions. This interlocking dynamic of action, perception, and exploration leads infants to recognize that they can plan and direct their actions and movements. It also enables them to focus on relevant information and to differentiate subtle similarities and differences between objects and actions, to tap into the varied affordances offered by objects, and to engage others in their actions.

The perception-action cycle begins very early and carries forward throughout our lives. It continually and reciprocally shapes our options for cognitive, perceptual, and social learning.

As the researchers noted: "Exploring and learning about the world are intertwined.... A more motorically mature and actively exploring baby likely elicits more opportunities for interaction, richer contacts with novel aspects of the environment, more joint attention, and more exposure to referential language. In turn, learning is attuned to affordances during manual or oral exploration."[50]

~~~~~~

The benefits of having acquired alternative problem-solving methods may emerge most clearly when we are faced with novel situations. Student pairs of online problem solvers who had been instructed in a only single shared problem-solving procedure achieved higher accuracy in solving routine problems; in contrast, pairs instructed in two different problem-solving approaches excelled in solving novel problems. A comparison of the communications between the pairs of students showed that those who were instructed in two different problem-solving approaches devoted more time to explaining and elaborating possible solution approaches than did those who learned only a single method. For the students who learned two methods, the additional time spent explaining their reasoning may have detracted from their routine problem performance but enhanced their flexibility of approach to nonroutine, more novel problems.[51] (This finding might bring to mind our earlier discussion, in Part 3, of the value of reflective verbalization in innovative thinking.)

Variable responding is often crucial to the discovery of new modes of thinking and acting, and taking part in novel activities may itself be intrinsically rewarding and engaging. Variability, together with either deliberate or implicit comparisons of our actions, may also allow us to extract perceptual and conceptual invariants in our problem-solving spaces. Discovering such invariants is an important route to problem-solving, as we saw in the checkerboard problem in Part 2. Additionally, identifying invariants and abstract patterns can leave us better prepared for unexpected future combinations of features or events.

So how can we better introduce productive variability into our creative processes? One simple approach is to *slow down*. Our habits and well-learned routines are performed quickly and with little effort. Deliberate variation may require a wider margin or greater leeway in time and space. Given some extra time, sometimes even just a few seconds or minutes, new alternative approaches or classifications can emerge. Sometimes we make sudden habitual judgments that, given only a moment's reflection, would seem ungenerous or unduly narrow.

> For a given level of expertise, as one responds more rapidly, behaviors
> may become more repetitive and predictable. Thus, to increase the vari-
> ations in one's daily life, slow down.[52]
>
> —Behavioral scientist Allen Neuringer

Paying attention in the moment and explicitly attuning ourselves to new
ways of categorizing our experiences and making nuanced distinctions—
showing *mindfulness*—may promote desirable variation and engagement.[53]

Musicians in an orchestra, just before playing a well-rehearsed familiar
piece, were asked by their conductor to play in one of two ways. They were
either asked to "Think about the finest performance of this piece that you
can remember, and try to play it that way" or, instead, to "Play this piece
in the finest manner you can, offering subtle new nuances to your performance."[54] The musicians themselves more strongly enjoyed playing the ren-
dition in which they were invited to offer new nuances and they thought
that their orchestra played better. This was not only a subjective judgment.
Independent trained musicians who were asked to evaluate the two performances by listening to audio recordings also rated the quality of the new and
nuanced version significantly more positively.

As one of the performing musicians observed, "I felt like I was successful
because I was creating—not trying to recreate."[55] Attuning our attention to
our habits, including our creative skills, may enable us to notice subtleties
that open the way to greater newness, expressiveness, and change.

> Asking each individual musician to find and add subtle nuances to [his
> or her] performance led to an aggregate performance that was more
> than the sum of the parts.[56]
>
> —Social psychology professor Ellen Langer and colleagues

Another approach to encourage useful variation is to deliberately and
explicitly adopt and spell out the constraints that we must work within.
Perhaps paradoxically, finding new variations may be easier when we are
restricted in the range of options we can exercise in some dimensions, so
that we are seeking to vary within a narrower class or set of classes of behavior. Adopting constraints—deliberately imposing them on ourselves—may
"restructure existing problem spaces in ways that make them ill-structured,
thus incrementing variability and facilitating creative solutions."[57]

Recall the field study we introduced in Part 1 with an expert practitioner of traditional Chinese ink painting who was asked to create two sets of large paintings on the theme of the four seasons. In one of the two sets, this noted and very experienced painter of traditional Chinese landscapes was asked to incorporate into his work 15 random lines generated by the experimenters. The work incorporating the random lines took almost twice as long to create and was judged to be more lively and dynamic than his more traditional style of paintings, which were judged as exhibiting more simplicity and better composition.

The artist discovered that the works constrained by the introduction of random lines were more exciting than his previous ones. He remarked, "Creating from random lines, I have to incorporate the others' world into my world. . . .. This is not just myself. I get serious about drawing in this way. Yes. I am highly motivated with this way."[58]

In this situation, the newly introduced constraints within which the artist worked were specific to the particular piece (unique lines and combinations of lines that needed to be incorporated into the painting) and were largely "bottom-up." But constraints may also be more far reaching and general and result from a more deliberate top-down choice. Artists may choose to work without traditional paintbrushes (Jackson Pollock), with a limited palette such as only primary colors (Piet Mondrian), to include everyday "found objects" (Robert Rauschenberg), or to avoid representation of objects altogether (Agnes Martin). Artists may set themselves novel and changing task constraints; recall Claude Monet's relentless efforts to capture the elusively ephemeral effects of light.

A third approach to finding and sustaining variation in our thinking is to encourage experimentation, both in ourselves and in others. Active experimentation is essential to uncovering and successfully forming our creative ideas, often surprising us along the way. We need to express or articulate our ideas or emerging thoughts *in the world*—outside of ourselves and for one another—as this allows us to see "where we are in our thinking" and to move forward to next steps. Prototyping, sketching, strumming, doodling, writing phrases, code, or calculations and admixtures of these allow us to see and understand both where we are and what we might have missed.

~~~~~~

 Thought Box: *Plunging in and Acting to Think*

By plunging into action we may better discover or articulate our goals. Sometimes we are not yet fully sure of our creative direction or where we should turn next. Action, then, may be a way of promoting or uncovering bottom-up suggestions for articulating or prompting new possibilities. The dancer and choreographer Twyla Tharp speaks of this process as "scratching"—actively and openly exploring and pulling together sensations, actions, emotions, and concepts by altering one's environment, intense reading, poring through archives, and receptively absorbing sounds and sights.[59]

By capturing snippets, phrases, and promising images and having sundry tools ready to hand we gather valuable raw material that we can return to during our phases of "scratching." These troves encourage us to playfully "mess about" with materials to discover/uncover possibilities. Ideas often do not all reactivate at once. They need help from one another. Novel relations among ideas, especially, may be rather "weak" and require more support from other ideas and from our environments.

Tharp came to videotape her lone improvisational sessions in the studio so that she would not need to remember them as she generated them. She found that trying to remember interfered with the very loosening of control that was pivotal to her improvising. "For me, scratching for ideas became a technical scheme of improvising (generating ideas), getting them on tape (retaining), watching the tapes later on (inspecting), and finding a way to use them in a dance (transforming)."[60]

Through their tangible sensory presence, our experiments of all sorts, may lead us to discover relations between components or gaps or conflicts between elements. Although initially we may be quite unaware of these relations, they may become much easier for us to "find" (perceive) once we have generated a physical externalization of our thoughts. The same may apply to many other experimental instantiations of economic, social, and political change. Often such change can profit from concrete prototyping and experimenting, including at a local or small-scale level. Our tools matter too, and experimentation here is crucial, especially in the case of newly emerging relatively untried and uncertain technologies. Experimentation may both jumpstart creativity and provide informative guidance for our next moves.[61]

A fourth approach to introducing greater variability into our creative thinking may be to *form a practice of variation itself*: intentionally adopting a questioning attitude toward when and if we should repeat. Is the situation we are now in one where we should do what worked before, or might we best try something different? If we do something different, how different

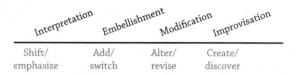

Interpretation	Embellishment	Modification	Improvisation
Shift/ emphasize	Add/ switch	Alter/ revise	Create/ discover

Figure 4.5 PICTURING A CONTINUUM OF VARYING IN OUR THINKING AND ACTIONS. Improvisation lies on a progressive continuum ranging from interpretation and embellishment through modification and improvisation. As we move from interpretation to improvisation we make ever more extensive changes, drawing increasingly more intensely on our concentration and imagination, potentially radically transforming the original starting point.[62]

should it be? Should we shift our emphasis? Perhaps we should find a different tempo? Or a surprising gesture? Ask an open-ended question? Should we omit a step or subtract something?

Drawing an analogy from the world of music, there are many ways to vary a melody. But the same is true for our actions both large and small. As depicted above in Figure 4.5, our everyday actions and creative efforts can be seen as situated on a continuum of improvisation. Not all new directions are dramatic. Sometimes productive variability arises from the subtle and slight.[63]

MAKING AND FINDING COLLECTIVELY

We improvise collectively in what we do, in how we do it, and in how we interpret and make sense of what we and others have done. In an in-depth field study of two companies, researchers identified three broad classes of improvisation.[64]

Behavioral or process innovations involve innovating how activities are pursued, such as the sequencing of actions or microactions. For example, one product development team regularly visited retail stores to compare the packaging used by its competitors for similar products. On one occasion, the team opted to look at not just similar products, but also dissimilar products but with similar packaging. This extension and improvisation on their usual practice unexpectedly ignited new ideas for them.

Another form of organizational improvisation involves the creation of new physical structures that are not part of an original design or plan, termed *artifactual productions*. These emerged through "ongoing actual interaction with the specific materials and behavior of the product itself."[65] The impromptu development of a new cover to enhance the safety and performance of a product that the team was designing illustrates this type of improvisation.

A third type of improvisation is initially conceptual. In *interpretive productions* team members recategorize or reframe events, changing their meaning and evaluative implications—including events that might otherwise appear as mistakes or flaws. In one case, there was an exceedingly high level of inconsistency in the performance of a particular product component, even though all components met or exceeded specifications. Engineers knew that this inconsistency was unavoidable. The wide range in performance raised the possibility that customers who initially received an exceptionally well performing part would be disappointed if they subsequently received an "average" (but still high-quality) performing component. An engineer suggested that the team be on alert for especially highly performing parts that, once identified, could be set aside to be specially offered to select customers, implying a new form of exemplary customer service.

Although planning and vision in an organization are undeniably necessary, in a constantly changing complex environment there are severe limits on what can be planned without the plan itself becoming obsolete or unwieldy. Groups or organizations, just like individuals, should actively make use of the perception-action cycle. Organizations, too, can make and find, iteratively transitioning between goal-directed thinking and action on the one hand and being receptive to the consequences yielded by those actions on the other. In organizations as in individuals, direction may gradually emerge through active experimentation and revision. The precise and ultimate strategic direction of an organization, then, may not be something that was ever explicitly spelled out in the mind of any one person or group of persons but that unfolds over time, as individuals act, evaluate the consequences of their actions, act again in accordance with the new information in hand, and evaluate once again.[66]

In an extensive analysis of the planning practices of 656 firms, researchers found that effective strategic planning involved both formal planning and what is known as incrementalism.[67] Formal planning involves deliberate and linear thinking processes. Here, the goals or ends to be achieved are specified first, followed by the route or means to attain them. In contrast, in incrementalism, the ends are seldom stated in formal documents or announced, and, if they are, they are stated in broad, general, and nonquantified terms. In incrementalism, the means to an organization's goals are allowed to develop and evolve over time, in response to learning by the organization and individuals within it.

> In improvisation, implementation is a form of instantaneous explora-
> tion. Implementation becomes a source of discovery (i.e., idea genera-
> tion) so that problem setting and solving feed continuously upon each
> other through anticipatory feedback.[68]
>
> —*Business management professors William Doll and Xiaodong Deng*

Improvisation involves both goal-guided making (intentionality and planning) and finding (observing, interpreting, and receptively responding). Improvisation is not random but is grounded in both our prior experience and aims. "The improviser is aware that his/her novel actions may deviate from the controls of previous routines without abandoning the purposes those routines seek to achieve. Thus, the deliberate two-way interaction between work planning and work doing and the novel ideas it creates is the hallmark of improvisation."[69]

One way for individuals and organizations to create and learn collectively is through improvisation, but it may not always prove beneficial. Improvisation often offers the benefits of context-specificity and rapid real-time respon-siveness. But these benefits are counterbalanced by potential downsides. It is possible that improvising may lead to a lack of generalizable knowledge or procedures. Nonsystematic search or information gathering may cause us to overlook possible valuable opportunities. While improvisation allows for rapid responses to newly emergent opportunities, it may also lead to unin-tended distraction or fragmentation of purpose and direction.[70]

Both planning or "making" and emergent, incremental changes or "find-ing" are necessary, but neither alone is sufficient. Improvisation is not invariably the best approach.[71] Sometimes "wise repeating" is best. At both the individual level and that of groups, teams, or organizations, dis-covering and realizing the best balance between making and finding with regard to our creative and change-inducing aims is a delicate, dynamic, and ever-changing, ever-renewing process.

> A strict insistence on purpose, consistency, and rationality limits our
> ability to find new purposes. Play relaxes that insistence to allow us to
> act "unintelligently" or "irrationally," or "foolishly" to explore alterna-
> tive ideas of possible purposes and alternative concepts of behavioral
> consistency. And it does this while maintaining our basic commitment
> to the necessity of intelligence.[72]
>
> —*Organizational theorist and professor James G. March*

Collective change, like individual change, is an integrative experiential learning process. It requires an intermeshing of thinking about our thinking (reflective learning) with concrete learning. We need to interlink our concrete experience with reflective observation, abstract conceptualization, and active experimentation.[73] We may differ, too, in the directness of our experience. Some people may have had immediate and concrete experience while others may have mainly secondary or vicarious learning. Or each person in a team may have different varieties of experience with a particular process or procedure.

Our team experiences, particularly direct team-based experience, may allow us to develop what is known as a group's transactive memory. **Transactive memory** is a form of group memory that is dispersed and shared across individuals. It involves identifying, communicating, and drawing on each member's unique knowledge and cooperatively sharing responsibility for learning and retaining team knowledge. Transactive memory distributes the "cognitive load" that otherwise would be placed on our individual memory, sharing the load across the wider team. It allows a team to "reap economies from specialization. A [transactive memory system] therefore enables a group or organization to better utilize extant knowledge and more efficiently learn or generate new knowledge and thus to reach higher levels of performance than a loose collection of individuals not embedded in such a system."[74] An important contributor to transactive memory involves the development of shared mental models. We will explore the role of transactive memory in team thinking and innovation more deeply in Part 5.

Beyond group or social memory, our material and symbolic environments merge into our efforts at collective improvisation and support shared memory. Expressing and elaborating our ideas in verbal and other material forms such as diagrams or sketches or models involves partially stepping outside of our immediate experience and making that experience the object of reflection for ourselves and others. Externalization in material forms allows others to play with ideas in parallel making-finding processes that can be revisited and returned to at different times and by different people. The objects themselves (diagrams, sketches, models) can change our idea landscapes but can also be a space and place for the convergence and interplay of the idea landscapes of others. Existing over time, they can be shared, juxtaposed, and combined with earlier and later ideas. These "provisional artifacts"—such as tentative models, partial storyboards, word clusters, or image banks—can help to capture and support the ongoing processes of collectively making and finding. (Recall our earlier discussion, in Part 1, of the valuable role of three-dimensional prototypes and electronic whiteboards to share information and emerging plans in effective creative product development.)

The making of partial and low-fidelity prototypes can, as we saw in Part 2, provide a sense of rapid and visible forward progress that can be shared. These and other modes of encouraging and signaling ongoing progress are essential to creative and innovative effort.[75] Minimally detailed or simple prototypes can allow us to test and share "abstracted" or "extracted" portions of an idea. They can allow frequent and low cost actions with more extensive and speedily received feedback.

Rapid partial prototypes also can reframe failure as acceptable and natural. They help us to concretely and actively deal with uncertainty during innovation. Encountering frequent feedback helps us minimize our over-responsiveness to failure and promote our ongoing intrinsic engagement. Together, the feedback, activity, and sense of ongoing progress emphasize our own and our team's creative competencies and confidence in making change.[76]

Our tools matter too. The interfaces with our tools, including the computer applications and computer programs that we use, themselves may make it easier or more difficult to create external representations of a certain type, including representations that are partial or rough approximations, and this might help or hinder the creative process. Our tools for creativity should not impose excessive cognitive or perceptual demands on us—or a rigidity of meaning—that interferes with our evolving thinking/acting. Where needed, the applications and tools that we and our teams use should afford *interpretation-rich* representations.[77]

Our collective making and finding endeavors may be spurred by playfulness, humor, and imaginative experimentation. A play orientation may encourage more figurative, circuitous, and elaborated ways of thinking. Two groups of MBA students asked to solve word puzzles but encouraged to think of the task as either work or as play generated quite different solutions. The solutions of the work-oriented students tended to be more mechanistic than those of the play-oriented students who were less literal and more poetic.[78]

Play provides us with brief times in between that encourage a "resetting" or refreshing of our mental landscapes, a release of tension, and an invitation to participation.[79] Humor and creativity are significantly positively associated with one another, in part reflecting shared characteristics such as risk taking, insight, cognitive flexibility with mild positive affect, and surprise.[80] Playful imaginative exploration—including in virtual online environments—may provide an impetus for creativity and act as a space that can welcome and sustain ambiguity and may stimulate nonroutine abstract learning in teams and organizations.[81]

OUR BRAINS AT PLAY AND
THE FLEXIBILITY-STABILITY PAIRING

> As in a kaleidoscope revolving at a uniform rate, although the figures are always rearranging themselves, there are instants during which the transformation seems minute, and interstitial and almost absent, followed by others when it shoots with magical rapidity, relatively stable forms thus alternating with forms we should not distinguish if seen again; so in the brain the perpetual rearrangement must result in some forms of tension lingering relatively long, whilst others simply come and pass.[82]
>
> —*Philosopher and psychologist William James*

We, and our brains, must continually "negotiate" between the partially intertwined polarities of flexibility and stability. Neither flexibility nor stability are always good; we need both under different circumstances, and cognitive control is essential in enabling us to move between them and to aptly balance them.

Evidence from studies of human and animal performance under different task requirements shows that there are complex dynamic interrelations and trade-offs in the brain between representational stability and representational flexibility. In Part 3 we briefly noted that the neurotransmitter dopamine plays an important role in cognitive control, with exquisitely fine-tuned levels needed to allow a "just right" balance between too much control and too little—between too much stability and too much flexibility.[83] The dopaminergic system is complex and highly dynamic, with "multiple pathways innervating multiple brain regions," and it "constantly regulates itself to maintain equilibrium both at the molecular and at the systems level."[84]

Within the prefrontal cortex (the more anterior regions of the frontal cortex), dopamine supports the active and stable maintenance of goal representations in our short-term working memory. Here dopamine is important to *cognitive stability* and so has an important influence on our distractibility and the ways in which we attend to and act upon goal-relevant or goal-irrelevant information. Elsewhere in the brain, however, specifically deep within the midbrain in the complex set of structures jointly called "the striatum" (including the caudate nucleus and the putamen), dopamine is important to *cognitive flexibility*. In the striatum, low levels of dopamine or its restricted availability lead to inflexibility and excessive persistence; we may then fail to adjust our goal and task representations to changing circumstances.[85]

The complex interrelations of dopamine to cognitive flexibility and stability can be seen in occasional paradoxical trade-offs in behavior. Sometimes increasing dopamine enhances our performance of one task or aspect of an activity because it shifts our flexibility closer to optimal levels. Yet this same increase may be detrimental to another activity or task component because it shifts our flexibility outside of already optimal levels toward excessive distractibility and over-responsiveness to new competing options.

The benefit of increased *flexibility* may (depending on context and circumstance) carry with it the cost of increased distractibility or failing to maintain task goals and rules stably in mind. But, similarly, the benefit of increased *stability* may (depending on context and circumstance) carry with it the cost of inflexibility or failures of updating our goals or the task requirements as needed. Additionally, individual differences in our longer-term or stable baseline levels of dopamine may affect whether increasing dopamine levels is beneficial or instead is detrimental to performance.[86]

Earlier, in Part 1, we saw several examples of how positive emotion, or mild positive affect, increased the cognitive flexibility of participants. Brief presentation of positive words or pictures compared with neutral or negative ones increases momentary flexibility of cognitive processing. Mild positive affect can also lead to enhanced insight during problem solving.[87] Dopamine may be an important contributor to such enhanced flexibility. It has been proposed that the influence of positive affect on cognition arises from a momentary (brief or "phasic" rather than long-lasting or "tonic") increase of dopamine release in the midbrain, where dopamine is first generated. The dopamine is then propagated forward to other brain regions, including the prefrontal cortex. This influx of dopamine is thought to allow for the updating of representations in prefrontal cortex, in turn enabling more flexible behavior.[88]

Brief phasic increases in dopamine have been conceived as providing a "gating" signal, leading to the updating of our short-term working memory and facilitating a switch or change in our subgoals or immediate plans. Transient release of dopamine from midbrain regions provides a signal to prefrontal cortex as to when it should accept new input. When the "gate" is open, the contents of short-term working memory relating to our current task or goal representations (context representations) can be appropriately updated. When the "gate" is closed, the contents of short-term working memory are protected from potentially incoming distractions.[89] Recent evidence using converging neuroimaging approaches supports this gate-keeping role of dopamine in updating sub-goal representations. At any one moment we may be open to new input at one level of abstraction but not at another, allowing for stability with respect to some of our subgoals, and plasticity with regard to other subgoals.[90]

Dopamine has been found, along with other neuromodulatory systems, such as that involving the neuromodulator noradrenaline/norepinephrine, to play an important role in the interplay between exploration and exploitation.[91] Dopamine in particular has been associated with a predisposition or trait to be open to experience. Involving pronounced receptivity to a broad range of sensory, perceptual, and symbolic forms of information, openness to experience is closely linked with general tendencies toward innovation, originality, and creativity.[92] Across time, openness to experience may extend both our skills and our aptitude for flexibly meeting novel challenges.[93]

The "exploration theory of dopamine" proposes that not only are we motivated to reduce the experience of uncertainty to levels that we can manage but that we are also "motivated to increase the experience of uncertainty to an *interesting* level—in other words, to a level at which some previously unknown reward or information may be discovered. Thus exploration is used not only to transform the unknown into the known but also the known into the unknown."[94]

~~~~~~

⎡C C⎤ **Creativity Cross Checks and Queries**
   ⎢ / ⎥
   ⎣C Q⎦

Questions to encourage reflection and connections to your own work and practice:

⇒ What is making—and what is finding—in your creative and change processes? What prompts you to change (or pause) between making and finding, and finding and making, again?
- Consider this: "When improvisation is restricted to the ability to 'think on your feet,' managers [and we] risk confusing improvisation with random moments of brilliance and conclude that either you have this ability or you do not. There is, however, much preparation and study behind effective improvisation."[95] What preparation and study might you and your team better undertake to maximize the benefits of your improvisation?
- Does your preparation include an understanding of *both* activity and receptivity?

⇒ When do you decide to "stay" (exploring deeper where you already are) and when do you decide to "go" (exploring farther afield, where you have yet to go)?

- What leads you and others to repeat behaviors or to perform routine actions, and what leads you to vary or to perform novel and unprecedented actions?
- Have you looked for subtle signs that you or your team may be too strongly pulled toward already familiar ideas and options?
- Are you giving yourself the times and imaginative spaces to notice and attune yourself to nascent novelty in all sensory and experiential realms? As one choreographer and dancer observed:

> The challenge for both dancers and choreographers in embarking on the generating phase of a new work is often *how to find oneself in a movement territory one has not felt oneself in before*, and the daily frustration is a recognition of: 'oh here I am again'! For the dancer in a busy touring company the previous work can have become so engrained in the body that its answers remain the most readily accessible, rising to the surface to offer solutions to new questions.[96]

⇒ The artist Jocelyne Prince observes, "A lot of what we do in glass, as opposed to thinking about skill and mastery, is think about dialoguing with materials in terms of their properties. 'Properties' could be synonymous with 'agency'—what agency does the material have?"[97]

- What does it mean to think of your materials and process as having "agency"—where does the initiative for your creative action originate?
- When might it be best not to think in terms of skill and mastery?
- How do you listen for, and become aware of and respond to, the unexpected potential and *autonomy* in your materials?
- What makes for positive or welcomed surprise in your endeavors?

⇒ When do you "plunge in"—finding the motivation and direction you need in the plunging action itself? Or are you more of a "wader"— gently and steadily reimmersing yourself in your creative momentum?

- What are the "invariants" in your creative process and your beginnings? That is, what things are nearly always there?
- Do you understand your own (and others') beginnings?

⇒ Do you reward yourself and others for varying and experimenting?

- Do you give yourself (and your team) enough time and leeway to begin and to begin again?
- How do you prototype in parallel?
- How early do you look for definite progress, and is it too soon?

⇒ How could you change your tools to be more creative? That is, what aspects of your working/playing process might be in your way?
  • Do your tools allow sufficient play for ambiguity?
  • How well do you understand all that your tools can do?
  • Do you change your tools to open new idea landscapes?
⇒ How do you think in and through your doings? When do you let "the work" take the lead? As contemporary painter Alex Olson describes her process:

> It [painting] becomes a lot of call and response, and reading the work and responding to the work in the moment. It's very important for me to play in the studio. I place a lot of weight on thought letting the work take the lead. And play and invention. I can't pre-think things. I think a lot of the thinking comes through working and doing. They're intertwined. Creativity comes while making and doing. I can't separate it from the material and the work.[98]

  • How do you read and respond to what you are making and finding?
  • Do you allow alternative possibilities and interpretations to coexist, stretching the temporal windows of openness to newness?
  • When do you prethink and when do you play (too), and are you giving both their opportune moments?

Part 5

Past to Future, Future to Future: Innovating Together Over Time

Thinking prompts

- How can roles, specializations, and routines support innovation?
- How can we make the best creative use of our collective experiences and know-how?
- Why and how are heedfulness, shared mental models, and situational awareness important in team adaptability?
- What prompts or enables second-order problem solving?
- How can we best simultaneously develop both routine and adaptive expertise?

Suppose that you were a coordinator of students helping them to move into their university residences (dormitories) at the beginning of the academic year. Over a three-day weekend, you and your colleagues are responsible for overseeing and coordinating the moving of 10,000 students into a dozen residence halls. How might you facilitate a smooth and agreeable process for these many students and their families? What interactions and interdependencies of the broader environment might you anticipate? What might you and your colleagues learn from one year's moving-in weekend to the next?

A four-year ethnographic study of the moving-in routines in such a large-scale setting revealed surprisingly substantial changes.[1] One year, to reduce traffic jams and bottlenecks, the coordinators negotiated with the city and each of the residence halls to synchronize an effort whereby the city police would partially close traffic on some of the streets so that traffic was one-way. They initiated a new "drop-off" policy in which each student and his or her family were given 30 minutes directly in front of the residence hall during which they could unload the student's belongings. A new satellite parking lot was designated in which parents could park their vehicles after the unloading. Routines, over time, continued to be refined and improved. Another coordinated effort involved the university's central administration and local vendors, whereby the vendors were assigned to a single nearby designated area in which to sell room furnishings to the students without impeding traffic flow within or around the residence halls.

Here positive change gradually emerged over time—with each apparently minor innovation supplementing and complementing later ones. Similar ongoing adjustments and responsive organizational improvisations were observed in a two-year study at a large international software company.[2] The company introduced an online customer service database for tracking the problems that customers reported with their software. The database was populated with records of particular customer-service incidents and details of how they had been resolved and closed. In introducing the new computerized database, some of the change initiatives were made deliberately by managers or by the customer service specialists themselves, but many other changes *emerged* without explicit intention and there were many unanticipated positive outcomes.

The database, for example, grew rapidly. It was discovered that searching through the extensive new record-system allowed efficient identification of similar problems encountered in the past, permitting the reuse of prior solutions to as many as half of newly arising customer-service issues. The electronic entry of customer incidents also unexpectedly provided a broader perspective on dynamic workload fluctuations, allowing everyone to see where more intense demands on services were occurring at a given time. Crucially, this afforded opportunities and an emergent social communication routine for collaborative proactive action in which colleagues could readily step in to support each other. The database also opened up unanticipated opportunities for teaching and vicarious learning by allowing unobtrusive sharing of experiences and expertise across individuals.

> By focusing on change as situated, it provides a way of seeing that change may not always be as planned, inevitable, or discontinuous as we imagine. Rather, it is often realized through the ongoing variations which emerge frequently, even imperceptibly, in the slippages and improvisations of everyday activity. Those variations that are repeated, shared, amplified, and sustained can, over time, produce perceptible and striking organizational changes.[3]
>
> —*Organizational theorist and professor Wanda Orlikowski*

In these examples and many other instances of evolving organizational change, each set of changes to an established practice provided the foundation for further more far-reaching but consistent change possibilities. Here and in other situations, modifications to an existing routine or procedure might be prompted by the need to *repair* a routine (amending it so that it would lead to the desired or expected outcome), or *expand* a routine (changing it to make the most of newly emergent opportunities). Modifications to routines might also be motivated by the broader *striving* of individuals, teams or organizations in which they continuously seek to reach ideals or challenging goals that may never be fully realized.[4]

> One can think of routines as flows of connected ideas, actions, and outcomes. Ideas produce actions, actions produce outcomes, and outcomes produce new ideas. It is the relationship between these elements that generates change.[5]
>
> —*Organizational theorist and professor Martha Feldman*

Change has many sources. In the moving-in study we discussed at the outset of this Part, change was emergent and incremental. In other cases, as in creative projects or more formal strategic change initiatives, the impetus and constraints for change may be less continuous or uniform, representing a more distinctive break from an organization's past practices and goals.[6] In still other cases, there may be fluid intermingling of sources of change, and a coexistence of the routine with the nonroutine.[7] Change in organizations may concurrently arise from multiple sources, ranging from the planned to the emergent and from the internally to the externally driven: "In most organizations, transformations will occur through a variety of logics."[8]

Organization is the attempt to order the intrinsic flux of human action, to channel it towards certain ends by generalizing and institutionalizing particular cognitive representations. . . . organization is a pattern that is constituted, shaped, and emerging from change. Organization aims at stemming change but, in the process of doing so, it is generated by it.[9]

—*Organizational theorists and professors Haridimos Tsoukas and Robert Chia*

In this Part, we take a deeper look at creativity and change over time and across people and places and spaces, from past to future and future to future. We first take up the many modes that remembering and knowing assume in the collective resources that we may draw upon in "organizational knowing and doing" in all of its forms. Then, just as we earlier devoted considerable attention to individual idea landscapes, we now look more closely at group and organizational idea landscapes and their contributions to the creative enterprise. Next we turn to learning to learn, focusing on adaptability and openness. We conclude with the sometimes surprising ways in which we as individuals and groups go about "imagining" futures and the closely tied overarching questions of values and goals in our change-making efforts.

ORGANIZATIONAL KNOWING, REMEMBERING, AND DOING

Let's begin by walking through a two-part experiment designed to compare the effects on creativity of direct hands-on experience versus indirect or vicarious team experience.[10] In the first phase of the study, students were divided into three types of teams, with teams given direct experience, indirect experience, or no immediately relevant experience. In the second phase, all students were unexpectedly given a new related creative task.

Students given the opportunity for *direct* experience learning were assigned to a team with two other students seated together at a table, provided with materials, and asked to build as many folded small-scale paper (origami) cows and milk buckets as they could in eight minutes. Students were explicitly encouraged to work as teams, with each person specializing in particular aspects of the overall production. After the eight minutes, the teams were asked to spend several minutes together discussing their processes and roles, including both what had worked well and what did not work well.

Other student teams were given *indirect* instead of direct experience. Rather than engaging in the origami activity themselves, these teams watched an eight-minute video of the origami task performed by a particularly well-coordinated and effective team. This was followed by a several minute period during which these students discussed what made the team they had watched work well or poorly together, and they jointly completed a questionnaire on that team's processes.

A third group of students was given neither direct nor indirect experience with the task. These students, in the control group, watched an excerpt on group decision making in a jury setting from the film *12 Angry Men*. Then they, too, jointly completed a questionnaire on what factors they believed helped the jurors work well together or had prevented them from working well together.

In the second phase of the experiment, the original origami materials were removed and the team members given new materials and new instructions. Now the teams were asked to develop as many creative origami prototypes as they could for a novel and original décor object with which to furnish or decorate a room. The teams were told that their paper décor objects should be recognizable and similar to some existing entity such as an object, animal, or plant. Again they were asked to function concurrently as coordinated three-member teams, with each member contributing to a particular aspect of his or her team's creations. Each team was allowed 20 minutes to complete a prototype using 20 sheets of colored origami paper, cellophane tape, a ruler, colored markers, scissors, and glue. A $20 prize was offered for the team that developed the most creative objects.

Which of the team types—those that earlier had direct experience, indirect experience, or no relevant experience—were found to be most creative when generating a new paper décor object? Which of the team types do you think relied least extensively on specific attributes or components of the earlier (cow and milk bucket) origami exercise? Why do you think so?

Two independent judges rated the prototypes of the paper décor objects for their overall creativity and additionally on such dimensions as the variety and novel use of materials, level of detail, and complexity. The team types did not differ in the *number* of prototypes they generated. However teams that had earlier gained *direct* origami experience demonstrated significantly higher creativity than was shown by either the indirect experience teams or by the control teams with no relevant experience. Yet indirect experience was also helpful: Creativity for the indirect experience teams significantly exceeded that shown by the teams in the control condition. That is, direct experience produced the highest level of creativity, indirect experience produced an intermediate level, and the teams with no relevant experience fared least well. The teams with direct experience also showed less frequent reliance on or repetition of the specific attributes or components of the earlier exercise than did the indirect experience teams.

These results underscore the contribution of earlier direct experience in enhancing a team's generation of creative prototypes and products. But what is the basis of this beneficial effect?

One possibility is that actually working with particular people, even relatively briefly, fosters an understanding of our own and our teammates' specific strengths in knowing and doing. This proposed account focuses on the detailed knowledge of particular team members. A second possibility is that creativity is enhanced by learning more broadly about the nature of the materials, their potential and constraints, and the distribution of task demands. This alternative account suggests that direct experience encourages a less contextually specific mode of learning that could helpfully carry over ("transfer") to a new team or situation.

To tease apart these two possibilities the experimenters repeated the earlier experiment but with an important twist: some of the team members were *rotated* into new groups after the initial origami experience involving the cow and milk bucket; other team members remained in their original groups. Do you think that the creative benefits of direct experience would persist even when the team members were changed? Why or why not?

Intriguingly, the creative benefits of direct experience persisted, with direct compared with indirect experience leading to greater overall creativity *both* when the team members remained the same and when team members changed. The teams with the new members also showed more *variation* in their ideas—relying less frequently on their prior experiences in the paper-folding task with the cow and milk bucket than did the intact teams that had stable group membership.

Together these outcomes suggest that greater team creativity was anchored in a prior concrete hands-on/minds-on immersion that enabled more abstract and cross-situational learning about the problem context, its overall challenges, and relevant constraints. Additional support and clarification for such a cross-situational learning interpretation was provided by the responses of the team members to the questionnaires about their team process.

All students were asked how they had coordinated their team expertise and specialization. Drawing on this information, it was found that direct experience boosted creativity largely because of how it enhanced a system of team transactive memory—a form of collective memory that allowed team members to combine information, expertise, and perspectives regardless of whether they had worked together previously. Teams and organizations develop **transactive memory** for how knowledge is distributed and coordinated, including needed expertise and procedures for learning, remembering, and communicating team knowledge.[11] Asking the students to explicitly consider and reflect on their team coordination and specialization may have encouraged the development of a transactive memory system that supported team creativity and effectiveness even when individuals subsequently interacted with entirely new team partners.[12]

Immersion in new forms of relevant direct experience can offer us both the necessary skills and the motivation needed to innovate. But expanding our experiential horizons may itself demand innovative social thinking. Take the case of Toshio Okuno, a newly appointed plant manager of a Japanese soy sauce company facing an urgent need for innovation.[13] He found that the employees and all 17 group leaders at the factory seemed "trapped in a self-imposed prison of comfort with the status quo, reluctance to make dramatic changes, and the belief that dramatic change was neither needed nor possible."[14] What to do?

Finding that the group leaders resisted invitations to traditional routes of education and training, Okuno was inspired to create the *Tatsumaki* or Tornado Program. One day and without warning, as each of the 17 group leaders arrived at the plant, he told them they could not enter, nor could they communicate in any way with their workers for the next three days.

Over those next three days, Okuno took the group leaders to visit local supermarkets to see how the company's products were being displayed and sold. They visited local factories with problems similar to those they were experiencing and learned how these problems had been addressed. They attended meetings with people from their sales division to learn more about the interrelationship between the factory and the sales department.

The three days were agreed by everyone to have been a great success. The "Tornado" lifted the group leaders out of their insular habit-bound views and allowed them to directly experience new technologies and business practices including alternative ways of working. In two subsequent years, a modified version of the *Tatsumaki* program was implemented, where for three days the group leaders themselves decided what they would do and where they would go. For example, they went to a trucking company to learn how to better manage their fleet of trucks, and they visited a major user of conveyer systems similar to those that they used so as to help improve their bottling processes.

The Tornado program was a radical way to effectively bring about change. But what is a more typical trajectory of ideas and interactions of individuals and teams as an organization innovatively creates new products, processes, or services?

To more deeply understand the earlier phases of the generation of a new idea—beginning with its embryonic form, its amplification (development and expansion), and crystallization (refinement and application), and the possible overlappings of all these phases—researchers examined 10 substantial innovation projects undertaken by 10 different organizations.[15] The organizations were of varying sizes, including a biotechnology firm, research institutions, a software firm, food production companies, and a regional government. All of the projects were difficult to accomplish, different from the organization's existing products or services, or challenging to existing ideas. The projects ranged from large-scale information technology initiatives to the development of new probiotics and novel genetically modified products.

In-person semistructured interviews were conducted with nearly all of the project team members. Additional information was gathered from internal reports, project documents, and published papers. The researchers specifically focused on four fundamental questions relating to new organizational knowledge creation:

1. What are the contributing roles of individuals and of teams at different points in time?
2. How does more abstract "know-why" knowledge and more concrete "know-how" knowledge shape evolving knowledge creation?
3. What is the nature of individual and team interactions across the knowledge creation process?
4. How and when do explicit vs. implicit or tacit knowledge contribute to new product or new service developments?

In-depth analysis and categorization of the data revealed several pervasive patterns. The innovation process generally proceeded through multiple phases from knowledge generation to evaluation, expansion, and refinement, followed by a knowledge crystallization phase. This last phase involved both a process of increasing differentiation, or breaking knowledge down into smaller parts, and a process of integration, or meshing knowledge into a coherent whole.

As shown in Figure 5.1, there was considerable overlap in these phases. Overlappings were invariably observed between the knowledge expansion and both the later knowledge refinement and crystallization phases. There was also extensive overlap between other phases, with multiple feed forward and feedback loops.

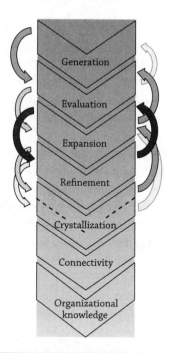

| THE INNOVATION PROCESS LEADING TO ORGANIZATIONAL KNOWLEDGE ENCOMPASSES MULTIPLE OVERLAPPING PHASES THAT RECIPROCALLY INFLUENCE EACH OTHER. | BEYOND THE INITIAL GENERATION OF IDEAS, INNOVATION INVOLVES SEVERAL SUCCESSIVE AND ITERATIVE PHASES. There are multiple and often overlapping phases subsequent to the initial generation of an idea for a novel product, service, or process. Realizing ideas into a concrete concept (crystallization) was subdivided into substages of knowledge differentiation and knowledge integration. Overlap was uniformly observed between the expansion and refinement phases, and frequently observed between several other phases. The curved arrows indicate the direction of overlap, and the darkness of those arrows indicates the extent of overlap, with darker arrows representing more extensive interrelations.[16] |

Figure 5.1

Charting the life course of larger-scale innovative ideas revealed differing primary contributions of individuals versus teams at different points in the multifaceted trajectory from initial idea inception to full integration and connection into group knowledge. When working independently of their teams, individuals contributed most extensively during the knowledge generation, expansion, and integration phases. Conversely, teams rather than individuals were most influential during the knowledge evaluation, refinement, and differentiation phases. Interactions were highly volatile among team members (as revealed by prolonged or emotional discussions) during the knowledge expansion and refinement phases, with moderate volatility during knowledge evaluation.

Reliance on tacit knowledge that was personal and not readily directly articulated followed a general U-shaped curve across time. Tacit knowledge contributed more to the innovation process at both the beginning and end of the process and less so in the middle phases. Reliance on explicit knowledge broadly followed the opposite pattern, with an *inverted* U-shaped curve of low contributions early and late and greater contributions in middle phases of knowledge evaluation, expansion, and especially refinement.

An organization's knowledge of its procedures (know-how) and background context (know-why) together with its shared organizational emotional experience all contribute to innovation. A survey of 103 firms from a diverse range of businesses—including manufacturing, retail and wholesale trade, transportation, and finance—showed significant positive associations between a firm's innovativeness and organizational memory.[17]

Innovativeness was positively correlated with measures of the firm's explicit organizational knowledge of product features and customer preferences, market conditions, and competitive strategies. Innovativeness was also positively correlated with the firm's *procedural memory*, involving agreed-upon methods for approaching such issues as assessing customer needs and product development efforts. Equally important, firm innovativeness was positively correlated with the organization's *emotional memory*—including the extent to which the organization enables people to acknowledge, share, and represent organizationally related emotional memories through symbols, stories, and participatory gatherings and ceremonies.[18]

Explicit knowledge sharing was significantly positively associated with both innovation quality and innovation speed in a survey study of senior managers of 89 high technology firms in China's Jiangsu Province, including companies specializing in information and communications, chemicals, petrochemicals, plastics, and electronics.[19] The effects of tacit (implicit) knowledge sharing on innovation quality and speed were relatively less strong but were also positively related to innovation quality. Tacit knowledge had a large effect on operational performance, including customer satisfaction, firm responsiveness, and asset management.

Several further contributions of organizational knowing, remembering, and doing to innovation are highlighted by survey findings on the organizational working and creative knowledge processes of 44 US design firms.[20] More than three-quarters of the design firms surveyed indicated that they had developed their own process approach to innovation. The approaches the firms had arrived at tended to have "fuzzy phases," with guideposts or recommended practices for each phase, rather than strictly or rigidly defined steps, "gates," or requirements. Such a flexible approach helps to keep attention focused on the particular needs and opportunities that each project presents rather than detracting attention (and motivation) to meeting predetermined checklists that may become too external and too distant from the situated project at hand.

Many of the design organizations had a relatively flat hierarchy, with rotating project leadership and sometimes dual leadership on projects. Creative projects were often widely "practice spanning"—including team members from multiple disciplines with varied expertise and interests. These diversely constituted teams provided individuals with ongoing challenges to both their current skills and knowledge and offered myriad opportunities to extend and refresh their own and each other's idea landscapes.

Beyond individual or group tacit and explicit knowledge, organizational memory exists also in our working-thinking environments, including the physical, symbolic, and technological artifacts that surround and support us.

Research Highlight: *Externalizing Our Group Idea Landscapes*

Firms and organizations have both physical and symbolic representations that carry and guide memory and interpretation A one-year empirical study of automobile production examined the carryover benefits of efficiency configurations from one working shift to another. Involving detailed study of the production of some 190,000 cars, the research revealed strong similarities in production performance across shift changes in personnel.[21] Remarkable correspondences in efficiency and quality were observed across successive shifts even though the people in each shift were different. This suggests that rather than residing entirely or exclusively in the knowledge and skills of specific workers, many of the plant's productivity or quality gains became "embodied in the physical or broader organizational capital of the plant."[22]

Ideas are inflected and reflected in physical artifacts. Who communicates with whom, and whether they are physically in the same space, and how often they communicate with one another or even know one another all may shape how the development and refinement of a product or process occurs. A research investigation of the development of several forms of computer software showed that the design of the organization behind the software development—how closely coupled and directly interactive the participants and their goals were—was reflected in the product design itself.[23]

Loosely coupled organizations produced software in which the components were more independent and modular, with changes in one part of the software program having fewer direct and indirect impacts on other parts of the program. As the researchers concluded: "The search for a new design is constrained by the nature of the organization within which this search occurs. . . . Managers of the innovation process must strive to understand the influences on their design choices that stem from the way they are organized. These influences are seldom explicit, but are a result of the interplay between a firm's problem solving and information processing routines, and the space of designs that must be searched to locate a solution."[24]

Technologies can help us to organize and productively access both tried-and-true and novel ideas. We can sometimes draw on technology to help provide apt reminders in the creative process, allowing for "wise repeating" of approaches or solutions that have previously worked well for our organization.

This was the precise function of a custom-built computerized project design search tool named Sweeper.[25] Sweeper allowed search through the myriad project files of a multinational firm that designed and manufactured metal and other packaging for food, beverages, and aerosol products. Explicitly developed to encourage creative concept reuse within the firm, Sweeper searched through large numbers of electronic project files looking for existing matches to the "musts" and "desirables" of a new project's specifications (e.g., a given new product must be recyclable, easy and obvious to use, have a shelf-life of at least three years, and require no changes to the glass finish). Sweeper was written to prioritize returning concept matches that met newly added or unique requirements for the project at hand. This served to increase the potential for uncommon matches by deemphasizing common requirements that were shared across many products. Sweeper yielded a succinct summary of the matches it found, including diagrams, solution principles, and design concepts.

Sweeper was not seen as a *substitute* for initial idea generation but rather as a case-based *supplement* or instigator of new idea directions that efficiently drew on the past experience of the firm. The ideas provided by Sweeper often "did not work by directly inspiring [totally] new ideas, but by diverting designers onto a new train of thought, enabling fresh and new ideas"—particularly sparking ideas about "how-to" enact or improve something already under consideration rather than entirely novel options.[26]

GROUP IDEA LANDSCAPES

Ideas relevant to a group or team effort often arise at varying times and may be spatially separated or distant from one another. Just as individual minds need an idea landscape in which various ideas or fragments of ideas, strategies, and their interrelations can meet, meld, and contrast, so too teams and groups need an ***idea intersection space***. A shared idea landscape enables us to access ideas and approaches together in time in order to integrate them or to recombine them in new ways.[27] We depict this basic idea in Figure 5.2.

Team mental models are key components of our group idea landscapes. As we saw in Part 1, mental models are cognitive representations that help us reason about the world; they allow us to have a shared basic understanding about how events or processes will likely unfold. We can take steps toward building more inclusive and accurate team mental models.

One approach—shown to be effective with teams of computer science students charged with developing a supermarket simulation application—is to begin by asking each person on the team to write down his or her particular take on the problem that the team is facing.[28] Then the team gets together to compare notes. They identify diverging interpretations and talk through a series of questions: What are the goals of the project? What are the implicit and explicit problem constraints and requirements? This helps the team develop a preliminary shared mental model of the problem and goal. Next the team moves into a phase of seeking possible solutions. All participants begin by writing down their answers to a series of questions. What is a possible strategy for solving the problem? Are there any difficulties with this strategy? What is an alternative strategy? What is the best alternative and why? A similar iterative process is used first to select the preferred solution approach and then to develop subgoals related to the problem constraints and requirements identified earlier.

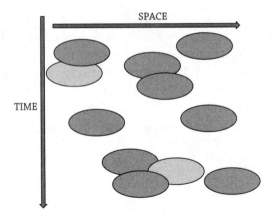

CREATIVELY COMBINING AND RECOMBINING IDEAS REQUIRES THAT THEY MEET IN AN INTERSECTION SPACE.	INTERSECTION SPACES FOR IDEAS. Forming novel combinations of ideas depends on their co-occurrence in a given space and time. This may require revisiting an idea from an earlier time or place (lighter shaded oval) together with other ideas (darker shaded ovals). An idea that earlier was premature or incomplete may, at a later time, meet with other ideas or circumstances that catapult it into a novel realization. Ideally, promising ideas are kept sufficiently active (perhaps through open goals) so that they do not become forever submerged beneath awareness in our group idea landscapes.

Figure 5.2

We have both individual and collective mental models of the world and the creative challenges we face. Mental models allow us to work things through in our minds.

Testing mental models with each other and in our own actions can enhance our ability to detect unforeseen features or relations. One way to test mental models is through mental simulation. Recall the example earlier of breaking a small birthday candle into three pieces. In mentally simulating breaking the birthday candle into three pieces, some people forgot about the candle's wick. Not everyone forgot about the wick: it depended on the person's mental model.

Encountering new and diverse types of information can often be a source of innovation. But the fate of new information that we, as a team or an organization, encounter is deeply influenced by our existing knowledge, skills, and capabilities. There are parallels between how organizations and how individuals depend on their prior learning and knowledge in order to absorb and interpret information. Our learning is rooted in what we already know and guided by what we deem important, including our goals.

> Innovation is not invention alone, in that it involves the orchestration of different forms of knowledge, not just from science and technology but also from entrepreneurial know-how and the institution of markets.[29]
> —*Innovation processes and systems expert Davide Consoli*

The ways in which teams and organizations evaluate, receive, and integrate new "external knowledge" depends on their dynamic ability to recognize the *value* of new external information, assimilate it, and apply it. This capacity of an organization to productively absorb new information, known as *absorptive capacity*, applies not only to concepts but also to skills and metaskills or "skills of skills," such as learning to learn.[30] Appreciating the potential value of new information is something that may not come easily or automatically and needs to be fostered.[31]

An organization's absorptive capacity depends on the depth and breadth of learning and prior knowledge of individual members; crucially, however, it also relies on its ability to *interconnect* information across individuals and subunits. Both substantive or technological "know-how" and more transactive "know-who" (individuals or roles) contribute to absorptive capacity. "Integrative processes are among the most important transactive events in groups because they manufacture new knowledge for the group—and so for all the group members."[32]

Cross-fertilization of ideas or interdivisional exchange of knowledge within an organization can ignite a positive chain reaction of innovation. When the international manufacturer and retailer IKEA decided to produce most of its product catalogue images using computer-generated imagery (thereby reducing environmental, logistic, and other costs associated with traditional studio photography of individual objects and entire rooms), it deliberately and ingeniously supported cross-pollination. All of the photographers had to learn the new computerized three-dimensional image-rendering process and, contrariwise, all of the three-dimensional artists had to learn photography. As someone inside IKEA explained, "This process [was] absolutely what made for an increase in quality—both in 3D *and* photography. . . . There's been a real merge. It's been astonishing, really."

Here, cross-fertilization involved individuals and units with closely aligned and readily identifiable convergent goals. But cross-fertilization may also span (or leap across) apparently widely disparate organizational divisions. Consider this chain of events: "A breakthrough in [General Electric's] Medical Systems business, with relatively little modification, led to a method by which an aircraft engine can transmit continuous information about blade speed, engine heat and other relevant data about its in-flight performance well in advance of any possible safety situation. This innovation, in turn, catalyzed an important new development with respect to a self-monitoring system for use with heart pacemakers."[33]

Individuals and subunits that span formal and informal organizational boundaries—such as equipment or material suppliers, downstream product or service users, and research institutions including universities and government laboratories and agencies—all enhance an organization's capabilities for interconnectivity. Connections and prior knowledge also provide the potential for increasingly forward-looking predictive or anticipatory knowledge, including proactive seeking and exploration. Longer-term trusting collaborative relations and information sharing within, across, and beyond an organization are essential for fueling and sustaining distributed problem solving and innovation.[34]

The deepening and extension of an organization's idea landscape can shape both the capability of the firm or group to innovate and the speed or efficiency with which it is able to do so. Analyses of more than two decades of patent data of 83 firms in the biotechnology and pharmaceutical industries demonstrated that firms which devoted more resources to their own in-house basic research and that also collaborated more extensively with scientists at universities showed faster innovation and produced inventions of more importance.[35] The invention benefits were greatest when in-house research intensity and collaboration with university scientists were *combined*. Firms with more external collaboration showed a higher pace of innovation, but the benefits for the speed of innovation were enhanced if the firm also had strong internal R&D, perhaps because the external connections helped to extend the idea landscapes of the local firm with regard to problem solution search.

From a broader perspective, absorptive capacity may likewise be important in a regional grouping or a cluster of interrelated organizations.[36] Firms or a cluster of firms may differ in how receptive they are to information exchange and in how extensively and readily they seek external knowledge. Firms with greater internal knowledge and innovation emphases may be more likely to make connections with external knowledge sources because the outside information is more readily accessed and assimilated into their idea landscapes.

A structured questionnaire and interview study of 32 wine producers in Chile's Colchagua Valley showed that firms with higher absorptive capacity interconnected significantly more often with external knowledge sources.[37] Firms with high absorptive capacity (evidenced by a combination of the technical training, length and breadth of industry experience, and the type and intensity of the firm's R&D) had more extensive connections with research institutes, business associations, suppliers, and consultants. Firms with higher absorptive capacity were additionally more likely to be the sources of knowledge shared with other firms, including providing them with assistance in problem solving and quality improvement.

Some firms never reached a minimal threshold of absorptive capacity. The gap in their skills and knowledge relative to other firms left them essentially isolated from knowledge flows with other local wine producers. Geographical distance on its own was mostly unrelated to the broader patterns of information exchange, with other characteristics of the firms assuming a more influential role than how physically close the firms were to one another.

Examination of the dynamics of knowledge exchange within the Colchagua Valley wine-producers revealed that physical proximity was, however, influential in the face-to-face exchange of *tacit and fine-grained knowledge* between pairs of firms, or "triads" of firms. Across a period of four years, the firms throughout the valley became increasingly interconnected. Both the number of mutual ties increased and the number of isolated firms substantially decreased. Additionally, new links often formed between two firms each already separately connected to a third firm. Nonetheless, on the whole, firms that were comparatively highly connected remained highly connected and firms that were peripheral tended to remain peripheral—perhaps reflecting the costs of a limited ability to apprehend the value of, and put to use, information relevant to innovation.[38]

These interactions in shaping an organization's absorptive capacity are diagrammed, in schematic form, in Figure 5.3.

Organizations and their idea landscapes may need to span multiple kinds of distance. In addition to *spatial distances*, which influences opportunities to meet face-to-face, organizations may have differing configurations of units, subunits, or unit membership. Such *configurational distances* channel opportunities for who can work together. Organizations or groups may concurrently experience *temporal distances*, with team members spanning multiple global time zones, which can impact their opportunities for simultaneous collaboration.[39]

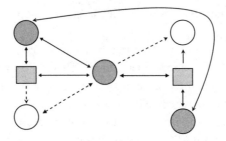

| AN ORGANIZATION'S INNOVATIONAL ABILITY DEPENDS ON ITS ABSORPTIVE CAPACITY. | ABSORPTIVE CAPACITY AND INNOVATION IN ORGANIZATIONS. Organizational innovation is influenced by both a firm's internal research and development resources and its interchange with external sources of knowledge. Organizations lower in absorptive capacity (shown as circles in white) often are less likely to provide knowledge or information to others (indicated by unidirectional and weaker dotted arrows rather than bidirectional solid arrows). Such organizations may also be unable to benefit from information even when it is available because they lack the knowledge threshold to apprehend the value of, and put to effective use, information relevant to innovation. Firms higher in absorptive capacity (shown as circles in gray) exchange and benefit from information both from other firms and from different sources, such as research institutes, suppliers, and consultants (represented by rectangles in gray).[40] |

Figure 5.3

Teams dedicated to new-product development, for example, may be geographically and otherwise separated or find it challenging to have frequent face-to-face meetings. For creative teamwork that relies heavily on improvisational problem solving, such dispersion may prove to be a barrier.

A questionnaire-based study of 299 team members of 71 software development teams from two large Italian technology consulting firms explored this issue.[41] These teams varied in size from 3 to 10 members. Questionnaires provided measures of team improvisation, creativity, and measures of the distance between team members. Three types of distance were assessed: spatial dispersion, configurational dispersion, and the degree to which team members were seen to be readily reachable, were nearby, and were accessible for spontaneous face-to-face meetings (termed "cognitive dispersion" by the researchers).

Team performance was evaluated by team leaders, and was based on their team's track record of producing high-quality work that met all client requirements. Performance of the software teams was significantly positively correlated with their level of team improvisation, but team performance was not directly influenced by any of the three measures of team dispersion. Instead, team dispersion influenced team performance through its effects on improvisation. Teams that were relatively closer together (spatially, configurationally, or cognitively) and also improvised relatively more often significantly outperformed those who were not nearby or were nearby but did not improvise. Simple proximity alone was not sufficient to lead to higher performance: Proximity *in combination* with an improvisational approach led to higher-quality software. Indeed, improvisation in teams that were spatially or configurationally dispersed led to poorer performance outcomes.

Why might this be?

One explanation is that teams that are located together spatially or configurationally may have a richer and more nuanced contextual understanding that supports effective improvisation and creative action. Collaborative innovation may require a collective or shared mental model—"a pattern of heedful interrelations of actions in a social system."[42] In **heedfulness** the actions and thinking of a group or team emerge based not entirely on habit but on a "heedful" monitoring and comprehending of an unfolding dynamic situation. Each person acts in a way that converges, supplements, or assists with the overall collective effort.[43]

Heedfulness is not solely an effort at paying attention.[44] Rather it is this combined with an active *taking care* and staying in touch with new information and its immediate and broader implications—for ourselves, for others, and for a collective envisioning of a larger unfolding joint enterprise.

> Without the strong potential for heedful interrelating—not just cooperation, not just commitment—but heedfulness it is no fun at all to try and create a really new product.[45]
> —*Innovation experts and professors Deborah Dougherty and C. Helen Takacs*

Heedfulness contributes to our shared team mental models. Heedfulness also promotes situational awareness. Team *situational awareness* involves not only the perception of changing aspects of our local environment but also how and which of those changing aspects relate to team goals and integrating this information to forecast and anticipate future developments.[46] Heedfulness, team mental models, and situational awareness are fundamental contributors to the multifaceted adaptability of our creative and innovative team processes.[47]

ADAPTABILITY AND OPENNESS

You are a director on a film set and you and your crew have just spent half of the day getting ready to pull a particular "picture car" for a simulated drive through a location for filming that day. As the grip crew are hauling the car up toward the set, the tow rig mechanism unexpectedly and irrevocably breaks. What do you do?

This incident, based on a participatory researcher's field notes of an actual film shoot, was first met with an immediate flurry of discussions, where it was determined that they would need to modify the planned shots for the day.[48] The person responsible for the towing, or the "key grip," promptly called everyone together with the following scene change instructions: "Okay, new deal, now the Technocrane is coming to me, and we are shooting scene 17." This flexible change capitalized on the fact that the specialized camera crane was already set up to be used later in the week but could be readily repurposed to be used now. The unexpected event prompted a rapid reorganization of the team's filming schedule—yet consistent with their longer-term plans.

The film crew was both adept at dealing with such surprises and accustomed to doing so; surprise was almost a daily routine for them and was mentioned in almost every interview with the participant researcher who informally interviewed crew members. This particular incident also epitomizes the process of *bricolage* or "making do by applying combinations of the resources at hand to new problems and opportunities"—or, more broadly, an emergent action that draws on existing and ready-to-access materials or capabilities.[49] The crew called upon the material, cognitive, and social resources that were already present and available, including their knowledge of planned future tasks, to fittingly deal with the newly emerging obstacle to moving forward with filming.

Where surprise, whether positive or negative, happens almost daily, teams build up repertoires that will allow them to meet and embrace the unexpected. These tools are not just material but encompass sociocognitive resources including "collectively held knowledge about how a task is performed and how activities advance."[50] Flexibility and adaptability are partially based on a prior widely debated, and agreed upon, collective provisional understanding of workflow expectations.

In another situation involving the film crew, a camera operator with the specialized skills needed to operate an aerial camera unexpectedly did not arrive for the shoot on the day that the aerial filming was scheduled. The executive director and camera crew discussed their options, and the cinematographer asked several members of the crew if they were able to operate the aerial camera. He also inquired about their flexibility in assuming other roles. After determining the crew's capabilities, several of the camera operators shifted roles, enabling the filming to continue on schedule. By reevaluating assumed constraints and tapping into shared hidden resources in their overall knowledge and skills, the camera crew successfully overcame the temporary setback.

The individual members on a team and the overall composition of a team equally contribute to its ability to adapt to unexpected or unstructured change. A general predisposition to be receptively welcoming of variety and of the opportunities inherent in novel situations, or of being "open to experience," may facilitate the needed unlearning of an earlier routine or rule-based process.[51]

Consider how openness to experience played out in an experimental scenario. Undergraduates in an upper-level management course were asked to take part in a computerized military simulation in which they needed to make judgments about the threat levels posed by different unidentified aircraft and decide how to respond to those threats. The students were told that they would need to learn, based on experience and feedback, how much to "weight" each of the different characteristics of the unidentified aircraft, such as its altitude, speed, range, and angle of approach. After each trial they were given feedback comparing their decision to the correct action. Partway through the experiment—and unknown to the students—the rule for weighting the aircraft characteristics changed, first after 25 trials, and then again after a further 25 trials.

Students who scored higher in openness to experience on a personality assessment questionnaire, or who were generally characterized as broad-minded, imaginative, and willing to try new things adjusted more readily and more successfully to the unannounced changes to their environment. In contrast, individuals high in aspects of conscientiousness, particularly those who scored high in the dependability aspects of orderliness and dutifulness, adjusted more poorly to the unexpected changes.[52]

It is important to note that prior to the unexpected changes in their environment, the individuals with different personality characteristics performed similarly. It was only *after* the unforeseen changes in their environment that strong personality-related differences, such as differing levels in openness to experience, were found to influence performance. These findings were obtained even after taking into account measures of general ability or intelligence. The benefits of openness to experience in adapting to rule changes in our external environment may reflect a greater readiness to move beyond highly automatized ways of making decisions.[53]

Change itself places higher demands on adaptability. The findings from the aircraft simulation study support the importance of personality characteristics for an *individual's* adaptability to change. Is there a corresponding role of personality characteristics in *team* settings?

To address this question, students were randomly assigned to three-member teams and were asked to assume different but complementary roles during a three-hour computerized simulation of a team-based version of the enemy aircraft exercise.[54] In this virtual simulation, it was possible to closely count the number and forms of interactions between team members and how the patterns of interactions changed in the face of unexpected events, such as a deliberately introduced technical communications breakdown between part of the team at a point just past halfway through the exercise.

Teams that had higher aggregate (summed) openness to experience, higher levels of conscientious achievement (e.g., higher perseverance and self-efficacy), and also lower levels of conscientious dependability (e.g., a lower need for order and higher spontaneity) showed a significantly greater ability to adapt readily to a new role structure. They also showed significantly better postchange decision making. After an unanticipated disruption to their routines, teams whose members collectively scored higher on openness to experience, higher on conscientious achievement, and lower on conscientious dependability made better decisions.

The personality composition of the group greatly shaped the team's flexibility in adaptively modifying their roles. This, in turn, was associated with improved team decision making. In contrast and paralleling the earlier findings with individuals, the team personality composition had little influence on team performance *prior* to the unforeseen change. For groups as well as for individuals, higher levels of openness to experience was associated with greater capabilities of adapting to change, including "unlearning" no longer applicable procedures and the learning of new routines or new processes.[55]

Teams with comparatively higher aggregate levels of openness to experience and higher overall emotional stability may be more adaptive in the face of change because they can more flexibly and directly confront problems or group tensions. They may also be more welcoming of alternative views, in the process extending their idea landscapes and the creative possibilities they can consider.

Let's look at a study of students randomly assigned to work interdependently together in 5-person teams for a 13-week academic term. Analyses revealed that higher team openness to experience and emotional stability were especially influential in how well the teams handled team conflict, which in turn substantially enhanced the team's project performance.[56] Openness to experience itself has many facets (e.g., openness may relate to ideas, values, or actions), and each of these facets might differentially impact aspects of a group's performance and process. It may be beneficial to try to ensure that teams include at least some members who are comparatively high in openness to experience whether as assessed by personality inventory questionnaires or based on extensive and varied past observations and peer reports.

The impetus for change, whether originating internally or externally, in individuals and in groups does not enter a vacuum. It always meets with preexisting beliefs, knowledge, attitudes, and routines that may be closely interconnected and interdependent, requiring modifications in both explicit understanding (know-what) and more implicit procedures (know-how). Successful change may involve *intentional unlearning* of previous routines and developing new knowledge and awareness at individual, group, and organizational levels.[57]

What factors might influence large-scale organizational unlearning and learning? Take the case of the introduction of a new organization-wide information technology system in a government-owned Australian energy industry corporation with approximately 5,000 employees.[58] The new system replaced multiple older, less integrated information systems and the change affected nearly all employees (for 20 percent it had a major impact, and for 67 percent the change had some impact on their daily routines). Analyses of the online survey responses of 189 companywide employees with first-hand experience in implementing the changes revealed seven key factors that contributed to the success of the change initiative.

Five of the seven factors related to the individual's responses to the change across time and two involved organizational-level factors. A key individual factor prior to introducing the new system was whether individuals had positive expectations related to the forthcoming change, such as how well they understood the need for change and how well prepared they felt they were (*positive prior outlook*). Whether they were apprehensive, anticipating that the change would be difficult, and how comfortable they were with the prior system (*feelings and expectations*) were also influential early on. During the actual information technology system change the individual's support from their colleagues and management together with his or her level of job experience emerged as important (*positive experience and informal support*). Following implementation of the new system, how well individuals understood the rationale for the change and how well they were adapting to the new system (*understanding the need for change* and *assessment of the new way*) were crucial. The two most influential organizational factors were the perceived success of how the company had handled prior change initiatives and the quality, timeliness, and applicability of organizational communication and training for effectively enacting the current change (*history of organizational change* and *organizational support and training*).

The interrelations among these five individual and two organizational factors are diagrammed in Figure 5.4.

The importance of intentional unlearning for organizational change was similarly emphasized in a study of the hotel industry in Spain that was aiming to improve awareness of environmental sustainability and to develop policies and actions to achieve more sustainable environmental impacts.[59] Telephone interviews using structured questionnaires were conducted with 127 owners or CEOs of hotels varying in size from as few as 10 to 49 employees to as many as more than 500 employees; approximately half of the hotel companies had between 50 and 249 employees. Analyses revealed that an unlearning context had a significantly positive effect on the company's progress, relative to their competitors, in using less polluting processes and products, developing more effective waste management, and enacting an environmental policy. An intentional unlearning context was associated with perceived improved organizational outcomes, including customer satisfaction, and the development of new and improved products and services.

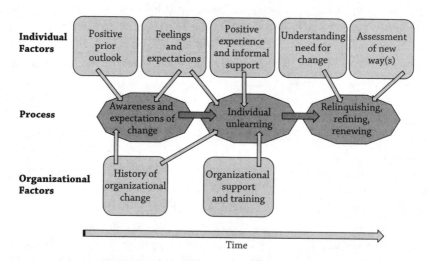

Figure 5.4 FACTORS SHAPING ORGANIZATIONAL CHANGE ACROSS TIME. Organizational change may follow a process from expectations of change through individual unlearning and broader organizational renewal. Large-scale change may be influenced by organizational history, including prior change efforts, and by organizational support as well as by a number of individual cognitive, affective, and experiential factors across time.[60]

The unlearning context was characterized by three main dimensions. One dimension involved *individual-based responsivity and reflection*. This dimension tapped the extent to which employees try to reflect on and learn from their own and others' mistakes, are readily able to identify problems and new ways of doing things, and incorporate suggestions and critiques from others. *Individual-based awareness and action* was a second factor. This second factor involved the degree to which employees recognize that current forms of reasoning and problem solving are inadequate, acknowledging the value of changing their attitudes and behaviors. In addition, *management-based emergent understandings* were crucial, particularly the extent to which management is open to new ideas and new ways of doing things, initiates innovations, and collaboratively solves problems.[61]

Openness to new ideas and new ways of doing things is critical at both the individual and group level, and can especially contribute to encouraging divergent discussion and healthy robust debate.[62]

~~~~~~

Research Highlight: *Ideas Need Both Diversity and Receptivity*

Both diversity and receptivity in our idea landscapes are important. Students at an East Coast American university were first asked to generate possible alternative uses of a common object for five minutes. The students were then randomly assigned into pairs, each with a partner of different ethnicity, and were asked, together, to generate additional novel uses for the same object for 15 more minutes. All pairs included one student who was Caucasian (all Caucasian students were born in the United States), and one student who was of Asian descent (95 percent of Asian students were born in Asia). Earlier, all of the students had completed an online survey assessing their multicultural experience, including questions such as the amount of time they had lived outside of their country of birth, the number of foreign languages they spoke, and their favorite foreign cuisines and favorite foreign musicians.[63]

Pairs that were high in multicultural experience were more creative than those low in multicultural experience. Over and above the creativity of the individuals and several individual difference factors, multiple regression analyses revealed a significant influence of the *combined multicultural experience* of the pair. Students who were high in multicultural experience and who, in addition, were paired with students who likewise were high in multicultural experience showed significantly greater team creativity than did students who were in pairs that were not both high in multicultural experience. Teams with high multicultural experience pairings generated significantly more ideas, ideas of greater novelty, and ideas from a wider range of different categories, thereby demonstrating significantly greater cognitive flexibility in moving across different ways of thinking. When each student in a pair was high in multicultural experience they were creative beyond the sum of their parts, resulting in *superadditive* levels of creativity, that were higher than would be expected by simply adding together their individual results.

We know from survey outcomes based on employees in a range of Irish and Australian industries that small to medium-size groups that were more open to cognitive diversity—characterized by group members' efforts to both freely express and fully understand suggestions—were significantly more likely to develop especially creative and novel ideas. The generation and incorporation of new knowledge was especially strongly affected by the group's ability to weigh multiple approaches against each other, debating ideas, and working disagreements through to resolution. Comprehensive discussion and extensive debate provide an important idea intersection space for diverse proposals to meet and play off of one another, increasing the potential for the emergence of greater novelty and creativity.[64]

When we face relentless or severe pressures arising from limitations of time, space, or other human or material resources, our ability and that of our teams to be and remain openly adaptable to change may be directly or indirectly undermined.[65] We may be forced to resort to reactive "patching" or "workarounds" of a situation. Such first-order problem solving may monopolize all of our resources, leaving little opportunity for second-order problem solving attempts to resolve, remove, or prevent the underlying causes.[66] How we respond to situations that allow for **first-order vs. second-order problem solving** may cumulatively improve or impair our individual and collective capabilities.

Second-order problem solving often requires noticing recurrent patterns, and moving up in our thinking beyond the current single situation we are in. Such detail stepping to a more general level may enable us to identify and address recurrent problematic issues and could be seen as a form of exploratory search at a *process level*. Searching in process space presupposes that there is motivation to do this, yet sometimes the positive immediate feedback from first-order frontline problem solving may paradoxically make second-order problem solving less likely. First-order problem solving is frequently more tangible, direct, and efficacious in the short-term and so we may neglect opportunities to pursue longer-term solutions.

Second-order problem solving also may require sufficient resources—including time, people, or communication options. Organization and team culture play a role too. Engagement in second-order problem solving efforts is more likely to occur when there are positive (encouraging) expectations about how proffered suggestions or diagnoses of problems will be handled.

Innovation often requires a certain amount of "slack" or discretionary allocation of resources to allow experimentation in the face of uncertainty. *Organizational slack* refers to any resources that are above and beyond those strictly necessary to achieve an aim accompanied with some discretion with regard to the allocation of finances, time, effort, space, and/or people. "Organizational slack is that cushion of actual or potential resources which allows an organization to adapt successfully to internal pressures for adjustment or to external pressures for change in policy, as well as to initiate changes in strategy with respect to the external environment."[67]

Yet slack does not mean a disproportionate flood of available resources. Indeed, excessive time, financial, or other resources may lead to insufficiently careful or undisciplined selection of projects or unwarranted ongoing support of projects. Just as we have seen in our earlier discussion of constraints, the presence of the right level of resource constraints is a welcome incitement to creativity.

Consistent with this suggested influence of resources on innovative performance, research with two large multinational firms revealed that the relation between innovation and organizational resource slack followed the pattern of an inverted U. An intermediate amount of slack was associated with the greatest innovation. Either too little or too much slack was associated with decreased innovation.[68] Slack and the preservation of sufficient resources to allow responsiveness in the face of unexpected shortfalls has been found to be important in increasing not just exploration itself but also in fostering an organization's development of second-order competence in exploration—that is, learning to explore.[69]

Think, for a moment, about the different types of resource availability that might be involved in planning the productions and promotional marketing for an upcoming season of a nonprofit professional theater company.[70] Along with more or fewer financial resources (such as cash reserves at the close of the fiscal year), the company may have more or less flexibility and also more or less intense demands on their personnel or human resources (for example, the number of full-time artistic staff as compared with directors, designers, and actors hired for a specific show). Additionally, their operational capabilities may be greater or fewer (for example, as indexed by unutilized theater seating capacity), and they may have stronger or weaker ongoing customer relationships. For instance, relative to a theater's overall expenses, some theaters may receive most (or little) of their revenue from regular subscribers.

All of these types of resources and their comparative availability may affect the ways in which the theater company considers and scouts its future creative options. Each of these varied types of resources may channel both its search scope and search depth, shaping just how innovative the upcoming seasons will be and the innovative variety across its seasonal schedule. Will the theater company create productions that are new to the world (world premieres), new to their market (regional premieres), or creative revivals of classics (e.g., a new production of a play by Shakespeare or Samuel Beckett)? How innovative will their choices be in regards to casting and design and conceptual approach?

If a theater has amassed resources that are especially hard to earn or to retain, such as many loyal subscribers, those resources themselves may tilt how the theater company and management thinks about different possible future directions. Some types of highly innovative productions, for example, may too thoroughly challenge some subscribers' expectations. All else being equal, an emphasis on maintaining its difficult-to-come-by and hard-to-replace loyal and steady patrons may reduce organizational adaptability and creativity.

There may be ongoing tensions between the need to make the most of what is already at hand, honing and refining approaches and talents, versus striking out into new promising yet riskier territory. One artistic director noted that the structure of rehearsal, fund raising, and the theater season itself can result in a mindset in which "The challenge each year [is] how to make the wheel slightly rounder."[71] In contrast, one managing director observed, "In terms of programming and taking risks, it's originality, exploration, and importance of a new idea. Imagination. Some new ideas are more important than others. There's new work, then there's *new* work."[72]

Consider the results of a survey study conducted in 2003 involving 163 managing directors of nonprofit US professional theaters. They had an average annual budget of $4 million and introduced an average of 14 new productions each year.[73] The study found that both higher customer loyalty and higher overall attendance were associated with *decreased exploration* (decreased risk taking, less experimentation, and an emphasis on a short-term view) and an increased reliance on "known and tried" approaches. Organizations, however, that also had *resources that remained flexible* more creatively and proactively deployed those resources, including financial resources, in the face of perceived external threats or demands, using the resources to actively counter the challenges.

A theater with a loyal and extensive subscriber base and few empty seats faces a classic exploration-exploitation dilemma. If the theater management and artistic director(s) opt to continue to pursue slight variations on existing approaches, this may appear to nicely preserve the status quo. However, this increasingly narrow "depth" of search will lead the theater to miss out on broader emerging opportunities, some of which may prove unsuccessful but others of which may yield essential longer-term benefits and organizational direction.

To circumvent this "either-or" situation, theaters can adopt various "either-and" strategies, both with respect to the plays or productions and their efforts to promote them. They might develop multiple theater spaces or venues, concurrently offering popular main-stage productions and trying out more experimental or innovative works in smaller spaces. Differentiated subunits or structural differentiation is another option. A theater company might use different subunits of actors for each production or host a resident company, producing "in rep" productions, with the shows changing but the actors cast in some plays that are traditional, others that are experimental. Using such approaches, theaters can provide audiences with a mix of new-to-the-world productions alongside novel reinterpretations of existing works as well as more traditional or tried-and-true productions. Paralleling these divergent creative efforts for their productions, divergent promotion and marketing initiatives could develop multiple rather than a single subscriber base, including crowdfunding, and tailoring different types of marketing approaches for particular audiences.

Despite the intuitive and logical appeal of adopting such a diversified approach, results from a follow-up study that examined the three-year financial data for a subset of the theaters from the 2003 survey raise some cautionary flags.[74] The financial data suggested that there were benefits from a *complementary pairing* of approaches to production and to promotion, with either "exploitation" for both or "exploration" for both, but only for the older and larger theater companies. Financial outcomes were better when, for example, highly experimental plays were paired with seeking a newer and perhaps untapped market using contemporary social media techniques and, conversely, when a more traditional play was coupled with marketing through established channels. Pairing an experimental or innovative production with traditional marketing had little effect on revenue.

Larger and older theater companies could achieve financial success through multiple means if they were using matched production-promotion strategies, with such multiple means based on different competencies. However, mixing the new and the tried-and-true in both their productions and marketing was financially beneficial only for older and larger theater groups and not for younger and smaller ones. This difference in outcomes may be because "smaller, nascent organizations lack the resources, capabilities, and experience required to manage the tensions and trade-offs that escalate when exploration and exploitation manifest within a single domain."[75] Smaller and younger organizations might struggle unsuccessfully with maintaining sufficient goal clarity when faced with the tug between innovation (scope) and elaboration/refinement (depth) within a narrowly circumscribed set of cognitive, physical, and financial resources.

Theaters, on average, have comparatively few full-time employees but often rely extensively on part-time directors, designers, and actors who typically are often invited for a specific production or season. This constant change in creative personnel substantially increases variation and organizational learning over time. In contrast, the administrative and marketing personnel in theaters tend to be stable across time, leading to the development of increasingly finely tailored subscription relations and strategies. For older theaters this may restrict their ability to explore emerging markets unless they grow in size, with an accompanying influx of new people with new perspectives and methods. Larger organizations might have sufficient flexibility in resources to concurrently pursue quite different aims but still maintain goal clarity and goal consistency within the separate pursuits. Paradoxically, however, these bountiful resources might lead them to be increasingly disinclined to implement and promote a more varied set of productions. There is clearly a need for approaches that provide both the capability and the motivation to spark and sustain continued innovation.[76]

ADAPTIVE EXPERTISE AND CONTINUAL SEARCH

To discover the history of possible surface water on the planet Mars, two identical planetary exploration robots were launched by NASA to land on opposite sides of the planet. Both successfully touched down in January 2004. The Mars Exploration Rovers (dubbed *Spirit* and *Opportunity*) were designed and equipped to characterize a diverse range of rocks and soils, take high-resolution images, and drive and navigate across the planet's surface. Each rover was in the hands of a science team of about 50 members. Each science team included scientists from a wide range of disciplines, including geochemistry, atmospheric sciences, geology, and soil sciences; also included was an interdisciplinary long-term planning group as well as engineers representing all of the rover's various instruments.[77]

In the first 90 days of the Mars mission, "the scientists operated in a co-located, real-time problem-solving manner, often in a large room with workstations for each science subteam. Communication was primarily conducted via face-to-face structured and informal meetings within and between subteams, taking advantage of the open room."[78] From the outset, the team progressively developed shared mental models. Multiple educational cross-training meetings with engineers and scientists ensured a deep understanding of both the scientific questions and the engineering challenges. The daily working process was one of continual variation, with an unrelenting stream of unexpected developments, new data, and newly emergent plans and subplans. The mission was remarkably successful from the beginning, providing many pioneering discoveries including evidence for the history of flowing liquid surface water.[79]

Researchers who later examined the team's communications, learning, and problem-solving processes across the first 90 days of the mission uncovered clear evidence of increased efficiency in the team despite the many ongoing and ever-new challenges. The meetings became shorter and the planning meetings became considerably condensed in length, with the average time decreasing from an already intense 8.5 hours to 2.0 or 2.5 hours per day. These efficiency gains point to the development of team *routine expertise*. The gains in efficiency were not due to a simplification of the tasks undertaken and occurred in the face of declining rather than growing essential rover resources, such as the availability of solar power and memory for on-board data storage.[80]

The increase in efficiency was realized even though the team continued to successfully overcome entirely novel challenges throughout the mission. This suggests that the team was developing adaptive expertise—a combination of acquired experience and skills in addressing both routine situations and novel challenges. **Adaptive expertise** involves learning not only how to perform procedural skills more efficiently but also how to *flexibly adapt* or *change those skills* to meet new situations. That is, adaptive expertise involves knowing how and when to use ("transfer") what was learned in the past and when to modify it or to invent a new procedure.[81]

Detailed scientific activity requests were conveyed to engineers and stored on a central server. Using these computer records, researchers assessed novelty as the number of new daily low-level activities that were logged and implemented in each Martian day (a day on Mars is about 40 minutes longer than a day on Earth). Routine expertise was assessed by counting the number of times per day that the scientists reused earlier plans as a template for specifying an activity. Adaptive expertise was measured by looking at the extent to which the scientists used plans from multiple time points in the mission, strategically drawing upon recent plans along with older plans. Variations in the amount of time that had elapsed between when a plan was first used and then later reused "implied that the scientists were constantly learning and choosing from the entire set of previously generated activities."[82]

In line with the notion that the team was developing increasing routine expertise, analyses of the first 90 days of the mission showed that the number of reused activities steadily rose over time until just past the midway point, after which it modestly declined and largely stabilized, suggesting a slower subsequent growth in routine expertise. In contrast, adaptive expertise, as shown in the variability of the "age" of reused activity plans, rose steadily and never declined across the 90 days. This implies that the scientists continued both to "wisely repeat" allowing for efficiency, even as they invented and introduced new combinations (innovation). Novelty (the number of new low-level scientific activities planned per day) neither increased nor decreased over the same period of time, suggesting that the team did indeed continually face an environment that was never fully predictable.

Analyses of change scores (difference scores from one time point to another) further revealed that routine expertise learning predicted subsequent learning. A similar pattern of learning building on learning was observed for adaptive expertise. The more the team varied at one time point (the previous day) the more it varied at a later time point (the next day). These findings suggest that exploration and exploitation are not always an "either/or" but can be an "either/and"—including intense innovative activities that involve high and continual levels of novel challenges.

Routine expertise is clearly often needed, but it is not enough and need not be isolated from adaptive expertise. The two can work in tandem, particularly in dynamically changing environments. At the individual and team levels, adaptive expertise may bear similarities to what is called *organizational ambidexterity*, or the ability, in parallel, to both successfully explore new opportunities and exploit existing capabilities.[83]

Although investing our team's attention and energy in novel exploration or conventional expertise appears to pull in opposite directions, it may be possible to concurrently develop increasing expertise in both directions. As diagrammed in Figure 5.5, it may be possible to discover an *optimal adaptability corridor* between efficiency (for example, relating to the automatic or habitual use of knowledge and procedures) and innovation so that both develop together, with different possible trajectories to this goal.[84]

Whereas routine expertise suggests procedural efficiency and the fluent application of acquired knowledge and skills, adaptive expertise involves flexible, innovative, and creative competencies within a domain. Like

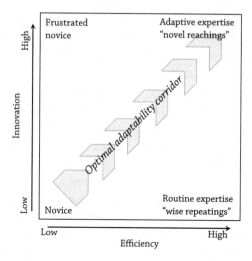

Figure 5.5

WE CAN PURSUE GREATER INNOVATION AND ENHANCED EFFICIENCY *CONCURRENTLY*—FINDING OUR OWN, OR OUR ORGANIZATION'S, OPTIMAL ADAPTABILITY CORRIDOR.	ADAPTIVE EXPERTISE AND THE OPTIMAL ADAPTABILITY CORRIDOR. Concurrently valuing and actively pursuing routine efficiency together with flexibility and creativity may allow the development of adaptive expertise.[85]

routine expertise, adaptive expertise is a lifelong process that requires ongoing practice and is as important for the beginning practitioner as it is for the seasoned veteran.

Organizational cultures may differ in the extent to which they both foster and require adaptive expertise from individuals and teams. Environments conducive to the development of team adaptive expertise are characterized by several features. Such environments involve a range of substantially different situations or variability in task requirements and contexts so as to allow for the abstracting of important commonalities. Environments that engender team adaptive expertise also promote shared and accurate knowledge and skills relating to how and why to apply the abstracted strategies, thereby demonstrating broad metacognitive capabilities and shared, updated mental models. A strong supply of intrinsic motivation rather than predominantly extrinsic motivation is likewise crucial. We need to continually see problem solving as not just an opportunity to apply previous knowledge but as a chance to forge new knowledge and skills and to find new perspectives and pursue new opportunities. Promoting an orientation toward our knowledge and capabilities that implicitly and explicitly recognizes the value of, and necessity for, ongoing exploration and continually renewed learning enhances both individual competencies and team mastery, especially in the face of difficulties and the unexpected.[86]

Continued active exploration and experimentation is particularly called upon in situations that involve ***ill-defined (versus well-defined) problem-solving***. Efforts at problem-solving in such ambiguous or uncertain contexts take many forms and are collectively referred to as "search." Search involves the deliberate accessing, recombining, and conjoining of knowledge and skills in pursuit of developing new products, services, or processes. More formally, search is "the controlled and proactive process of attending to, examining, and evaluating new knowledge and information."[87] The primary focus of searching, depending on context, may assume many directions, such as developing new markets or clients, finding new technology or processes, and identifying new sources of supplies or materials.[88]

Innovation is not confined solely to those who design products. Those who *use* products often adaptively modify the products. Users, including lead and intermediate users (those whose needs are "ahead of the curve" and so may forecast possible future markets), can also inform the search space as sources of innovation and insight.[89] Findings suggest that as many as 6 percent to nearly 40 percent of product users engage in developing innovative industrial and consumer products and spearheading process innovations.[90] Companies may expand their search and exploration processes through deliberate and systematic invitations for user innovation.[91]

Known for developing well-designed, minimalist, unbranded, innovative products, Muji is a Japanese manufacturer and retailer of a broad range of consumer goods ranging from furniture to kitchenware as well as health and beauty products, clothing, and stationery.[92] In one approach to search, Muji solicits ideas on specified themes (e.g., developing better and more comfortable seating solutions in homes). Both external users and internal designers suggest possible ideas in response to the theme, such as a floor sofa that would shape itself to one's body. Initially users may propose an idea; then others can comment on it online. If an idea is found to be promising, an internal product team specifies product characteristics, such as fabric and other materials. After soliciting further feedback from users, the product may be moved into production.

Researchers tracked the fortunes of 37 designer-generated and 6 user-generated furniture products at Muji from February 2005 through July 2009. They found that:

in the first year after introduction . . . user-generated products [sold] roughly twice as much as designer-generated products . . . five out of six user-generated products [were] represented in the top third of the best sellers among all 43 [furniture] products . . . The results [were] even more pronounced using aggregate sales data across three years: units of user-generated products sold three times more frequently than designer-generated ones.[93]

In this example, we can see parallel development and marshaling of ideas from both users and designers. We see a type of perception-action cycle, encompassing and welcoming feedback at multiple points. More broadly, actively seeking and incorporating user insights within an ongoing cycle of making and finding may be immensely mutually beneficial.

Similarly, search may be broadened through diversity within an organization itself. This might include individuals and teams located across geographical and cultural boundaries as well as spanning varied functional, technological, and/or educational backgrounds; it may also include the organization's connectivity to external knowledge sources, such as the expertise provided by suppliers and research institutes. Within an organization, intentionally encouraging people to rotate or circulate across subdivisions or projects in an organization may lead to the injection of new knowledge.[94] Across organizations, search may also encompass new forms of interorganizational idea "scratching" processes involving open innovation, innovation contests, or broadcast searches.

Research Highlight: *Innovation Contests*

We alluded, in Part 1, to the fundamental contribution of diversity to our collective idea landscapes and the potential of innovation contests or prize-based competitions to provoke innovation and creative problem solving. Such contests or competitions may promote a parallel search process among heterogeneous individuals with diverse motivations, differing skills, and various knowledge backgrounds.

To maximize the reach of an innovation contest, the central problem may need to be "recast" or transformed into a less domain-specific and less context-specific form. Casting the problem in a comparatively more abstract or generic form may enhance its attractiveness to nondomain experts, providing freedom to adopt procedures from other fields and allowing the application of divergent perspectives.

In a large data set of 166 science challenges involving over 1,200 scientists, innovation searches that were recast more abstractly and disseminated widely were shown to be helpful in removing barriers to entry for nonobvious individuals, including persons who might otherwise be in the "outer circle" of knowledge expertise and exchange.[95]

Recently, in a search for an effective approach to a "big data" algorithmic genetic sequencing problem, researchers rephrased the issue into generic terminology. The problem statement purposefully excluded domain-specific language and omitted context-specific information. For example, the problem statement referred to "strings" and "substrings" rather than "gene sequences" and "gene segments." The researchers also devised and communicated a specific scoring metric to reward computational solutions that had greater accuracy and higher efficiency (improved speed).[96]

Solutions were submitted by 122 individuals, from 69 countries, with 44 percent being professionals and the remainder students at some level. None of the participants were academic or industrial computational biologists. Participants could submit more than one solution, and a total of 654 solutions were submitted, or an average of more than five proposed solutions per participant.

Results showed that 16 of the 122 submissions outperformed the accuracy of one of the benchmark procedures, and 30 out of 122 outperformed a different benchmark procedure. Eight submissions "achieved an 80% accuracy score, which [was] very near the theoretical maximum for the data set."[97]

There were also clear improvements in speed. Solutions that were at least as accurate as the benchmarks ran 30 times faster than one benchmark and 175 times faster than a second benchmark.

Three independent computer science researchers who analyzed the submissions found 10 distinct elemental methods were used, in 89 combinations; the more the number of methods increased so did performance improvements. Overall, 30 different solutions were clear improvements over the "state of the art" computer methods.

As the researchers observed:

> Although the solvers were virtually devoid of domain-specific knowledge, abstracting the problem into general algorithmic and mathematical terms allowed a wide range of nondomain experts to address an important, complex problem. These contestants brought to the problem whatever skills and expertise they had

or could find, probably yielding a far more diverse tool kit than would be available locally, and generated substantial diversity in technical approaches. Accessing such diversity may be particularly important, as big-data biomedical analytics is a rapidly evolving field in which it is difficult to know a priori the kind, quality and breadth of expertise needed to produce an effective solution.[98]

Search may predominantly explore areas that are new in which a firm has relatively little current knowledge—that is, "exploration" or scope search. Alternatively, search may aim to reconfigure or recombine existing knowledge into new products, processes, or services, involving "exploitation" or depth search. Exploration search offers the promise of greater innovativeness and novelty because it widens the range and variability of the knowledge options considered but carries higher risk of failure or unproductive outcomes. Exploitation or depth search, on the other hand, makes search less risky, and more reliable, but decreases the promise of true novelty.[99] Scope search has been found to be associated with the development of new products that are highly innovative,[100] whereas depth search is associated with the introduction of a *greater number* of new products that are, however, *less innovative*.[101]

Not only the direction or scope of search but the timing of search in relation to a firm's or organization's competitors matters. From this perspective, search has also been conceived of as a "learning contest" with three types of search: *head start* or searching a new area first, *in synchrony* search or racing with competitors to create innovative products, or *catch-up search*, involving searching after competitors already have done so.

The search direction and momentum of an organization's competitors may lead to "racing behavior in which the focal firm searches simply to keep up with its competitors. In the extreme, competitors' achievements provide a continuously moving target for the focal firm, establishing a 'Red Queen effect' (i.e., the firm has to run just to stay in place)."[102]

An in-depth study over a 15-year period of 124 Japanese, European, and American companies that produced industrial robots systematically examined the effects of the timing of search on innovation outcomes. Researchers consulted three sources of data: trade publications and product catalogs, patent data, and interviews with industry participants including robotics executives, suppliers, customers, industry experts, and university scientists. To be considered an industrial robot "a product needed to be programmable to move a gripper or tool through space to accomplish a useful industrial task."[103] Robots varied on four dimensions, including repeatability, speed (maximum velocity), dexterity (degrees of freedom), and load capacity.

Innovativeness was based on a comparison of the average performance on these four characteristics of a firm's new products in a given year, with the average performance of industry-wide new products in the previous year assessed separately for those four dimensions.

The most frequent innovators simultaneously used *both* head-start search and catch-up search but not in-synchrony searching. This dual-pronged approach enabled these firms to enjoy the best of both worlds in that they introduced some highly innovative products together with a larger number of new but less innovative products. Higher levels of innovation may be fostered by the concurrent use of both head-start and catch-up search because "participation in both [learning] contests helps the firm use knowledge from one part of the knowledge domain to challenge accepted beliefs in another."[104] In other words, concurrent head-start and catch-up searches may create an enriched idea intersection space, with novel ideas meeting and melding with established expertise and knowledge.

OUR FUTURE-MINDED CREATIVE BRAINS

How do we think about our individual and collective futures? Engaging in mental contrasting is one form of future-related thinking that may influence our successful future goal pursuit, and (relatedly) our appropriate choice or selection of goals. As we saw earlier in Part 3, **mental contrasting** is a form of prospective thinking in which we first vividly imagine a desired and achievable future goal. Then we identify and envision current and real obstacles to achieving that goal. This process makes both our future and current goal-related circumstances simultaneously accessible to us in our idea landscapes. Mental contrasting has been found to lead to greater likelihood of achieving a desired goal than does either simply passively imagining a desired future state ("indulging"), or engaging in the process in the opposite order, first vividly thinking of present obstacles, and then the future goal ("reverse contrasting").[105]

The interspersing of perceptually simulating a not-yet-realized but desired future situation, with the perceptual simulation of likely intervening impediments to achieving the desired state, may assist us in moving toward our goals both emotionally and motivationally. Mental contrasting may lead us to engage in a *process simulation* rather than an *outcome simulation* and so provide us with more concretely helpful guidance as we move forward, "enlisting problem solving activities, such as planning, and regulating emotional states."[106] It may also help us to appropriately and readily classify current "obstacles" as being obstacles[107] and increase our time and effort in combatting obstacles—in part because they were anticipated.[108] Mental contrasting additionally can counteract our tendency to be excessively positive in our imagining of future events.[109]

Take the case of undergraduate students who were randomly assigned to receive (alleged) positive feedback on their potential for creativity (as purportedly based on a brief personality measure they had completed). Some of the students were asked to engage in mental contrasting, other students were not encouraged to mentally contrast, and still others were given only moderate positive feedback about their creativity potential. Students encouraged to engage in mental contrasting scored significantly higher on a set of verbal, spatial, and mathematical insight problems than did participants in either of the other groups. These results suggest that the improved insight performance was due to the perceptual-cognitive-motivational processes engaged by the self-regulatory strategy of mental contrasting, especially when this strategy was combined with a high positive expectation of success.[110] Prospective mental simulation may also enhance group interactions and decision making.[111]

Prospectively projecting ourselves forward into the future and concurrently vividly imagining possible roadblocks that we may encounter as we attempt to realize a desired future goal (large or small) may also facilitate essential detail stepping. This may simultaneously equip us with an abstract longer-term perspective and prepare us to take concrete steps toward realizing our longer-term goals.[112]

A good dose of optimism may carry us more buoyantly forward. Although optimism is very often seen only as a "bias," it is also a "buffer" and sometimes a very protective cushioning zone that can enable us to respond resiliently to setbacks or obstacles. When asked to characterize how optimistic others should be in different scenarios, most people do not say that they should be strictly "accurate" but that they should be *moderately optimistic*, with greater optimism recommended when the event is something the individual (or group) has chosen.[113]

Shifts toward and away from optimism may help to foster our *preparedness* for the future—shifting our thinking and attention toward goal pursuit or dealing with obstacles.[114] At a more distant point in the future, optimism may be stronger because our level of detail is more abstract; as "the moment of truth" arrives, our level of detail may shift toward concreteness.[115] Immediately prior to our performance we may experience an adaptive downward dip in our positive expectations, perhaps in part to buffer ourselves against negative affect and also because we become more aware of potential obstacles or snags in our environment or gaps in our preparations.[116]

Rather than a uniformly positive and exclusively optimistic approach, our adaptive flexibility may be best promoted by a predominance of positivity intermixed with a smaller but contextually appropriate addition of critique and skepticism. Research suggests that optimism predicts creativity either directly or through a mediating role of positive affect and that an excessive frequency of positive affect proves detrimental to creativity, perhaps reflecting inadequate or insufficient feedback or attention to feedback.[117]

When we plan our future-related activities imaginatively[118] or engage in complex creative activities such as developing and evaluating artistic designs generated in response to specified constraints,[119] we may, as we saw in Part 3, depend on our large-scale brain networks or subnetworks, such as the default-mode network (shown earlier in Figure 3.6). This network is often active during internally driven spontaneous and imaginative thinking. As we also saw in Part 3, complex creative and future-focused activities may invoke couplings between subnetworks of the default-mode network and the executive control network (shown earlier in Figure 3.5), which are important in effortful control and short-term working memory.

The neural networks and subnetworks that enable our different ways of imaginatively extending beyond our present circumstances support more than imagining our own possible future states. They equally support other critical forms of imaginative projection, such as vicariously empathizing with the experiences of others as well as conjuring imagined scenes that are not closely anchored in our prior experiences. Forming self-defining future projections[120] that are embedded in our experiential long-term knowledge and skills[121] may especially be associated with activity in the default-mode network.[122]

The representation of novel (hoped for or aspired to) future events draws deeply on our ability to richly remember and reconstruct the past. Yet "representing novel future events requires more than just a system that projects the past into the future."[123] Beyond rich experience-near recollection and beyond an ability to flexibly recombine previously experienced elements into novel configurations, we also need many other imaginative skills. We need, also, skills for "placing the [imagined] episode at a specific time in the future; thinking about one's own and others' future minds; judging the future episode on dimensions such as likelihood and desirability and altering it accordingly; inhibiting immediate impulses so that the future episode can be envisioned and actualized; and discussing the future episode with others."[124]

Creativity and change crucially depend upon the adaptive interplay of multiple abilities of our brains as we imaginatively anticipate the future and work with and build upon our pasts.

[cc/cQ] **Creativity Cross Checks and Queries**

Questions to encourage reflection and connections to your own work and practice:

⇒ Are you individually and in your creative/change teams, pursuing a mixture of both *exploring* possibilities (increasing the breadth or scope of your knowledge) and *exploiting* your existing capabilities (increasing the depth or specificity of knowledge)?
  - How do your search pursuits relate to your absorptive capacity?
  - Are your searches ahead of or after those of others?
  - How often are you exchanging ideas with suppliers, customers, and research institutes or other professional organizations?
  - Given the size and age of your organization, are you trying to do too much with too little, or are you doing too little with too much?
  - Are you casting your questions in terms that can reach beyond your organization, to those outside the inner circle?
  - Do you have a process to seek, find, and pursue promising innovative ideas from others?

⇒ How do new skills, procedures, or problem-solving approaches become known and aptly accessed by others in your organization, within and across units?
  - How often do you and others share reports and documents?
  - Do you have a variety of formal development and training programs, or information technology systems with which you explicitly share information and acquired experiences?
  - How frequently do you meet face to face with others in and across your organization?
  - How are lessons learned from positive and negative initiatives collected, shared, and exchanged?

⇒ "Learning tends to crowd out exploration . . . as firms grow large and search more, they will typically explore less, thereby making their search more reliable at the expense of variation."[125]
  - What things are "crowding out" exploration and search in your making and finding creative endeavors?
  - Should you diversify your learning to avoid crowding out exploration?

⇒ Are you, your team, or your organization privileging one phase or aspect of the overall ongoing innovation process?
  - Is your thinking about creativity and innovation too "front-end heavy"?

- Have you turned your attention to each of the phases or stages involved in your creative or change initiative?
- Consider this articulation, in regard to your own situation, of the many points at which innovation may occur beyond the research to prototype stages and into the pre- and outset-of-production stages:

> Much innovation occurs in the production stage. Moving from prototype to product can take years. It requires solving engineering design problems, overcoming production and component cost problems, building production processes, creating an efficient production system, developing and applying new production and product business models, educating a workforce, building a supply chain, financing scale up, actually scaling up production to fit evolving market conditions, and reducing all these steps to a routine. The initial innovation is often thoroughly reworked.[126]

⇒ To deal with the *expected unexpected*, incident response teams keep their vehicles well equipped with a variety of multipurpose tools and supplies.
- For you, and your team, what are the analogous equipment, tools, and protocols that you have at the ready to deal with surprise or unanticipated dynamic events?
- How do you cumulatively learn from past surprises?

⇒ Consider these two principles for innovating wisely: "Creative skill lies not just in doing something novel, but also in knowing how much novelty to pursue at what time." "New designers often want to reinvent the wheel because it's fun to try designing new things. But veteran designers know how to use [already existing structure] in clever ways to achieve their goals without taking on too much custom work."[127]
- How and why do you decide when to pursue a new direction rather than adaptively alter an approach used in the past?
- Do you aptly use "wise repeating"?
- Are your "novel reachings" timely?
- Do you recognize precedent as not only backward-looking but also *forward-facing*? In the words of one legal scholar:

> An argument from precedent seems at first to look backward. The traditional perspective on precedent ... has therefore focused on the use of yesterday's precedents in today's decisions. But in an equally if not more important way, an argument from precedent looks forward as well, asking us to view

today's decision as a precedent for tomorrow's decisionmakers. Today is not only yesterday's tomorrow; it is also tomorrow's yesterday.[128]

⇒ What are your *presuppositions* about creativity and change? Consider the following four perspectives of a university president, a novelist, a filmmaker, and a justice of the US Supreme Court, respectively. What aspects of these perspectives most resonate with you? What aspects might you better emphasize in your own thinking about the source and course of novelty and change?

- "Change is constant, endemic and necessary."[129]—President of Harvard University and historian, Drew Gilpin Faust
- "Young people—schoolboys and girls who are put up to this kind of pestering by their teachers—often ask, with youthful bluntness, 'Where do you get your ideas from?' My usual, perfectly honest reply is, 'I don't get them; they get me.'"[130]—Novelist, playwright, and critic Robertson Davies
- "I am not a documentary filmmaker, I happen to be a filmmaker who made a documentary. It tends to be that documentaries find you, even if you are not looking for them, and that is what happened to me. This documentary [*Gawah*, or Witness] found me and I had to make it."[131]—Writer, director, and filmmaker Gauri Chadha
- "Broad absolute rules don't really suit me, because I can always imagine—and do—the next case."[132]—Justice Sonia Sotomayor

Part 6

Ever-Renewing Goals and Keeping Our Aims in View

> *Thinking prompts*
>
> - How do our goals—and our orientation to our goals—shape our immediate and longer-term idea landscapes?
> - Why is feedback and our receptivity to feedback so crucial to our aims in view?
> - How might our environments (physical, social, technological, symbolic) be altered to better support our goal pursuits?
> - Where do your goals come from—and are they really yours?
> - How do we begin to make something new? How do we best begin, and why?

What makes us distinctively who we are over time? How and in what senses are we (or are we not) "the same" person, group, or organization across successive moments, weeks, and years? How do we continuously update and modify our interpretations of who we are and where we are going, particularly as generators of creative and innovative change?

A key part of the answer to these questions turns on our goals and values. In the immediate here and now we pay attention to, think about, and remember information that is related to our goals and values. Our values (overarching principles of what we regard as important and worthy of commitment) and goals (the ends that we aim to achieve) conjointly help us to know what is relevant, where to concentrate our energies, and how to interpret and anticipate our future. With time, this process cumulatively shapes our identity, including our capabilities and our further and future aspirations for creative growth and change.

One helpful perspective for tracing the interrelations between our individual and collective goals and values through time is offered by an understanding of autobiographical memory. How we carry forward what we have personally experienced—our accumulating self-related knowledge—shapes what we do and aim to do. Recall from Part 2 how the artist Patti Smith remembered walking as a young child along a river with her mother. Her vision of the "singular miracle" of a swan engendered in her a lifelong yearning for articulate voice. Seeing the swan called from her an urge for which she had no words: "a desire to speak of the swan, to say something of its whiteness, the explosive nature of its movement, and the slow beating of its wings."[1]

Our current goals, subgoals, and goal priorities together with our self-knowledge guide our attention and actions with little conscious effort. But when there is a change in the status of a goal that is important to us, an emotional or affective "triggering process" occurs. Changes in the status of our goals come in many forms. Perhaps we achieve a goal: the product is launched or the poem is published. Or we find that our progress toward a goal is blocked or suddenly recognize that there is a direct conflict among our goals. At this point we actively seek to understand this change in goal status from the broader context of our longer-term selves and our autobiographical understandings. We try to categorize anew the change in the status of our goal and to reprioritize our aims.[2]

As we try to work through our altered goal context, we may draw upon various aspects of our past and current knowledge, including both highly specific and concrete *experience-near* events and more general and abstract *experience-far* constructs and knowledge.[3] On a continuum of abstractness we may access our personal experiences and knowledge at any of multiple levels that interplay and support one another, with an admixture of our persistent past actions and routines, knowledge about what we care about and admire, and our perceptual and conceptual capabilities.

Just as we can think about the past in more specific, perceptually and emotionally rich, or more abstract and generic ways, so can we think about the *future*. In imagining the future, those events that are connected to our personal goals and values are more fully *preexperienced* and feel closer to us in time. The more a prospective future event is aligned with our values and goals, the more likely we are to have a "subjective sense of pre-experiencing the future."[4] Our preexperiencing may increase our motivation and effort and help us to concretely anticipate the steps we need to realize future outcomes.

In this final Part we begin by introducing a process we call *goal tuning*, which alerts us to each of the different phases of keeping our aims and their interdependencies in view. In the next two sections we see how initiating changes in our working and creating environments (physical, technological, social, bodily) can enable a shared and integrative understanding of progress toward our goals and of where we are in our making-finding cycles. We highlight—using examples from such varied domains as the temporally challenging world of scheduling and the creation of a new dance piece—the importance of searching within our methods of exploration themselves. Often we need to search within our search itself. Throughout we are reminded of the importance of varying and experimenting as we go to best unlock new insights and directions.

In our last section, "going forward," we consider broader connections and interconnections we have learned together throughout this book. We revisit our five thinking framework questions, with their many interweavings, to encapsulate the many ways that the thinking framework can help us all as we innovatively go forward.

> Aspiration and excellence are our essential guardians.[5]
> —*Neil Rudenstine, former president of Harvard University*

GOAL TUNING

We propose the process of goal tuning as a flexible conceptual guide alerting us to each of the different interrelated phases of keeping our aims in view. Goal tuning helps us to differentiate our choices and to be more resiliently adaptive and discerning in our change and creative endeavors.

Bang & Olufsen is a Danish company, founded in 1925, with the early and long-standing goal of designing and producing high-quality, well-designed, innovative sound systems. Although its products had won several international design awards and appeared in prestigious art and design museums, research showed that by the late 1980s the organization's goals had drifted to a new focus on exclusivity and luxury, where "the 'unobtrusive style' and the 'human side' of the products had been lost to 'marble and empty banqueting halls.'"[6] Company documents and interviews with people inside and outside of the organization pointed to an increasing form of disconnection or dissociation between the competencies of the company, how the company portrayed itself, and what the researchers described as a "blurring" of the company's identity and organizational purpose.

Recognizing the need to reorient and realign its beliefs about itself and its genuine distinctiveness, the company created two teams to work independently: one to gather survey evidence from four international groups of actual and potential customers and the second, a senior management team, charged with clarifying and characterizing the core features that distinguished the organization and its products from competitors.

The survey revealed that the company was recognized as developing products that create "harmony between aesthetics and technology"—including "'the immediate perception of technological excellence' (reliability, high performance, advanced research etc.)" and "'the emotional side of the product' (as reflected in the design, in the choice of material components and in the mechanical movements)."[7]

These outcomes led to the development of a rejuvenated, refocused, and coherent organizational mission that was firmly anchored in the company's long-standing distinctive strengths and existing capabilities, described as "a confirmation of the past and a guide for the future."[8] Technological excellence and emotional appeal were endorsed as guiding principles that provided coherence and direction throughout new-product design and all aspects of production, marketing, and distribution. This newly reaffirmed identity was focused *internally*, integrated into all aspects of the company, and never used in an explicit or direct manner externally.

Especially noteworthy here is the process engaged in by the company: "Organizational leaders did not try to counter discrepant perceptions through impression management, but questioned themselves regarding what attributes of the organization could be plausibly claimed as core and distinctive *and* at the same time meet the expectations of critical constituents."[9] Even when multiple aspects of an organization and its capabilities change, there are enduring, sometimes forgotten, and also newly emerging features of continuity that can be identified, underscored, and carried forward through a process of self-reflection and introspection. Organizations, like individuals, need to resist molding themselves to meet outside expectations and images that may be not only fleetingly ephemeral but also undermining of core strengths, creativity, and innovation.

Attention coexists with intention.[10]
—*Design expert and professor Pradeep Sharma*

Goals are ever-present and actively changing players within our idea land-scapes and sculpt what we are likely to notice and pursue. Here we specifically explore especially *longer-term goals* that shape our trajectories as individuals and groups over time and evolving internal and external circumstances.

Our goals differ from one another in many ways. To fully harness the creative energy and direction that goals can offer us, it may be helpful to guide our thinking through a set of five interrelated questions. First, how have we chosen and characterized our goals? Second, how well do our goals work or play together? Third, how pliable and responsive are our goals to unanticipated opportunities? Fourth, are our goals coming and staying in mind at the right times to guide our striving? Fifth, are we keeping track and adjusting our goals as needed based on ongoing feedback about our progress?

The processes of answering these questions invoke what we call *goal tuning*. This tuning encompasses processes of modification and continual adjustment to achieve maximal adaptive change and innovation. The ongo-ing processes of goal tuning involve five key interrelated components:

1. *Goal selection:* Identifying and committing to essential goals that uniquely characterize us now and well into the future.
2. *Goal synergy:* The ways in which our goals positively interrelate with one another to support and reinforce each other.
3. *Goal making/goal finding:* The ongoing interplay between what we intend (make) in terms of our aims and plans, and what we discover (find) in interaction with the world and with others while attempting to realize our aims.
4. *Goal activation:* The processes and factors that determine if our goals come to mind and remain in mind when we actually need them and are striving toward them.
5. *Goal updating:* How and whether our goals are refreshed and modified in appropriate ways as circumstances change.

These five components of goal tuning are summarized in Figure 6.1. We discuss each of these components in turn.

The processes of accepting or declining short-, medium-, or long-term aims together with our characterizations of those goals involve *goal selection*. With regard to our sustained creative and generative projects, goal selection concerns how many longer-term goals we have, of what type, and at what level of abstraction they are specified.

Goal selection is critical for many reasons. If we have too many or too widely disparate goals, our goals may compete and draw resources from one

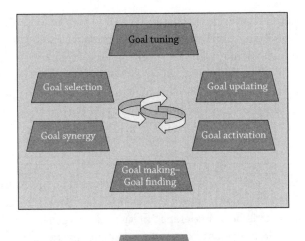

Figure 6.1 THE FIVE INTERRELATED COMPONENTS OF GOAL TUNING.

another—including our time and attention as well as emotional and material resources. Multiple disparate goals may also lead to decreased ongoing situational awareness regarding the current circumstances surrounding each goal, leading to problems with goal updating. Too many goals carry increased costs of coordinating projects and of shifting between different mental worlds as we try to reinstate different sets of relations and situational circumstances.

The goal-selection phase of goal tuning partially corresponds to what in goal implementation theory is called the *predecisional phase*. In this phase, as individuals or groups, we evaluate potential alternatives, including whether we choose to act or not to act. This phase has been associated with comparatively greater open-mindedness and even-handedness and leads to goal intentions. However, goal intentions do not automatically lead to actual goal pursuit. Planning as to when, where, and how the goal will be worked toward may increase actual goal pursuit. Appropriate goal selection can help in the later phases of realizing our goals by reducing our "second guessing" and minimizing possible conflict regarding what goals we should adopt.[11]

As we have seen, we may want a mixture of goals for newness together with goals for expanded or deeper learning within familiar or ongoing pursuits, excessively favoring neither "exploration" nor "exploitation." Additionally, goal selection requires appropriate balancing of both the *value* that we as individuals or organizations perceive in attaining a goal, and the *likelihood* or feasibility of reaching it.

Goal selection requires attention to the level of abstraction we are using: we need to conceive and articulate our goals at an appropriate level of specificity. Often this may lead to a midlevel characterization of our purpose and aims that avoids both hyperspecificity and overgenerality. We need to frame our goals in a way that is not too tied to a particular set of circumstances, as such hyperspecific goals may prove to be brittle or rendered obsolete in the face of change. But, similarly, we need to avoid overgenerality, as framing goals in an overly abstract or underspecified manner may render assessment of progress uncertain. Often, a midlevel of abstraction provides guidance in the form of flexible constraints that leave degrees of freedom for assimilating new information.

~~~~~~

 Thought Box: *Making New Structures/Places for Constancy Through Change*

Individuals and institutions often confront novel challenges that call for innovative responses. What are some of the parallels and possible linkages that we might draw among the following five very different ways of addressing challenges?

1. Sharing financial risk to support small-scale sustainable market gardening through Community-Supported Agriculture, where local community members pay a sum up front for a priority "share" of fresh seasonal produce. Or, alternatively, encouraging new technologies in developing countries through what are known as Advance Market Commitments (AMC). In an AMC, a sponsor or sponsors commit to a guaranteed price, in advance, for creating new technologies such as those that provide clean water or developing low-cost, as-yet-unavailable vaccines for neglected diseases.[12]

2. Reconstruing public libraries as "maker spaces" that simultaneously connect with the community and other maker spaces by providing resources, expertise, and mentoring for a wide range of creative

activities such as music recording, videography, computer programming, and three-dimensional printing and laser cutting.[13]

3. Creating new intersection spaces for cross-community and intergenerational sharing and teaching of skills and values through "Repair Cafés." Such cafes bring together people who like to fix things with people who want to have things fixed—concurrently placing less stress on landfills, keeping skills alive, fostering community sharing, and supporting a cradle-to-cradle product philosophy.[14]

4. Rethinking restaurant reservations as a "ticketing system," where you buy a ticket online for a table at a particular time. In ticketing, you are shown all the tables that are available at various times for a given evening and then pay a "deposit" on your selected table. Ticketing, rather than traditional or other reservation systems, can increase the transparency and efficiency with which both customers and the restaurant can see what tables are available, decrease no-shows, reduce demands on staff, increase the number of customers served, and potentially minimize food waste through enhanced predictability.[15]

5. Developing new forms of social enterprise "mixed-mission" business corporations, including what are variously known as benefit corporations (B corporations), public benefit corporations, or flexible or social purpose corporations to promote a firm's capability to responsively conduct its business in socially and environmentally responsible ways. These new entities differ in a number of aspects but each generally aims to offer for-profit corporations a more explicit way to seek or directly communicate goals beyond primarily shareholder interests and to achieve goal synergies across diverse stakeholders.[16]

Research Highlight: *Goal Specificity and the Interplay of Emotion, Concepts, and Perception*

Let's walk through a brain imaging experiment that demonstrates the close interplay of cognition, motivation, and emotion with what we see. The experiment shows how the *specificity* of our goals impacts what we see and feel, and whether we are likely to respond in more automatic or instead in deliberately controlled ways.[17]

During functional magnetic resonance imaging, participants were asked to examine a series of rapidly presented pictures in order to identify a particular target image—a photograph that had been rotated 90 degrees from its typical viewing position. All of the target images were photographs of a landscape or a building. On some trials, participants were given a specific goal or description of what to look for on that trial. They might, for example, be asked to "look for the rotated building." On other trials, participants were given a less specific description of what to look for as a goal. Here they were asked to "look for *either* a rotated building *or* a rotated landscape." To assess if participants could ignore irrelevant emotional stimuli, the target images were presented intermixed with both neutral and emotionally negative distractor images that portrayed highly fearful or violent scenes.

There was one further important "plot turn" in the experimental procedure. Unbeknowst to the participants, based on their earlier responses to a personality measure related to emotion and motivation, they were characterized as either low or high in harm avoidance. Some participants were low in harm avoidance in that they were of a generally confident temperament, likely to engage in risk-taking behavior, and tended to quickly recover from stress. Others, in contrast, were high in harm avoidance; these individuals had anxious and tense temperaments, tended to be risk-avoidant, and often were slower to recover from stress.

A key finding was that brain activity—in brain regions involved in more automatic and also more controlled processing—was affected by the *combination* of the participant's level of harm avoidance and the specificity of the goal he or she was pursuing. When participants were given nonspecific instructions of what they were to look for, those who were high in harm avoidance showed increased activation in the amygdala—an important emotional processing brain region—compared with those who were low in harm avoidance. Yet when participants had a more specific target to look for, amygdala activity did not differ between individuals who were high versus low in harm avoidance.

When participants could adopt a *specific goal*, everyone was able to effectively ignore the emotional distractors. In addition, when given the specific goal, the highly harm-avoidant individuals showed increased activity in the anterior cingulate cortex, a brain region especially important in exercising deliberate cognitive control and monitoring our own performance.

This study shows how our motivations—and in particular how we characterize our goals—shape what we see and feel and the mental control we can marshal for our goal pursuit. At a practical level, this study illustrates that if we can frame our goals with the right level of specificity, we may avoid becoming derailed by irrelevant events and stay focused on the task at hand.

There are costs to either being too specific or too general in how we think about our goals and projects. We can conceptualize our projects both as specific concrete acts and in terms of our broader overarching values. We can ignore neither. "Some individuals tilt their projects toward the specific act end of the hierarchy and others toward the values end" and there may be "a meaning-manageability tradeoff" in which focusing on concreteness and specificity enhance manageability, but if carried to an unremitting extreme, threaten to undermine meaning itself. The level of detail that we adopt in thinking about our goals may affect our motivation and how we perceive and evaluate our progress. If we are thinking at a more specific or concrete level and we think of our goal in specific terms, we may be especially sensitized to the *difficulties* in pursuing the goal. If, though, we are thinking at a more general or abstract level and we think of our goal in specific terms, we may be sensitized to the *importance* of pursuing the goal and be more adaptively resourceful in navigating obstacles. Effective value-steeped goal pursuit requires us to draw on "the ability and desire to flexibly alternate between the principled and pragmatic aspects of project pursuit."[18]

As we saw in Part 5, mental contrasting is one process that may help us with appropriate goal selection and may also boost our creativity. By vividly imagining an achievable future creative or change goal and then equally vividly bringing to mind currently existing or known obstacles, we may channel our motivational efforts and energized commitment in promising directions with prepared foresight. "The self-regulatory strategy of mental contrasting enables people to discriminate between their feasible and unfeasible desires, provides the strength to change what stands in the way of achieving the feasible, and gives the composure to let go of the unfeasible desires—to then re-engage in alternative pursuits."[19]

Another crucial aspect of goal selection is clarity. Well-defined and articulated goals were found, for example, to result in higher innovative performance among software development teams. At a team level, goal clarity indicates "a team's shared understanding of its goals and objectives."[20] We can use questions at a midlevel of specificity to clarify and fully articulate the relationships among our goals. For example, we may deliberately ask ourselves which requirements for a given project or undertaking support each other, contradict each other, or are mutually exclusive.[21]

Teams that have well-crafted purposes are much more likely to competently manage their own processes than are those whose purposes are either too vague and general or too specific and detailed.[22]

—*Organization and team dynamics expert professor Richard J. Hackman*

Goal selection and goals themselves are not just about efficiency or task-related progress. Goals also include our hopes for play, indirection, or surprise, and the way we move toward realizing various types of goals may differ. Depending on context, sometimes the lack of settling on a single goal or permitting multiple goals to merge and coexist without forcing an interpretation of a single goal or intent may be beneficial, especially for encouraging play and individual interpretation and responsibility. We don't always know the potential value of a process or outcome at the outset. We may profit from a phase of "goal babbling" in which we flexibly "try out for size" alternative courses of action.

It's also often the case that explicit instructions to "be creative" lead to higher creativity—so explicit and persistently consistent goal setting in relation to creativity and innovation is vital both for ourselves and others.[23] Even a momentary instructional cue to encourage creativity may enhance our ability to aptly notice more remote or distantly related analogies. Setting ourselves the clear goal of being creative enables us to *be* more creative, demonstrating that creativity isn't a single ever-present ability but is something we can purposefully boost in response to particular contexts.[24] Explicit goals for the generation of a high proportion of novel ideas, concentrating on suggesting ideas that are unlikely to be mentioned by other people, may also be beneficial, particularly in situations where we are highly committed to a project.[25]

Longitudinal research on teams has shown the motivational impact of shared vision for longer-term product and process innovation, with innovation fostering yet further innovation. "Shared vision appears to take a central role in the innovation process: Previous innovation effectiveness seems to significantly influence the degree to which teams subsequently share a vision regarding the purpose of the team and this enhanced sense of vision is ultimately tied to subsequent team innovation effectiveness."[26]

One source of constraints on goal selection is provided by *goal synergy*. "Goal synergy" refers to positive interactions or convergence among goals, sometimes involving the felicitous meeting of multiple constraints. When we focus on goal synergy, we try to take into account not just the number of longer-term creative or change goals we have but how our goals may interrelate with one another, including at various levels of abstraction. Adaptive movement between differing levels of detail in our goals requires that our abstract goals themselves be functionally integrated rather than being conflicting or incoherent. Such adaptive flexibility also depends on our continual receptive responsiveness to the current environment in an ongoing see-move-see or perception-action cycle.[27]

Let's consider the case of the Aravind Eye Hospital in southern India, founded in 1979.[28] In 2012, the hospital performed over 340,000 surgeries, most of them involving the removal of cataracts. In the same year, the hospital provided vision screening for over 10 times that many people. The surgeries have been remarkably successful, with a superb quality of care and markedly low rates of complications. The surgeries are provided regardless of an individual's ability to pay, with nearly two-thirds of the operations performed for patients who are billed below market prices and many receiving free treatment.

Given its outstanding success, the hospital has often been invited to consider expanding its organizational mission beyond that of offering surgical services to those suffering from cataract blindness to other vision-related health concerns, such as blindness prevention programs. "At a superficial level, such an upstream expansion in scope might seem to meet the stated mission of the organization, but when examined more closely does not fit the capabilities of the organization."[29] Prevention programs would be targeted beyond individuals with visual impediments toward, for example, families with children. A blindness prevention program might, for instance, encourage families to change the way they cooked and ate so as to make greater use of fresh local vegetables high in vitamin A. In contrast, Aravind's core purpose "is centered on delivering high quality surgical intervention rather than on mass-media prevention campaigns."[30] Instead, the hospital has chosen to add a second line of vision treatment by fitting prescription eyeglasses. This expansion in organizational scope is synergistic with the hospital's goals and longstanding identity of directly and immediately improving the quality of vision of individuals.

Goal synergy does not require that our goals be excessively similar to one another. Indeed, synergy may arise from the right type of *variety* in our goals. Engaging in projects with different goals can help us to refresh and move within our idea landscapes in ways that have unforeseen positive benefits.

If we think of our goals as members of a team, lessons learned from research on team synergy can help us. Individual members in a group may bring different functionalities or specializations, but these are likely to be optimally used only if the functionalities are *complementary* and there are strong processes that facilitate the integration and coordination of expertise and information in the group.[31] Even very "smart" teams may perform poorly when they are not encouraged to develop strategies for coordinating and integrating the contributions of all the team members. Being explicit and clear about the importance of integrating our goals and developing practices that make such integration more likely, may bolster our performance and creativity.[32]

Requirements come from different kinds of considerations and, as we have seen, live at differing levels of specificity. In the case of conflicting goals, it may be difficult to reconcile even key values with other demands. Take, for example, the case of developing and designing environmentally sustainable ecologically effective products, processes, or services. Even though undergraduate engineering students learned about and fully endorsed the value of "cradle-to-cradle" sustainability, research revealed that the students found it difficult to access the key skills and materials necessary to realize their sustainability goals.[33] Despite its central importance, sustainability may need to compete and work with other constraints and demands, such as client requirements, deadlines, and the limited availability of materials.

Sometimes the coactivation of several of our goals together may lead us to search for ways of meeting those goals with a single means. For example, we may attempt to concurrently address our time demands and our aim of eating healthily by choosing to have lunch at a place nearby that serves fresh seasonal food. Such attempts to simultaneously meet multiple goals through adopting a single means are neither invariably harmful nor invariably beneficial. However, attempting to find a single means to multiple goals can inadvertently narrow the range of options we consider for a focal goal. This may be particularly likely if our concurrently activated goals have only moderate feasibility or if the importance of our focal goal is not salient to us.[34]

Asking that a single means meet multiple goals for us has additional potential costs. Expecting that one particular activity address multiple, different, highly valued goals may detract from our experienced satisfaction in meeting those goals. Volunteers who strongly and equally endorsed two or more motivations for their volunteering activity were found, six months later, to experience *less* motivational satisfaction and also to have experienced more stress in relation to their volunteering than did volunteers who had a single highly important goal in volunteering (with their other reasons for volunteering assuming less importance).[35]

This difference in the outcomes experienced by more "singly-motivated" volunteers compared with "multiply-motivated" volunteers was not related to their total degree of commitment or to direct conflicts between the goals they endorsed. Perhaps expecting one activity to meet multiple highly valued goals attenuates our ability to notice, feel, or perceive *progress* to each goal. Or it may be that singly-motivated individuals experience *increased buffering* against challenges, setbacks, or stresses because less motivational urgency is associated with any one activity and is diversified across multiple roles or activities.[36]

From a broader perspective, as for other change endeavors, the motivations that initially prompt us to volunteer, for example, may be different from those that sustain us over the longer term. What we accomplish through our initial endeavors may feed back and amplify or build on each other through time. Longitudinal data indicate that there may be a cyclical process at work. In the case of volunteering, for instance: "Connection to community leads to volunteerism, which builds further community connection, which stimulates more volunteerism, which in turn leads to other forms of social action."[37]

At the organizational level, contradictory or conflicting goals may substantially undermine creativity and change initiatives. This is particularly so when the conflicts revolve around questions of more abstract goals relating to organizational identity or values, such as "Who are we?" In a study of US nonprofit professional theaters, researchers observed that although minor disagreements in the relative weightings of creative and marketing priorities may not be detrimental and may even be beneficial, major disagreements about organizational direction and purpose proved extremely harmful.[38]

But where do good goals come from in the first place? The process of discovering and successively clarifying our creative and change goals may itself require *goal making and goal finding*.

> We can treat *goals as hypotheses*. Conventional decision theory allows us to entertain doubts about almost everything except the thing about which we frequently have the greatest doubt—our objectives. Suppose we define the decision process as a time for the sequential testing of hypotheses about goals. If we can experiment with alternative goals, we stand some chance of discovering complicated and interesting combinations of good values that none of us previously imagined.[39]
>
> —*Organizational theorist and professor James G. March*

It is important that our goals provide us guidance without too rigidly dictating or specifying where we need to go. Individuals may vary in the extent to which their goals in a creative enterprise are fully conceived and conceptualized beforehand, versus how much their goals and creative efforts are guided by ongoing interactions with their materials: what they perceive and what unfolds in the world as they act within it.

A distinction has been drawn between *conceptual* innovators/artists and *experimental* innovators/artists.[40] Artists who are predominantly conceptual in their approach (for example, Pablo Picasso, Robert Smithson, F. Scott Fitzgerald) have clearer top-down ideas and tend to make sudden breakthroughs using those ideas. In contrast, artists who are predominantly experimental in their approach (for example, Paul Cézanne, Auguste Rodin,

Virginia Woolf) work more incrementally, by trial and error, and respond more to the "data" provided by their ongoing dynamic interactions with the world. There is empirical evidence that predominantly conceptual artists (painters, poets, sculptors) tend to make their most important creative contributions earlier in their career, at a younger age, than do artists who tend to be more experimental. Experimental artists tend to continue to innovate and produce radically new works many decades past the beginning of their artistic careers.[41]

Research on the processes underlying *productive failure* and *desirable difficulties* may also point to the value of experimentation, tinkering, and confrontation with where our assumptions lead us.[42]

> Always keep the goal in mind, but not as a destination. Keep it as a guide. You do not need to move toward it. In fact, you may need to pull away entirely and go in another direction, but the objective will remain with you. Those who are willing to just start making something no matter where those steps are leading will go much farther than those who timidly walk a direct line, because every step of the journey amounts to something.[43]
>
> —*Visual artist and professor Leslie Hirst*

Despite their importance and our commitment to them, goals are only one of the many constituents of our idea landscapes and so will fluctuate in their level of activation and prominence in our conscious awareness.

The relative activation level of our goals in our idea landscapes, or **goal activation**, varies across time and situations, including times when we are able to actively strive toward goal fulfillment.[44] We have seen (in Part 1) how open or pending goals can enable us to aptly notice novel relations or opportunities by attuning our attention, enhancing our readiness to absorb and understand. We have also seen, in our discussion of implementation intentions and prospective memory (in Part 3) that sometimes we need to postpone goal pursuit if the circumstances for goal engagement are not yet present. Forming implementation intentions at an appropriate level of abstraction may increase the likelihood that our postponed goals will come to mind—be activated—when an opportune situation for again pursuing the goal is at hand.[45]

Not only goal activation but also its converse, goal *deactivation*, is crucial to our innovative progress. Sometimes we need to let go of goals. At other times we need to "bracket" our goals or put them aside temporarily.

Goal deactivation, or intentionally or unintentionally letting go of a goal that we at the moment cannot pursue, can sustain our full mindful engagement in our current activities without rumination or excessive anticipation of upcoming activities. By decluttering our idea landscapes and bracketing future goals, we can also better sequence our current goals and subgoals. Bracketing our future plans and focusing on the present moment can set in play an immersive feedback cycle of positive emotion as we progressively move toward our creative aim. Bracketing can be facilitated by bringing to mind the contexts in which we should return to a temporarily set-aside goal; we might say to ourselves that we will take care of "item 2" from our to-do list later that day, on our way back from lunch.[46]

Perhaps counterintuitively, we should sometimes bracket our creative goals too. Especially if we have become blocked or stuck in a creative pursuit, temporarily "letting go of goals"—through goal deactivation—may release us to move into a different idea landscape. It may also enable us to avoid an overly narrow and too tightly controlled pursuit of a particular goal. Recall from our discussion of times in between in Part 3 that the interleaving of our creative tasks can be an especially effective way of sustaining our creative momentum.

Apparently paradoxically, if we're making *better* than expected progress toward a current goal, not infrequently the relative accessibility of *other* goals may increase.[47] When progress toward a given goal is satisfactory, we may become more likely to entertain a *reprioritization* of our goals. We may either then turn toward activities that (earlier) were slightly lower in our list of priorities, or we may opportunistically capitalize on new developments that happen to arise and come to our attention.

Such fluctuation in our priorities in relation to our goal progress has been understood in terms of the informational role of emotion in behavior and cognition. Positive affect, like negative affect, may be a *signal* that helps us to manage our priorities. But whereas negative affect tends to narrow and focus our attention on the specific factors that may lead to undesired consequences, positive affect tends to broaden our attention, encouraging us to scan both for new priorities (including identification of neglected matters that may later become threats if not dealt with soon), and new opportunities.[48] Expressed more broadly, emotion may comprise "a domain general mechanism for regulating effort allocation."[49]

We need to be continually updating and adjudicating between different possible courses of action and meeting different pending goals. Both better than expected progress toward any one of our goals and times in between may be occasions for the emergence of new configurations of priorities and aims.[50]

The importance of goal activation for comparatively shorter-term goals is illustrated by the phenomenon of "goal neglect." If our projects involve a very large number or complexly interrelated goals and subgoals or we have been interrupted, some of them are at risk of being neglected or lost from awareness. Such goal neglect occurs to everyone occasionally. In some cases goal neglect reflects a disconnection between *knowing* what is required and *acting* in accordance with it. In such cases we may be able to verbally state the task requirement or subgoal if asked, but fail to effectively bring the goal to mind when it is relevant. This may reflect difficulties in activating or maintaining the goal at the right time.[51] Forms of novel on-the-spot thinking that require reasoning about multiple components and their interrelations may be especially prone to goal neglect. After an interruption, we can prevent goal neglect by pausing at the time of the interruption to vividly picture where we are and then reinstating this picture once we resume again. Even briefly pausing to rehearse our current situation may allow us a necessary transition time in which to encode and later retrieve the goal memory.[52]

In *goal updating* we modify and refresh our goals based on our progress, feedback, and changing circumstances. Modifying, further articulating, refining, or abandoning goals on the basis of new information, feedback, or changing circumstances are all forms of goal updating. Goal updating involves recognizing problems and realizing that a change of direction or approach (sometimes large, sometimes small) may be needed.

> What makes Pixar special is that we acknowledge we will always have problems, many of them hidden from our view; that we work hard to uncover these problems, even if doing so means making ourselves uncomfortable; and that, when we come across a problem, we marshal all of our energies to solve it.[53]
>
> —*Cofounder of Pixar Animation Studios Ed Catmull*

Goal feedback in undertakings of creation and change has been shown to enhance creativity in several ways.[54] Feedback that is more specific, task-focused, and positive has been found to be especially beneficial, not only because it serves to clarify the creative objective but also because it may enhance positive affect and task engagement, which has the spillover effect of increasing cognitive and affective flexibility.[55]

More generally, feedback is an essential contributor to developing skilled intuitive judgments and to adaptively and progressively learning from our mistakes and "experiments." The ability to make genuinely skilled intuitive judgments—rather than simply having lucky intuitions—requires extensive *deliberate practice* and multiple related factors, such as adequate opportunities for feedback and learning from mistakes.[56]

Researchers used videotapes of baseball pitchers to provide college baseball players (batters) with rapid feedback on the accuracy of their judgments on whether the pitches that were shown would be within the batter's strike zone.[57] The videotape showed the delivery of the pitch and the release of the ball toward the batter. The task for the batters was to identify the type of pitch being thrown, but without the need to attempt to actually hit the ball with a bat. The use of videotapes made it possible to block out (or occlude) part of the pitcher's release of the ball in order to assess what information the batter acquired at different points in time.

Crucially this method allowed players to see hundreds of pitches with *immediate feedback* on whether their judgments were correct. The college players who were given this type of training in a series of ten 15-minute individual video sessions improved their actual batting proficiency. They showed significantly higher batting averages over 18 games after completion of the training than was shown by a comparison group of players who were not given the pitch-recognition training. This demonstrates the importance of immediate feedback in developing expert judgment.

Explicit and direct feedback may also help to guide our day-to-day change efforts, helping us to better achieve our goals. In one field research study, individuals who had already taken several actions to achieve a goal of electricity conservation in their homes received fine-grained graphic and social comparison feedback, which further boosted their progress toward their goals. Time-based feedback—provided through a web-based portal that featured consumption graphs and offered information about how a given household compared against similar households—substantially further reduced the participants' use of electricity.[58] Similarly, but in a rather different domain, students who were provided with a running total of their current overall grade status and more frequently accessed this information achieved higher course grades even after taking into account their initial grades in the course.[59]

As we have seen, one of the key functions of prototypes and mockups is to provide rapid and "real" feedback. Design firms use prototypes and feedback on prototypes extensively. One survey of US design firms found that 80 percent of the firms surveyed performed detailed design reviews on their prototypes throughout the process and 55 percent included field trials as a regular part of their design process in the later phases of a project.[60] Beyond product innovations, *process* innovations also depend on multiple coarse and more fine-grained laboratory tests and experiments, with iterative feedback across multiple phases from an initial idea to the final decision to move into production.

Attempts to measure an organization's goal progress must be at an appropriate level of specificity. The Nature Conservancy in the late 1990s provides a telling example.[61] Dedicated to advancing conservation of land and water around the world, the Nature Conservancy had for years relied on a simple metric of "bucks and acres" (total charitable donations and number of acres acquired). According to these measures, the organization was successful and on a decidedly upward trajectory. But grounds for dissatisfaction with this measure had been mounting within the organization. The number of acres protected by the conservancy did not necessarily translate into preserving biological diversity.

Advances in conservation biology compelled the conservancy to move up from its focus on comparatively smaller parcels of land to broader large-scale ecosystems. This reconceptualization of the organization's "acres" measure was accompanied by a rethinking of their "bucks" metric. Their first attempt to develop new measures of their performance was far too detailed. Pilot testing of the new performance measures showed that the proposed "ninety-eight point" system was excessively complicated and time-consuming. Going back to the drawing board, the conservancy recognized that they needed to find measures that were simple, based on data that were easy to collect as well as readily communicated. The measures needed to address progress toward mission, be formulated in a way that they could apply across all levels of the organization, and encourage units to focus on the highest-leverage strategies.

It was comparatively straightforward to develop good measures of the conservancy's capacity and activities. More challenging and time-consuming was developing good measures of progress to mission. The conservancy eventually arrived at two complementary measures: biodiversity health within its protected properties and "threat abatement," or the extent to which the organization was combatting human and natural threats to biodiversity health. In combination, these measures of goal progress helped the conservancy proactively focus on tangible outcomes aligned with the organization's mission.

As we saw in the case of the renewal of long-term focus and identity in Bang & Olufsen, feedback may also alert us to ways in which we may be off course from our overarching goals and ideals. This is another reason for encouraging questioning, greater openness, and transparency and establishing clear ways of recognizing, recording, and reporting failures or breaches of standards or ideals. Alerting us to our driftings, evasions, injustices, or off-course actions may be one of the important feedback functions of organizational advocates or an ombuds office. Advocates or ombuds offices, as well as alternative processes or institutions to promote social justice, may help us to establish or reestablish what should have been the case in the first place. Feedback and feedback-generated dialogue may promote change toward our *already held ideals*.[62] Feedback is essential to better align our everyday actions with both our current overarching and our more newly formed aims.

Goal updating is often a natural evolution from both goal feedback, and our goal making/goal finding, but may also be necessitated by changes in our internal and external circumstances. *Strategic renewals* may exemplify goal updating at the organizational level, with ramifications throughout the organization. "Strategic renewal includes the process, content, and outcome of refreshment or replacement of attributes of an organization that have the potential to substantially affect its long-term prospects."[63]

Among individuals and organizations, goal updating often arises from changing idea landscapes that offer new opportunities, including reinterpretations of identity and the reemergence of earlier technologies and processes. Today we may see this, for example, in the renewed vitality of craftsmanship related to a resurgent interest in a wide range of products and processes, including mechanical watches, fountain pens, organic winemaking, and vinyl records.[64]

Finally, better than expected or substantial progress toward our goals may itself be the instigator of our goal updating.

> After people attain the standard they have been pursuing, those who have a strong sense of efficacy generally set a higher standard for themselves. The adoption of further challenges creates new motivating discrepancies to be mastered.[65]
>
> —*Social cognitive theorist and professor Albert Bandura*

ENVIRONMENTS FOR FLEXIBILITY AND CHANGE

The emergency department in what we will refer to as "City Hospital" is an urban teaching hospital that sees on average over 300 patients a day.[66] The waiting room was often crowded and—given the long and unpredictable waiting times—as many as 30 percent of the patients arriving there left without even being seen. But it was not only the patients who found the situation stressful and ineffective. Doctors and nurses often did not know one another, or whose patient was whose, and frequently could not find one another when needed. They reported that it was difficult to communicate quickly and to follow up on their actions; they felt isolated from the bigger picture and rationale of a patient's care and had little coherent or integrated information to permit the effective prioritization of treatment plans.

Yet six months later many things had changed. The hospital redesigned the emergency room process and space into a "pod system." Each of the five pods or stations was in a separate physical space, with its own dedicated computers, supplies, counters, and beds. Each pod was staffed by one attending physician, at least one senior resident physician, and usually three nurses, including a nurse who was designated as the "pod lead." Newly arriving patients were now assigned to one of the pods on a "round robin" or quasi-random basis, and the pod team was responsible for all aspects of that patient's care.

Researchers interviewed and extensively observed the emergency department physicians and nurses after the change to the pod system. They also analyzed 160,000 (deidentified) electronic medical records representing all of the patients seen in the emergency department over the 18 months following the change. The total time per patient in the emergency department was reduced, on average, by two to three hours—a dramatic improvement on the previous average of eight hours. And there were more than quantitative changes.

Observations and interviews underscored several far-reaching effects of the new pod organization. The pod structure allowed teams to work in closer physical proximity and permitted greater personal interaction among team members. Team members could now more spontaneously and rapidly improvise in helping one another and prioritizing processes. The new structure promoted a greater sense of shared responsibility for the patients in the team members' pod and increased motivation arising from a sense of greater autonomy and mutual accountability. It also strongly improved communication and feedback and created a shared focus.

The process of moving through an episode of care now could occur in parallel for multiple patients. The nurses and physicians interacted constantly, improvising to adjust expectations and treatment plans. As one of the medical residents explained, "So much of what we do changes minute to minute. [The pods] allow us to interface with each other in the whole closed-loop communication. That really matters in what we do because priorities change constantly."[67]

Notably, although the *roles* in each pod remained constant, the *individual doctors and nurses* in the roles changed continually over the course of a day; indeed, over the course of as few as five hours all of the nurses and physicians in a pod might have changed. Additionally, individuals seldom worked together in the same pod more than briefly: interviewed physicians and nurses estimated that they worked with another person in the same pod only once or twice a month.

Yet despite such continual flux, the new organizational structure enhanced all aspects of the goal-tuning process: goal selection and prioritizing (for example, allowing for more effective time prioritization), goal activation (enabling within- and across- personnel communication of changing needs), goal synergy (problem solving together), goal updating in a rapidly changing environment, and goal making and finding, as in improvisational and on-the-spot decision making.

The newly implemented pod system at City Hospital exemplifies one innovative approach to the tension between the need for plasticity (change and adaptability) and stability (constancy) and the crucial role of the physical environment. The pod system provided a way to structure working and physical space such that both dynamic change and constancy in goals and goal pursuit were accommodated with minimal effort and minimal deliberate conscious intervention. Such "team scaffolding" may become increasingly important as a growing number of organizations in areas such as banking, data processing, and information technology move into 24-hour multishift schedules.

The new spatial arrangements at City Hospital are an especially vivid example of the ways in which our physical environments have carryover effects onto our social and knowledge interactions and change initiatives. But equally dramatic examples may be singled out in quite different domains, providing both parallel and divergent examples of the importance of the implicit and explicit boundaries on the flow and exchange of ideas in our idea landscapes.

Let's turn, for instance, to an experimental initiative in rural India, aimed at creating a new shared space for the exchange of ideas and information among widely dispersed small-plot cotton farmers.[68] Using already existing and available low-cost technology, particularly simple mobile phones, the pilot experiment in Gujarat, India, enabled cotton farmers to obtain and share current information about climate and crop conditions. For decades, the government had offered an agricultural informational program on recommended practices, yet fewer than 6 percent of the rural farmers reported having used the public extension agent's service, in part because of the high costs of travel and time away from their work to receive information.

With the new information distribution method, the farmers did not need to leave their fields; they could now access information in a timely manner close to where they needed it and while they were working. The new approach to distributing information also provided unprecedented opportunities for iterative and peer-based idea exchange and comparisons and reduced the farmers' reliance on suppliers with conflicting interests. The novel low-cost interactive voice application, called *Avaaj Otalo* (voice porch or voice stoop) was explicitly designed to be as accessible as possible to individuals who were semiliterate or who could not read or write.[69] To use the service, farmers called a toll-free hotline, asked questions, and received answers via recorded messages. Callers could also listen to the answers to questions posed by other farmers and respond to them. Additionally, they automatically received weekly information delivered through automated voice messaging about weather forecasts and pest planning, the content of which was guided by expressed concerns of farmers from a weekly random poll.

More than half (58 percent) of the farmers in the experimental group used the new agricultural consulting service. Based on the advice received, they purchased fewer hazardous pesticides and relied on more effective ones. They also diversified their crops, including planting significantly more of a riskier but more profitable crop (cumin). These outcomes suggested greater exploration and search on the farmers' part.

Despite the many differences, the mobile phone informational service has several parallels to the hospital pod example already explored. The interactive voice application enabled greater shared situational awareness together with timely and continual updating about unexpected rapidly changing events. The agricultural information change effort was designed to be highly responsive to where the participants were located and their particular constraints (e.g., that they tended to be tied to the land at certain times, they were not highly mobile, and their work was subject to unpredictable changes in weather and crop-related factors). Yet this was an extremely low-cost intervention, especially compared with the traditional educational approaches, which offered much less flexibility and far less opportunity for bottom-up calls for information in a time-sensitive manner. Although the interactive voice application did have drawbacks (for example, it did not allow for in-person demonstrations or face-to-face discussion), like the hospital pods it provided an *integrative knowledge and skills hub* that extended the capabilities and options of the participants.

A third, again different illustration of the contribution of our environments in supporting the collaborative interchange of knowledge—in this case across a highly distributed science community—is provided by the Large Hadron Collider Computing Grid (LCG).[70] One of the world's largest computing grids and dedicated to particle physics, the LCG spans 170 computing centers in 34 countries. Researchers observed and conducted semistructured interviews with physicists and computer scientists in the UK Particle Physics Grid who help to process data from the Large Hadron

Collider particle accelerator at CERN near Geneva, Switzerland. To examine the scientists' collaborative working processes, researchers collected team and individual data from 2006 to 2008; they reviewed documentation and subscribed to its main online mailing lists.

Notably, here everyone on the teams was working toward very high-level goals (aiming to discover possible new subatomic particles), and they used intermixed controlled planning and improvisation throughout. The team members recognized the importance of detail stepping. They saw the need for abstract ideals and having, as they expressed it, their "heads in the clouds" with respect to keeping the big picture aims in mind. Equally, they saw the need to be mindful of concrete and interim events on a day-to-day basis because problems and problematic situations continually emerged that could not have been anticipated, requiring improvisatory "make-do" approaches to move forward.

Other prominent characteristics of their collaborative science environment and idea intersection spaces were widespread trust (general recognition that everyone does their best and is knowledgeable) and acceptance of *failure* as part of the process of getting things done. There was a meritocracy of ideas with parallel development of different approaches to solving problems, as everyone was situated in his or her own environment with its peculiar context-dependent difficulties and needs. These characteristics were combined with pervasive "retrospective sensemaking" as the physicists and computer scientists struggled to understand what was causing a given phenomenon or to identify the source of a particular data pattern.

The actions and decisions of the scientists on a day-to-day basis intermixed spontaneity and planful deliberate action. Experimentation and improvisation were valued. They were, though, consistently guided by, on the one hand, intermediate and longer-term aims and, on the other hand, an ongoing situational awareness and heedfulness—coupled with a deep tolerance for inevitable imperfections and errors. A combination of well-articulated longer-term goals and clear milestones and deadlines provided both forward impetus and essential feedback.

EXPLORING, EXPERIMENTING, EMBARKING

Beyond searching for innovations in any one particular product or service, our search for useful variation and change may encompass broad cross-situational aspects of our environments, including explorative search as to which tools or methods we use in our creative efforts themselves. The development of thinking scaffoldings and design heuristics that were explored in Part 2, such as design by analogy and biologically inspired design, are examples of "search within search" tools, or searching within methods of exploration themselves.

Increasingly, sophisticated computing and information technology approaches continue to uncover new possibilities for all stages of the design and exploration process. One recent approach that can serve as an illustration involves a process of *coabstraction*.[71] In coabstraction, a computer program begins with a collection of three-dimensional objects and then extracts a "spectrum" of possible alternative abstractions of the three-dimensional objects. The coabstraction method allows for the creation of multiple alternative three-dimensional forms at similar levels of abstraction while still maintaining sufficient detail to permit the ready identification of the object.

Testing with a group of 74 participants of varying backgrounds revealed that, consistent with the researchers' hypothesis, fully or completely abstracted models were more difficult to identify and to match to the original (nonabstracted) objects vs. models created by the coabstraction method. Both the matching accuracy and speed of participants were significantly higher with coabstraction.[72]

The coabstraction approach recognizes that we do not necessarily form a *single* abstract representation of an object but rather *multiple* ones at different levels of detail. This approach nicely coheres with developmental and other evidence that we encode and form representations of objects and events at differing levels of abstraction, in parallel or concurrently.[73] Coabstraction additionally benefits from our powerful abilities to notice distinctions and to gather information by comparing and contrasting.[74]

Moving from product to process, computer and information technology likewise may provide unique insights into human interaction, allowing novel, personalized interventions. In the realm of higher education, for example, meta-data on the patterns of digital communications between students in a first-year university course allowed charting of the dynamic unfolding patterns of peer learning interchanges between students and how these interactions correlated with the students' course performance.[75] Across two academic semesters, researchers analyzed 80,000 interactions of 290 students as they used digital communication channels for posting and exchanging course information and questions (for example, an e-learning platform, a collaborative electronic work space, and live interactive Internet text messaging).

Compared with students who performed less well in the course, better-performing students initiated information sharing *earlier* in the term and *persisted* in such sharing across the term. Better-performing students demonstrated more stable, frequent, complex, and longer

information-sharing chains. As shown in Figure 6.2, the information sharing of higher-performing students involved more than the simple one-step
relaying of information; their patterns of information exchange took advantage of both the convergent and divergent sharing of information. Students
who sought out and shared information early were more effective in finding
and maintaining learning partners; delayed and less focused search resulted
in weaker and less stable online learning relationships.

Beyond pointing to the importance of peer learning and involvement,
these findings highlight the often overlooked opportunity for strategic
instructional or pedagogical interventions. These interventions could guide
or scaffold less experienced or academically disadvantaged students in the
use of digital and peer information-sharing technologies, especially *early* in
their courses.

More broadly, we can ask what best leads to the creation of supporting and
stretching idea-intersection spaces in all of our endeavors. How might we
better foster our own and our team's education and learning efforts, not only

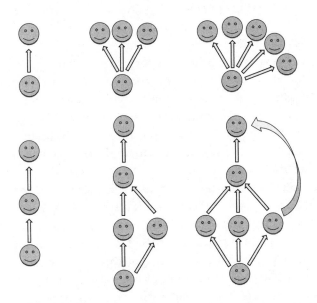

Figure 6.2 PATTERNS OF ONLINE COURSE-RELATED INFORMATION
EXCHANGE AMONG STUDENTS. Shown schematically are the online information
cascades of students initiating, receiving, or relaying course-related information.
Students who subsequently performed better in an introductory university course
showed more varied and multiple-path information exchanges that were also
initiated early in the course (bottom row). Students who performed poorly in the
course (top row) tended to rely on simple one-to-one or one-to-many broadcast
exchanges initiated only later in the course.[76]

in face-to-face or in-person interactions but also in online contexts? And how do we take into account "beginnings"—acknowledging the importance of the *temporal domain* as a pervasive part of our environments, especially the new habits we establish early?

The need for effective exploration and search within the temporal dimension of our environments is especially prominent in the complex case of scheduling. Scheduling is a multifaceted enterprise, with multiple stakeholders and dynamically changing constraints, that requires both top-down control and spontaneity. Consider this scenario, involving a passenger train station.[77]

After arriving at the end of the day, passenger trains remain during the night at a train station. To avoid blocking incoming and outgoing trains, the trains are assigned to a shunting track. During the night the trains may be washed and cleaned, requiring access to the washing equipment, and for their outgoing morning journey the trains may need to be reconfigured with other rail coaches, possibly on a different track. To plan these movements, planners must assign drivers and also train shunters to connect and disconnect the rail coaches. The planners must further be ready to accommodate unexpected events, such as the need for maintenance work on a shunting track or delays in trains arriving at or leaving the station.

One approach to providing more support to this complex planning process involved subdividing the larger planning objective into four basic assignment tasks: a track-finding algorithm to find a free track or combination of free tracks; a driver/shunter assignment to assign tasks to the drivers/shunters; a train unit matching algorithm to associate incoming coaches with outgoing coaches; and a routing algorithm to route the train to its shunting track using the shortest feasible route.

Computerized interventions here might assume differing degrees of control and different amounts of human intervention. At the most automatic level, a "control" algorithm could be executed that successively performed *all* of the subtasks for all of the trains, with a user's input only at the outset of starting the control algorithm. With a more intermixed type of control, the algorithm might provide alternatives from which the planner could choose. For example, the track-finding algorithm could evaluate a range of tracks and provide the five best options, with the planner then selecting one and the routing algorithm thereafter automatically executed. At a more fully deliberately controlled level, the planner might work mostly manually but for some subtasks could choose to let the algorithm search for the solution. For instance, the planner might select both the track and the train driver but then use an algorithm to choose the route.

Empirical results implementing these advanced planning options suggested that the computerized support helped to decrease cognitive load for human planners for comparatively more simple problems but *not* for more complex problems. Perhaps for complex problems, the computerized planning system interfered with well-learned problem-solving patterns of the planners. Additionally, the system may have shifted the mental load on a planner from *creating* a solution to *evaluating* a proposed solution generated by the algorithm.[78]

More generally, search within the process space in the challenging case of schedules of all kinds is not just a matter of determining an "ideal" schedule but of scheduling that allows for flexibility, negotiation, and communication.

> Scheduling is not only a "production process," in which a schedule is created or adapted, but also a "service process," in which information is collected and delivered, interests and trade-offs are discussed, and constraints or commitments are negotiated. Thus, alongside schedule-focused criteria, the functioning of the schedulers and the way in which scheduling activities are executed are important factors in determining scheduling performance.[79]

Our final two examples draw our thinking about creativity and change first nearer, into, and around our bodies through an illustration of search in the process of choreographing a new dance and then briefly extend it out to the far-reaching scale of international economic and environmental policy innovation.

Imagine that you are a choreographer of a contemporary dance troupe. You are scratching about for new ideas. How might you communicate possible new ideas to the dancers? How might they communicate with you?

Wayne McGregor and the dance company Random Dance were observed and examined in detail to discover the working processes of a choreographer as a new contemporary dance piece was being developed. This study revealed a diverse set of approaches to the communication of evolving or nascent ideas.[80] Over a course of eight weeks the dance troupe worked on an emerging dance piece. They created in the absence of both the specially commissioned music and the set (both of which were yet to be created), with music available but not explicitly used to generate dance phrases.

The communication of intentions was much more than verbal and was physically diverse. The choreographer often concurrently used speech with its own emphasis or phrasing together with touch and gestures, other vocalizations, and dance itself including changes of position. These *multimodal communications* allowed touch to coexist with vocalization or words to coexist with gesture, permitting new meanings to emerge from their combinations.

Words and syntax were used to convey forms, general tempo, mood, and the manner in which a role was to be performed. Intonation or prosody was used to convey especially subtle nuances of shape, tempo, and mood. In addition to designating forms, gesture was employed to modify forms and illustrate the dynamics of form. To incite, correct, or reshape a posture or movement and to show a pivot point, the choreographer often used touching. Touch was typically used not to denote or describe a movement or dynamic but rather to change the way the dancers moved.

"In a physical context such as dance, where the structures being created are dynamics of form and position, it is natural to see touch used as a tool for sketching, shaping or correcting."[81] Calling out phrases, and vocalizations such as "N'yahh uh oom" or "Tri dah day" were used to convey information about form and feeling or to help the dancers remember the dynamics of a phrase. Dancing itself was used to imitate a form, often in an idealized manner. The concurrent use of these many combinations and forms of communication over a creatively focused period of only five minutes is shown schematically in Figure 6.3.

Although the choreographer did spend a portion of the instructional time using his own body to display the dynamics and structure of a move, either dancing with or facing the troupe while they reproduced the move, such *showing* occurred only about 7.5 percent of the time. Almost a third

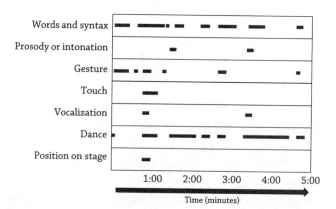

Figure 6.3 THE MANY FORMS OF COMMUNICATING WHILE CREATING A NEW DANCE. While developing a new dance piece, a choreographer used seven different types of physical communication extensively, often employing multiple approaches concurrently. Shown is a schematic of the combinations and forms of communication used over a five-minute period.[82]

of instructional time (30.5 percent) was devoted to *make-ons*—a process whereby the bodies of specific dancers were used, so to speak, as "creative material" with which to show the dynamics and form of a phrase or move.

Most of the instructional time (62 percent) was used in *tasking*—in which the dancers were presented with particular problems or tasks to work on, usually requiring them to create and sustain mental imagery. They might, for instance, imagine themselves moving a heavy bell about while encircling it with both arms, or imagine the feeling of being caressed on the shoulder. Or they might evoke, through gesture, the skyline of Manhattan. Throughout, the dancers strived not only to think of the concepts to be conveyed but also to closely integrate those concepts with emotion, perception, and action.

The process of *tasking* enables dancers to discover ways in which to represent a given concept or experience. If the dancer generates a novel possibility through such tasking, he or she learns new moves and the choreographer can see new things that the dancer can do.

> By assigning the dancers problems to solve they stretch their repertoire more effectively—they discover new ways of moving themselves . . . if a movement originated as a solution to a problem, the dancers are likely to imbue it with greater feeling, affect or quality—what some call greater intentionality; they will find the phrase easier to remember; and they will have intellectual "anchors" that can serve as reference points in the phrase later.[83]
>
> —*Creative cognition researcher professor David Kirsh and colleagues*

In *making on*, the dancers and choreographer engage in an embodied conversational back-and-forth dialogue. This process leads to uniquely individuated movements and phrasing as an emergent combination of what the choreographer intends and the dancer realizes. The explicitly and purposefully intended moves of the choreographer meet with the implicitly subtle differences of accents and emphases that arise as the dancers, in their own way, attempt to make real that intention in the physical world. The dancers accomplish this with their own particular bodies, with all their particular strengths and capabilities, quirks and qualities. Like tasking, making on is a "mechanism for fostering novelty. In a make on, [the choreographer] uses another dancer's body in place of his own. The phrase that emerges invariably reflects something of the personal style of the dancer and something of the body style."[84]

From the perspective of search, tasking is an especially individuated approach that recognizes the varied idea landscapes of the dancer
and dancers across time. It calls upon the dancer's imagination and rich
experience-near memories, including private or idiosyncratic notions and
the perception-action cycle. Tasking has the further benefit of drawing on
the self-generation of an idea or action, with self-produced ideas leading
to enhanced memory for those ideas through what is known as the generation effect.[85] Although tasking has the highest potential for generating truly
novel outcomes, it is also more risky, with some tasks yielding little or no
direct benefit for the evolution of a creative piece. By contrast, showing is the
least risky but also the least generative of fully novel ideas, with the likely
benefits of "making on" falling in between.

Asking two or more dancers to recall and enact a given phrase or movement may be a form of parallel prototyping. Parallel "making on" can open
the way for detail stepping and effective comparison and contrasts, where
various dancers each recall and especially express and embody particular
aspects of a more general phrase. By relying on multiple instantiations of a
given dance phrase, this process can also invoke a form of distributed or collective memory and thinking.

The creation of a new dance piece, as in the creation of any work of art or
design, faces clear trade-offs between reliably repeating with smaller variations vs. engaging in more risk-laden experimentation and searching farther
afield. Our best creative endeavors find an optimal adaptability corridor that
contextually permits both wise repetition and novel exploration.

We close this section by briefly and suggestively drawing an analogy
between our five-part iCASA thinking framework and recent calls for a new
economic or environmental policy mindset that is driven toward *experimentally discovering* policy innovations. In complex adaptive systems, especially
involving common-pool resources in fisheries, forestry, and irrigation, contributing players and stakeholders are involved at multiple scales, small,
medium, and large. Various players interact and communicate (including
across information networks and through monitoring systems) both nearby
and farther away in time and space. Given this complexity, the policy design
process should take advantage of a multilevel trial-and-error approach,
"involving an effort to tinker with a large number of component parts . . .
Those who tinker with any tools—including rules—try to find combinations that work together more effectively than other combinations."[86] The
approach begins open-mindedly, from a position that is relatively agnostic
about what works and what does not work. The new policy mindset leans
toward being *diagnostic* rather than *prescriptive*—seeking particularly
to empirically identify local constraints and bottlenecks. It emphasizes

experimentation in all of its forms together with evaluation and receptivity to feedback and searches for contextually modulated adaptations and unique opportunities for change. The mindset recognizes the importance of encompassing a wide range in level of detail, such that there is no "one-size that fits all." Although it may seem difficult to imagine an experimental approach to very large-scale economic policy, this may in part depend on how narrowly or rigidly we understand "experimentation" and "search."

> What, then, does it mean to be a macrodevelopment economist and an experimentalist at the same time? There is no contradiction here as long as "experimentalism" is interpreted broadly, and not associated solely with randomized evaluations. Experimentalism in the macro context refers simply to a predisposition to find out what works through policy innovation. The evaluation of the experiment need be only as rigorous as the policy setting allows. Some of the most significant gains in economic development in history can in fact be attributed to precisely such an approach.[87]
>
> —*Economist and international development expert Dani Rodrik*

GOING FORWARD

We invite you, going forward, to treat our thinking framework just as we have seen Alice Munro does as she reads a story:

> I go into it, and move back and forth and settle here and there, and stay in it for a while. It's more like a house. Everybody knows what a house does, how it encloses space and makes connections between one enclosed space and another and presents what is outside in a new way.[88]

We invite you to live with the thinking framework as though it were a volumetric space, like a house, where you can move about, and feel at home in various rooms, looking out, pausing, acting, sharing and learning with others, and richly experiencing within and without.

The thinking framework is a structure (not simply a list) because it allows us to organize and relate many ideas, including new ideas. The thinking framework is a type of structure for integrating and interrelating the many moving "parts" of our idea making and finding, thus forming something that is greater than the sum of their parts: creating a space/home for our making-finding creative and change efforts.

Going forward in our individual and collective efforts for creativity and change, the thinking framework is meant to provide us with greater options and interconnected options for beginning anew, staying on course, and restarting or changing direction in our thinking/making/creating because we understand more about the strengths and limits of contributors to our thinking and how they interplay.

Let's briefly return to the five questions of the thinking framework that we asked at the outset. In particular, let's now consider how several broader themes that we have encountered throughout this book could be incorporated into the framework, realizing that much of what we have learned does not fall neatly under a single question but may span two or more of the framework's questions.

Q1: What ideas are competing for your attention and awareness—and how are you helping to form and *re*-form them?

Q2: Are you aptly zooming in and zooming out?

Q3: Do you allow room for both spontaneity *and* deliberateness in your thinking?

Q4. As you think, are you using the full interplay not only of concepts but also of sensing, feeling, and well-chosen action goals?

Q5. How do you invite your environments and your "thinking tools" to creatively partner with you?

Based on what we have learned, we invite you to think of the thinking framework as a pathway to:

• Encourage us to be more understanding of our own thinking/making/creating process and the processes of others, asking us to be more patient with our own and others' thinking, more tolerant of the apparent indirection and waywardness of thinking, and more ready to notice when we should just let "thinking run" by itself and when and how we should intervene. [Think of Q3—together with Q4.]

• Enrich our awareness of the myriad ways in which we can zoom in and zoom out in our ideas and making: choosing, adjusting, extracting, and combining abstractions; stepping up and stepping down into the densely packed realms of our experiences in all their sensory-perceptual, emotional, and motivational complexity through analogy, prototyping, mental simulation, and reflective verbalization. [Think of Q2 together with Q4 and Q5.]

• Help us to value our times in between and our open goals: once we recognize a snag or a gap we can stay attuned and on "automatic" lookout for ways to address it; we do not get stymied by that one thing (the snag or gap), and may continue working and playing and experimenting elsewhere without dwelling on it yet also neither dismissing nor diminishing the snag or gap. [Think of Q3 and how it bridges to both Q4 and Q5.]

- Recognize how we create and update shared mental models, and the ways that motivations, emotions, and perceptions meld with concepts when we are "heedful" of each other in our creative endeavors. [Think of Q1 concurrently with Q5 and Q4, and also Q2 and Q3.]
- Be ever cognizant of the immense permeability (and reliance) of thinking on our environments, and how thinking emerges in our bodies in action, in our ongoing making and finding (the perception-action cycle); environments have more than literal dimensions: they can seep into our thinking *processes* as well as into the *content* of our thinking. [Think of Q5, and then Q1, and then Q4 with Q2 and Q3.]
- Attune us to emotion and motivation as "informational aids" for our thinking and making; motivation is neither simple nor one-dimensional but rather multifaceted and changing; reimmersion in our creative endeavors brings its own momentum. [Think of Q1 and Q4, concurrently.]
- Harness the creative energy and direction that goals can offer us through the process of goal tuning, including understanding our goals at different levels of specificity and being tolerant of our need, at times, for "goal babbling"—experimenting to find our next steps or next direction that is in keeping with our values over time. [Think of Q2, then Q3, then Q4, then Q1, or other orderings?].
- Be more understanding of what our brains do for us and how they do it: our brains are highly collaborative and interconnected and dynamically responsive to changing contexts and goals. The brain is exquisitely attuned to our interconnected need for flexibility *and* stability. [Think of Q5, together with Q4 and Q1.]
- Sensitize us to the forms and timing of our encounters with information and our sharing and exchange of thoughts and ideas: as organizations (and individuals) we may develop our "absorptive capacity"—a receptive network of concepts and ideas and an open orientation to experience that enables us to see value in new ways of doing and thinking. Teams and organizations have knowledge and memories too (procedural, emotional, transactional) of what they have experienced directly and what they have observed/experienced indirectly. [Think of Q1 in conjunction with both Q4 and Q5.]

- Equip us with ways of understanding, adopting, and changing constraints: deliberately choosing and altering our own constraints—questioning our constraints as a way to open up opportunities and aptly channel our efforts and attention. [Think especially of Q2 and Q3 in interplay.]

- Point to how learning to vary introduces degrees of newness and awakens our attention; how variation allows us to use what we already know but extend it, cumulatively expanding our repertoire of action/thought possibilities by providing "rewards" (reinforcement, encouragement, incentives) and opportunities (occasions, invitations) to try out variations in the tried and true and to try again differently. [Think of Q5 as an entry to Q1 and Q4.]

- Remind us to neither overvalue nor undervalue newness, asking ourselves how much "newness" is needed here: should we wisely repeat, shift our emphasis, offer a new interpretation, or begin afresh? We keep good strategies and approaches alive and part of our idea landscapes by not letting them become completely submerged with "new" input. [Think first of Q3, and then of Q1 with Q4.]

- Move us beyond views of creativity as simply bursts of insight and avoiding a too exclusive emphasis on the "front-end" processes of idea generation: ideas are formed and constructively shaped and modified across time. Our creative persistence ("staying the course") is itself flexible and takes many forms over and across time, revising, reenvisioning, returning to our projects in different frames of mind and at different times, allowing for successive unfolding and greater precision/definiteness of our ideas and not asking for too much certainty or too much "resolution" too soon. [Think of all of the framework questions: what seems to be about Q1 broadens into and implicates Q3, and Q5, and Q2, and Q4.]

Thinking works across time from milliseconds to minutes to hours, days, weeks, years, and decades or more. On all of these time scales our minds, brains, and environments are continual partners in our idea worlds. Thinking is an ongoing lifelong discovery process: our thinking about thinking changes our own thinking and that of others as we grow and edge forward, questioning and requestioning, making, finding, and making again.

We trust that the thinking framework that we have developed and explored here will provide us all with new conceptual leverage as we individually and collectively reach toward our futures—making and finding our way toward ever more equitable, freedom-enhancing, truth-seeking, and enduring ways of working, playing, and creating together.

~~~~~~

 Creativity Cross Checks and Queries

Questions to encourage reflection and connections to your own work and practice:

⇒ What aspects of your creative and generative goals could benefit from "goal tuning"?
  - Do you feel fragmented across too many goals?
  - Are your "aims in view" clear?
  - Are your goals (individual and team and organizational) delineated at a level of detail that allows both making and finding?
  - Are your goals flexible guides?
  - Are you demanding too much or too literal a type of progress from each step you take?
⇒ Do your goals have sufficient "elbow room"?
  - How could you articulate your goals to yourself and others in ways that allow creative envisioning with sufficient but not excessive leeway? In thinking about your answer, consider this advice:

    Great team leaders . . . tend to use words about team purposes that are just a bit ambiguous, and they are likely to draw on stories, analogies, and metaphors to get the point across. Such linguistic devices, far more than any specific quantitative objective, encourage members to project their own interpretations onto what is being said and to develop their own images of the end states that are sought. Good direction for a work team is clear, it is palpable—but it also is incomplete.[89]
  - What are the advantages and disadvantages of the following approach of a major retailer, as captured in their one-page employee handbook for new employees, that stated:

    Welcome to Nordstrom. We're glad to have you with our Company. Our number one goal is to provide outstanding customer service. Set both your personal and professional goals high. We have great confidence in your ability to achieve them.

    Nordstrom Rules: Rule #1: Use good judgment in all situations. There will be no additional rules.

Please feel free to ask your department manager, store manager, or division manager any question at any time.[90]

⇒ Goals are not always readily dismissed or abandoned; unmet goals tend to persist or remain active for some time. This goal inertia underscores the importance of not adopting unnecessary, inappropriate, or "cluttering" goals.

- What are your strategies for setting aside goals?
- Clean breaks may be needed so you are not dwelling on goals that you should relinquish or let go of and to remove strong environmental cues to the goals. Do you find and make for yourself separate spaces (and times) where the cues surrounding you are predominantly creativity-related?
- To help you let go of a goal, have you tried mental simulation, imaging yourself in a different time or place?

⇒ Our innovations and change efforts do not always have the impact and reach that we anticipated, and sometimes ideas that are clearly good in theory are subverted or distorted in practice.

- What are your processes for checking that your innovations are indeed moving you toward your goals?
- Is your change effort targeted at the right level of a potential problem? Does your attempted change encourage and provide resources for creatively adaptive second-order problem solving?
- Does your change effort offer opportunities for the development of new group idea landscapes that are creative problem-solving idea-integration spaces? How could you make "pods" in your organization?
- "Experience should be used explicitly as an occasion for evaluating our values as well as our actions."[91] Do you make the space and time to "detail step up" and "detail step down" in your evaluations of your change and creative efforts?

⇒ Creativity and innovation require an ongoing collaboration among people, spaces, tools, and ideas.

- Are your tools collaborating well with you? Should you give your tools more of a voice, or a different voice, in your creative search?
- When are you introducing and intermixing novel exploration and wise repetition into your collaborations?
- Do you give your ideas the temporal spaces they need? What is the "tempo" of your making/finding and making again?
- Are you using "know when" and "know why" (as well as "know how" and "know what") to aptly contextually modulate when you

change your degree of control and when you alter your level of detail?

⇒ Are you prototyping widely enough: across not only objects or products, but also timescales, processes, and experiences? Consider this observation from a partner at IDEO, "In many ways, prototyping *is* the process. Increasingly, we're prototyping all aspects of a new venture—the technology, the business system, and the human experience—starting on day one."[92] Is making and finding an integral part of *all* of your creative processes and change initiatives?

This guide offers brief elaborations on selected key concepts and ideas encountered in this book. Like the "thought boxes," the guide is intended to prompt and provoke insights into our creative thinking processes and the dynamics of change and innovation.

abstraction. In the process of abstraction we focus our attention on certain aspects of an object, situation, event, or process, and temporarily ignore others. Abstraction enables us to categorize objects, actions, and experience by grouping them on one or more dimensions and setting aside other aspects. There are many degrees of abstraction. Think of a healthy pine tree: it is a living thing, a plant, a softwood, and an evergreen; it may also be a white pine or a red pine. From alternative perspectives it might be part of a windbreak, a source of timber, a food source for birds, or a means of producing resin or pine tar. For different purposes and goals we might choose to focus on any one of these abstractions. Abstraction applies to concepts but also to our emotions, motivations, and perceptions.

action or goal identification. Any action and intended action (goal) can be thought of at many levels of abstraction. As you are reading this entry, many things are going on at once. You are moving your eyes across the page, comprehending a sentence, and trying to better understand a concept. Each of these is a description or identification of your action or goal. Relatively lower levels of action or goal identification typically concern *how* an action is done (e.g., moving your eyes across the page). Comparatively higher levels of action or goal identification often concern *why* an action is done or the effects of an action (e.g., trying to better understand a concept). Identifying our actions and goals at the right level of abstraction for a particular context allows us to be more mentally flexible and creative.

adaptive expertise. Individuals or teams who develop greater and greater skill in a relatively narrow area or field, leading to increased efficiency and automatization in solving familiar problems, are exhibiting routine expertise. In contrast, individuals or teams show adaptive expertise when they exhibit not only routine expertise but also a capacity for flexibly extending that expertise to novel contexts, leading to increased efficiency *and* increased innovation.

affordances. Affordances are pairings of an object or situation with an intended or possible action. An affordance signals or makes salient opportunities for us to take action. A handle on a cup affords holding the cup, and could (depending on the design) afford the stacking of cups within cups. A tree branch may afford swinging for a young child but not for a heavier adult. The symbolic representations we use also carry affordances, making it easier or harder to think through a problem (e.g., a topographical map may facilitate our ability to find a less steep downhill route).

associative cuing. Associative cuing is the prompting of an idea, or the noticing of a relation, often spontaneously or with little effort. Associative cues gently jog our thinking in different directions (beneficial or harmful) and can take the form of the words we hear or encounter or things we see and touch. A visual pattern might evoke a sense of dynamic rhythm, or weaving grasses in the wind might evoke the idea of oceans. Associative cuing is based in the highly distributed, connected, and overlapping nature of our mental representations. Associations vary in their strength and semantic remoteness, with more remote associations often generating greater creativity. Associations can involve perceptions, emotions, motivations, or actions and may be about objects or relations.

biologically inspired design. Biologically inspired design, also referred to as *biomimicry*, or *biomimesis*, is a creative process that draws on analogies from biological systems to identify novel solutions to challenging problems in engineering, computer science, architecture, or other fields. Biologically inspired design involves emulating natural models, systems, and processes to solve human problems.

control dialing (degrees of cognitive control). This is a metaphorical expression we use to designate altering or adjusting our degree of cognitive control in our concepts, emotions, perceptions, and motivations/goals. Adjustments or changes in our degrees of mental control may be deliberately selected or indirectly or directly induced through our environments. No one point on the continuum of cognitive control (deliberate to spontaneous to automatic) is invariably appropriate across all contexts. It is possible to be overcontrolled as well as undercontrolled, and we typically move repeatedly between greater and lesser degrees of cognitive control during our creative pursuits.

creativity. There are several dimensions to creativity. Beyond the often noted dimensions of novelty and usefulness, creativity is frequently generative and influential: "generative [in] that it leads to other ideas or things; influential [in] that it expands a domain or area of knowledge ... changing the way other people look at, listen to, think about, or do things like it."[1] Another important and overlooked dimension of creativity may be cohesiveness. "Novelty and usefulness alone may not sufficiently measure creativity, especially at the abstract conceptual level. Many suggest that the wholeness, clarity, elaboration, or *cohesiveness* of an idea must also be considered."[2]

Although many propose distinctions between creativity and innovation, such as suggesting that creativity involves the generation of ideas and innovation involves the application or realization of ideas (including also adapting ideas in use elsewhere), the view of creativity that we develop throughout this book does not propose such a sharp distinction. Making and finding and the perception-action cycle apply to both creativity and innovation. Generating, forming, refining, and successively realizing our ideas continually interplay and iteratively inform each other.

default-mode network. The default-mode network is a set of functionally connected brain regions with "hubs" that densely connect widely distributed regions in the brain. A "fundamental function of the default network is to facilitate flexible self-relevant mental explorations—simulations—that provide a means to anticipate and evaluate upcoming events before they happen."[3] The default-mode network is often active during *times in between* and has been found to contribute to remembering our personal past (autobiographical memory), imagining events or scenarios that may occur in the future, and thinking about the thoughts of others. The name "default mode" derives from the initial discovery that this interconnected brain network was often active "by default," active even when research participants during brain scanning did not have a specific task that they were to be performing. For a schematic depiction, see Figure 3.6.

design (designing). "Designing is a process of trying out *meaning-establishing moves* ... An initial idea, a 'frame' of meaning, is posited and put into play in the design *process*. But then the designer enters into a 'frame experiment,' a 'dialogue,' with the materials of the situation. In the process the designer makes tentative operational moves and the materials 'talk back,' to the designer, constraining and shaping subsequent moves." Design can be seen as having three key properties: it is opportunistic, exploratory, and incremental, requiring that earlier and later decisions cohere with one another. Design is opportunistic in that "it is not performed using a fixed set of operators applied in an ordered way. Design is a process wherein various design activities occur in an opportunistic manner, either top-down or bottom-up." Design is exploratory because "typically, the initial description of the solution is incomplete and/or ambiguous and/or inconsistent." The incremental nature of the design process often calls for reversing or refining earlier decisions both within an individual and across a design team.[4]

design fixation. Design fixation is the "sometimes counterproductive adherence to a limited set of ideas in the design process."[5] Design fixation may be unwittingly prompted by the provision of examples or samples. Considering multiple examples rather than only one or two may help to counteract design fixation.

design heuristics. Design heuristics are useful approaches or cognitive strategies to speed up or facilitate the generation of ideas during the design process. They help to "take the designer to a different part of [the] space of potential design solutions. Design heuristics are transformational strategies that take a concept, such as a form, and introduce systematic variation. Each heuristic requires specific features within the design problem in order to be applicable, and produces a changed concept altered in a specific fashion."[6] Design heuristics are a powerful type of *thinking scaffolding* that prompt us to vary our levels of specificity and our degrees of cognitive control.

detail stepping (levels of specificity). This is a metaphorical term we use to designate altering or adjusting our levels of detail or specificity in our concepts, emotions, perceptions, and motivations/goals. Adjustments or changes in our level of detail or abstraction may be deliberately selected, or indirectly or directly induced through our environments. No one level of the continuum of detail (abstract to midlevel to specific) is invariably appropriate across all contexts. It is possible to be too abstract as well as too detailed and we may move repeatedly between greater and lesser levels of specificity during our creative pursuits. To counteract an excessive valuing of abstraction and to underscore the remarkable contributions of concrete particulars throughout our creative processes we use the term "detail stepping," rather than abstraction stepping.

empathic design. This approach to creative design involves engaging in experiences that are explicitly intended "to help a designer empathize with customers under a variety of conditions, including non-ideal physical usage environments (e.g., noise or moisture) or strenuous user-product interactions, including physical, cognitive, or sensory-related situational disabilities."[7] The empathic design approach encourages both changes in our level of abstraction and induces us to fully draw upon the interplay of our feelings, sensations, and motivations.

environments (physical, social, symbolic, temporal). Our environments span time and space, and encompass the physical, social, and symbolic aspects of our experiences. Our creative and change efforts are dynamically shaped by our environments and depend on representations in multiple modalities (e.g., written symbols, two- and three-dimensional diagrams and objects, spoken words, intonation, or gestures).

executive control network. A set of functionally connected brain regions, with "hubs" that densely connect widely distributed regions in the brain, the executive control network as its name implies is comparatively "top-down" and important to the flexible control of attention, short-term working memory, and the tracking of our goals. It is primarily active during cognitively demanding activity such as novel problem solving, effortfully following complex rules or reasoning, and in resisting distraction or unhelpful habitual responses. For a schematic depiction, see Figure 3.5.

experience near/experience far. These two terms designate a dimension referring to the relative proximity of our autobiographical knowledge to specific or "one of a kind, one of a place" events that we have experienced. Representations that are experience near are more concrete and often unique; representations that are experience far are more abstract and cross-situational or general. We need immersion in the rich sensory-emotional particulars of our experiences yet we need, too, to travel across and combine them using abstractions, stepping down and up throughout our creative processes.

first-order versus second-order problem solving. First-order problem solving may involve a temporary "workaround" or problem-solving efforts that address an immediate problem or problematic situation but without necessarily addressing the longer-term, potentially systemic factors that gave rise to or caused the problem. Such second-order problem solving may require us to move up in level of abstraction out of the immediate context of a problem and change our degree of cognitive control to ensure that our immediate responses are not repeatedly or counterproductively automatic.

goal activation. Goal activation and goal deactivation refers to whether our goals come to mind (or can be held in abeyance) when we need them and in appropriate circumstances. Goal deactivation is important in allowing us to appropriately focus on the task at hand, without intrusions from goals that we hold but cannot at the moment pursue. Thinking that your home refrigerator needs repairs during a project meeting is likely an example of an insufficiently deactivated or bracketed goal. Keeping all of the task-relevant goals and subgoals activated in mind is a crucial contributor to successful complex reasoning and creative problem solving.

heedfulness. When teams work with one another heedfully, they interact "with each other carefully, critically, willfully and purposefully rather than habitually or without heed." "The more heed that is reflected in the pattern of interrelations, the greater is the capacity of the organization to comprehend unexpected events that evolve rapidly, because people are attuned to connecting and sharing ideas."[8]

iCASA thinking framework. See integrated Controlled-Automatic, Specific-Abstract thinking framework.

idea intersection space. "Idea intersection space" is a term we use to inclusively refer to opportunities for the coactivation and conjunctive emergence of ideas in a shared time and space. Idea intersection spaces may occur both within an individual and in groups and teams and are crucial in allowing cross connections, relations, and patterns across ideas to be noticed and articulated.

idea landscape. A term we use to refer to the relative ease of bringing to mind ideas (or intimations of ideas), from the past, present, or future, allowing them to newly form and emerge into our awareness. The landscape consists of "peaks and valleys," with information at the peaks currently within our conscious awareness and information in the valleys not currently readily accessible to us. At any one moment, some of our experiences may be *available* but not necessarily *accessible* to us (for example, in the tip-of-the-tongue phenomenon, we know a given fact or name, but are temporarily unable to effectively retrieve it).[9] Even in our short-term working memory, some ideas may be more directly accessible to us than others.[10]

ill-defined (versus well-defined) problem solving. "Sometimes the problems we face are well defined, such that the initial state of the presented problem, the desirable goal state, and the operators to implement the necessary steps to achieve the goal state are clear." Frequently, though, problems are ill defined. "When confronted with ill-defined problems, such as problems that require 'insight,' there is a lack of clarity regarding the goal state and the steps to be taken, and the solver frequently reaches an impasse in which he or she is very uncertain just how to proceed in approaching the problem."[11]

There is a clear temporal component to whether a given problem is more or less well structured, and some parts of a problem might be well structured but others not. As Herbert Simon—who proposed this distinction—incisively observed, "There is merit to the claim that much problem solving effort is directed at structuring problems, and only a fraction of it at solving problems once they are structured."[12]

implementation intentions. Implementation intentions involve acting deliberately at one time so as to do something more spontaneously or automatically at a later time. Implementation intentions are a form of strategic automatization in which we anticipate future contexts in which we will act to pursue a pending goal. They take the form "if situation X is encountered, then I will do Y." In implementation intentions, "the mental representation of the anticipated situation (specified in the if-component of the plan) becomes highly accessible when implementation intentions are formed.... This heightened accessibility leads to fast and accurate detection of good opportunities in which to act because people are 'perceptually ready' to encounter these opportunities."[13]

incubation. Incubation is one form of *times in-between* that allow productive fluctuations in the ideas that are readily accessible to us. Incubation typically involves "taking a distracting break when running into a dead end (impasse) in the solution process, and then returning to the problem, [which may prove] more efficient than working continuously for the same net duration."[14] Depending on the content of the problem and its complexity, as well as the type of intervening break, the benefits of a phase of incubation may partially be due to the forgetting or dissipation of misleading or incorrect structurings of a problem space or to the influx of new helpful cues or information.

innovation. See **creativity.**

integrated Controlled-Automatic, Specific-Abstract (iCASA) thinking framework. The thinking framework that forms the basis of this book. The iCASA framework emphasizes that ideas (concepts, emotions, perceptions, and motivations/goals) always occur in a multidimensional space with one key dimension of levels of specificity in representational content and another key dimension of degrees of control in mental processes. A central tenet of the framework is that our ability to reach, access, and use ideas in each of the four interrelated constituents of thinking (concepts, perceptions, emotions, and motivations/goals) is embedded within both our wider experiential environment (physical, social, and symbolic, extended across time and space), and dynamic brain functions and structures supporting mental representations and processes.[15] For a schematic depiction of the iCASA thinking framework see Figure 1.10.

intrinsic motivation and forms of extrinsic motivation. Although it is common to dichotomize extrinsic and intrinsic motivation, there is a continuum in the degree to which motivation is extrinsic. Some forms of extrinsic motivation, especially identified or "self-directed motivation," although extrinsic are characterized by a strong sense of autonomy. Identified or self-directed forms of extrinsic motivation are often crucial to creative endeavors by helping us to persist even when our work is not immediately stimulating or rewarding but is nonetheless essential to our creative goals. Intrinsic motivation and identified motivation "may work in a complementary fashion . . . Intrinsic self-regulation promotes a focus on the task itself and yields energizing emotions such as interest and excitement, whereas identification keeps one oriented toward the long-term significance of one's current pursuits and may foster persistence at uninteresting, but important, activities."[16] We may also be high in *both* intrinsic and extrinsic motivation at the same time.

making and finding. A concept that we use to broadly encompass dynamic alternations between phases of our *top-down* goal-directed efforts to create or effect change, and the comparatively more *bottom-up* open receptivity to the perceptual and other consequences our actions exert on our environments. Making (intending) and finding (discovering) is related to the perception-action cycle, but it is more explicitly focused on our creative and change endeavors and may also apply to our efforts to clarify and articulate our goals themselves.

mental contrasting. Mental contrasting is a problem-solving strategy in which people vividly bring to mind a desired future state *together with* current obstacles or impediments to the realization of that desire. Mental contrasting may be a way to help us discriminate between feasible and unfeasible goals.

mental simulation/perceptual simulation. Mental or perceptual simulations are imagined "workings through" of a possible future situation or actions. Although simulations are often visual, they may also involve other senses such as auditory, motoric, spatial, or kinesthetic imaginings. Such simulations are valuable ways of imagining and testing our ideas and the relations among ideas, and can substantively extend the ideas that we discover through tangible prototyping.

mind wandering/task-unrelated thinking. "Mind wandering" refers to thinking that is not directly linked to our here-and-now context or to "stimulus-independent" thoughts, images, and plans. Such thinking (frequently reflecting a decrease in our degree of mental control) may lead to task mistakes or stumblings in the short term. Yet, it can be beneficial in the longer term by helping us to anticipate upcoming situations with greater mental flexibility, a wider range of options in mind, and more tangible advance preparation.

perception-action cycle. This term, proposed by neuroscientist Joaquin Fuster,[17] refers to the continual dynamic interchange between our actions and our perception of what our actions have accomplished in the world. Our perceptions of the external environment guide our actions, and our actions lead to consequences; these, in turn change what we perceive and what our next moves might be. Cycling between acting and perceiving our environments (physical, social, symbolic) is fundamentally built into the ways our brains use, process, and extend our understandings and insights.

reflective verbalization. Reflective verbalization involves a process of asking ourselves or others to draw back from our creative endeavor, as if we are naïve, and to explain what we have done, and why or how we have done it. "A 'naive' person is a person who asks relevant questions out of curiosity, for instance open questions of the form why?, where?, what for?, how?, etc., without contributing directly to the content of the solution."[18] This process of explicit articulation can uncover new possible directions and insights.

representations. Broadly speaking, a representation is a re-presentation of one or more aspects of an object, event, process, or relation. Representations vary in their level of specificity or abstraction, and may be partial or ambiguous. We rely on both mental (internal) and environmental (external) representations and their combinations throughout our thinking and acting.

salience network. A set of functionally connected brain regions, with "hubs" that densely connect widely distributed regions in the brain, the salience network is important in directing and shifting our attention to important (salient) information of all forms. The salience network "initiates dynamic switching between the central-executive and default-mode networks, and mediates between attention to endogenous [internally-generated] and exogenous [externally-generated] events."[19] For a schematic depiction, see Figure 3.7.

sensemaking. "Sensemaking" refers to the ways in which teams, groups, and organizations collectively try to interpret their environment and arrive at shared understandings and projected actions. "Sensemaking is about labeling and categorizing to stabilize the streaming of experience.... If the first question of sensemaking is 'what's going on here?' the second, equally important question is 'what do I do next?' "[20]

thinking scaffoldings. This is a term we use to broadly designate any intentional queryings and quarryings of our thinking processes that are intended to help bootstrap (that is, "scaffold") our idea generation processes. They include formal design heuristics, reflective verbalizations, analogical search, and databases/tools for extracting and identifying promising ideas or directions.

times in between. This is our term for comparatively brief interludes or transitions between more focal intentional activities. Times in between can be brief, on the order of minutes. During times in between we often spontaneously experience shifts in the formation and accessibility of our ideas, including the accessibility of our goals, allowing the emergence of new perspectives or possibilities.

transactive memory. Transactive memory involves "the cooperative division of labor for learning, remembering, and communicating team knowledge."[21] This cooperative information sharing can be based on team roles, or on particular individuals. Developing transactive memory "involves the communication and updating of information members have about the areas of the other members' unique knowledge. Each member keeps track of other members' expertise, directs new information to the matching member, and uses that tracking to access needed information. . . . In this way, team members use each other as external memory aids, thereby creating a compatible and distributed memory system."[22]

PART 1

1. See, for example, Draganski, Gaser, Busch, Schuierer, Bogdahn, & May, 2004; Kempermann, 2008; Scholz, Klein, Behrens, & Johansen-Berg, 2009; Taubert, Villringer, & Ragert, 2012; Zatorre, Fields, & Johansen-Berg, 2012; for an extended review of the role of our environments in brain plasticity, see chapters 10 and 11 of Koutstaal, 2012.
2. The "timekeeping without clocks" experiment that we discuss over the next several pages is reported in Tseng, Moss, Cagan, & Kotovsky, 2008a,b.
3. Table 1.1 provides a schematic overview of the "timekeeping without clocks" experiment reported in Tseng, Moss, Cagan, & Kotovsky, 2008a,b.
4. Crane, Winder, Hargus, Amarasinghe, & Barnhoffer, 2012, p. 182.
5. Altmann, & Trafton, 2002; Eitam & Higgins, 2010; Fuster & Bressler, 2012; Kirsh, 1995; Klinger, 2013; Marsh, Hicks, & Bink, 1998; Moss, Kotovsky, & Cagan, 2007; Patalano & Seifert, 1997.
6. Tseng, Moss, Cagan, & Kotovsky, 2008a, p. 218.
7. P. P. Carson & K. D. Carson, 1993.
8. Wallas, 1926.
9. The study of the Chinese ink painter is reported by Yokochi & Okada, 2005.
10. The distinction between information that we know and is *available* to us, but may not (momentarily) be *accessible* to us was introduced in Tulving & Pearlstone, 1966. On the tip of the tongue experience, see, for example, Brown & McNeill, 1966. Our short-term working memory is typically 4 (plus or minus 1) items, or fewer, especially if the items are difficult to tag with words. Earlier estimations of short-term working memory being 7 (plus or minus 2) items were overestimations that included support from long-term memory, see Cowan, 2001; Nee & Jonides, 2014; Olsson & Poom, 2005. On variations in accessibility even within our short-term working memory, see Nee & Jonides, 2014. The metaphor of idea landscapes also is broadly based on the concept of our knowledge being represented in the connections and activation levels of neural networks. For a recent review of this perspective, see McClelland, Botvinick, Noelle, Plaut, Rogers, Seidenberg, & Smith, 2010.

11. The cartoon was created by David Waisglass and Gordon Coulthart, and originally published in 1993, as part of the syndicated newspaper cartoon, FARCUS.

12. The schematic depiction in Figure 1.3 is broadly based on Gabora, 2010.

13. See, for example, A. Clark, 2001, 2008; Duncan, 2010; Eccles, 2006; Miller & Cohen, 2001; Rubin, 1995.

14. See Conway, 2009; Dehaene & Changeux, 2011; Dehaene & Naccache, 2001; Eitam & Higgins, 2010; Horga & Maia, 2012; Maia & Cleeremans, 2005; Oberauer, 2009; Tulving & Pearlstone, 1966.

15. See, for example, Desroches, Newman, & Joanisse, 2009; Koutstaal, 2001.

16. For an analysis and review of the different ways that collective knowledge can be created and sustained, see Hecker, 2012. On the contribution of such factors as conversational turn-taking and social sensitivity to a group's "collective intelligence," see Woolley, Chabris, Pentland, Hashmi, & Malone, 2010.

17. Hackman, 2002, 2012.

18. DeChurch & Mesmer-Magnus, 2010a,b; DeFranco, Neill, & Clariana, 2011; see also Hinsz, Tindale, & Vollrath, 1997.

19. Weick, Sutcliffe, & Obstfeld, 2005. On the contributions of material objects to sensemaking for individuals and groups see Stigliani & Ravasi, 2012.

20. G. Klein, Moon, & Hoffman, 2006a, p. 71; see also G. Klein, Moon, & Hoffman, 2006b.

21. Weick, Sutcliffe, & Obstfeld, 2005, pp. 411 and 412.

22. G. Klein, Moon, & Hoffman, 2006a.

23. Battilana & Casciaro, 2012; Jain & Kogut, 2013; Leung & Chiu, 2010.

24. L. Cohen, 1992/2003, p. 340.

25. Munro & Awano, 2006, np.

26. See, for example, Atman, Chimka, Bursic, & Nachtmann, 1999; Atman, Yasuhara, Adams, Barker, Turns, & Rhone, 2008; Guindon, 1990.

27. See Wetzel, 2014; Wetzel, Anderson, Gini, & Koutstaal, in preparation.

28. Guindon, 1990, p. 320.

29. The schematic depiction in Figure 1.6 is adapted from Guindon, 1990.

30. The philosopher and psychologist William James spoke of "vicious abstractionism" to refer to a tendency to move too far away from concrete particulars and get lost in concepts and abstractions that are too simplistically extracted from and no longer anchored in our real experiences, including the experiences that gave rise to the concept in the first place. See William James, 1909/1978.

31. On solving the remote associates problems through insight or systematic search, see, for example, Bowden & Jung-Beeman, 2003; Subramaniam, Kounios, Parrish, & Jung-Beeman, 2009; Vartanian, 2009; see also K. A. Smith, Huber, & Vul, 2013. Although the remote associates task is often characterized as a convergent task, because there is (typically) a single correct answer, engaging in the word triplets task can call upon *both* divergent (more associative/inductive) and convergent (more analytic/deductive) thinking processes. In practice, creative thinking involves admixtures of divergent and convergent thinking processes, *together with* several other processes such as conceptual combination, analogy, mental imagery or perceptual simulation, and problem restructuring.

See, for example, Abraham, 2014; Benedek, Könen, & Neubauer, 2012; Gabora, 2010; Gilhooly, Fioratou, Anthony, & Wynn, 2007; Lee & Therriault, 2013. On the early distinction between divergent and convergent thinking, and other contributors to creative thinking, see Guilford, 1960. For a classic treatment of the associative bases of creativity, and an early introduction of the remote associates task, see Mednick, 1962.

32. Crump, 2013, p. 122.
33. The study on varying degrees of control in the operating room is reported in Moulton, Regehr, Lingard, Merritt, & MacRae, 2010.
34. On the interrelations between cognition, emotion, and motivation see, for example, Bechara, Damasio, & Damasio, 2000; Damasio, 1996; F. Dolcos, Iordan, & S. Dolcos, 2011; Fuster, 2006; Mesulam, 1998; Most, Chun, Johnson, & Kiehl, 2006; Pessoa, 2008; Pourtois, Notebaert, & Verguts, 2012.
35. For the research on thinking warmups see Chrysikou, 2006; Wen, Butler, & Koutstaal, 2013.
36. See Kaplan & Simon, 1990, and the Research Highlight "The 62-square checkerboard problem" in Part 2.
37. Lewis & Lovatt, 2013.
38. Colzato, Van den Wildenberg, & Hommel, 2013, p. 1012.
39. The recent study is reported by Wei, Yang, Li, Wang, Zhang, & Qiu, 2013. For more on the default-mode network see Figure 3.6 and accompanying discussion.
40. Woo, Chernyshenko, Longley, Zhang, Chiu, & Stark, 2014; Zenasni, Besançon, & Lubart, 2008.
41. See, for example, Carver, 2003, 2004; Forgas & George, 2001; Forgas & Eich, 2012; Schwarz & Clore, 1983.
42. See, for instance, Baas, De Dreu, & Nijstad, 2011; De Dreu, Baas, & Nijstad, 2008; Fong, 2006.
43. Rego, Sousa, Marques, & Cunha, 2012; Shrira, Palgi, Wolf, Haber, Goldray, Shacham-Shmueli, & Ben-Ezra, 2011. See also Amabile, Barsade, Mueller, & Staw, 2005; Forgas & Eich, 2012.
44. Isen & Daubman, 1984; Hirt, Levine, McDonald, & Melton, 1997; Kahn & Isen, 1993; see also Akbari Chermahini & Hommel, 2012; Ashby, Isen, & Turken, 1999; Binnewies & Wörnlein, 2011; Bonnardel, N. & Moscardini, 2012; Davis, 2009; Sakaki & Niki, 2011.
45. Baumann & Kuhl, 2002.
46. Estrada, Isen, & Young, 1997.
47. Okuda, Runco, & Berger, 1991; Vosburg, 1998.
48. Chermahini & Hommel, 2012.
49. See, for example, Chermahini & Hommel, 2012; Cools & D'Esposito, 2011; Davis, 2009. For an overview of research on the influence of motivational intensity on cognitive scope, see Harmon-Jones, Gable, & Price, 2013.
50. George, 2011; George & Zhou, 2007; Oettingen, Marquardt, & Gollwitzer, 2012.
51. Bledow, Rosing, & Frese, 2013.
52. Carnevale & Isen, 1986.
53. Rego, Sousa, Marques, & Cunha, 2012.
54. George, 2011.

55. See, for example, Bittner & Heidemeier, 2013; Higgins, 2000; Zhu & Meyers-Levy, 2007.

56. The idea of "pre-mortems" was proposed in Klein, 2007, and is discussed in Kahneman & Klein, 2009; see Kahneman, 2003, for a broader discussion of the "availability heuristic" in decision making; see also Roskes, De Dreu, & Nijstad, 2012, and our discussion of mental contrasting in Part 5.

57. Onarheim, 2012; Rosso, 2014; Stokes, 2009; M. Weiss, Hoegl, & Gibbert, 2011.

58. For the student speech anxiety reinterpretation study described in the following paragraphs, see Brooks, 2013.

59. Keynes, 2009, p. 102.

60. The benefits of a brief period of walking, whether indoors or outdoors, on creative idea generation were experimentally demonstrated by Oppezzo & Schwartz, 2014.

61. See, for example, A. Clark, 2001, 2008; Eccles, 2006; Kirsh, 1995.

62. Hunkin, 2013, np.

63. The study of how and when design teams used their environments is reported in Jang & Schunn, 2012.

64. Kozlowski & Ilgen, 2006, p. 85.

65. Gino, Argote, Miron-Spektor, & Todorova, 2010; Kozlowski & Ilgen, 2006.

66. Furr, Cavarretta, & Garg, 2012; Lakhani, Jeppesen, Lohse, & Panetta, 2007; Terwiesch & Xu, 2008; we consider innovation contests and competitions in Part 5.

67. On the perception-action cycle, see Fuster, 2006, 2009; Fuster & Bressler, 2012.

68. Clark, 2008, p. xxviii.

69. Figure 1.9 is broadly adapted from Fuster & Bressler, 2012.

70. Fuster, 2009, p. 2063.

71. See, for example, Badre & D'Esposito, 2007; Desai, Conant, Binder, Park, & Seidenberg, 2013; Mesulam, 1998.

72. Curlik & Shors, 2013; Kempermann, 2008. Recent findings also suggest that neurogenesis in adult humans may occur in the striatum, a subcortical region of the forebrain, including the caudate nucleus and putamen; see Ernst, Alkass, Bernard, Salehpour, Perl, Tisdale, Possnert, Druid, & Frisén, 2014.

73. Draganski, Gaser, Busch, Schuierer, Bogdahn, & May, 2004; Scholz, Klein, Behrens, & Johansen-Berg, 2009; Zatorre, Fields, & Johansen-Berg, 2012.

74. Mackey, Singley, & Bunge, 2013.

75. Mackey, Whitaker, & Bunge, 2012; Mackey, Singley, & Bunge, 2013.

76. Wilkin, 2006, np.

77. R. Smith, 2008, np.

78. Curlik & Shors, 2013; Kempermann, 2008; on the importance of engaging in novel challenging activities, see Tranter & Koutstaal, 2008.

79. Aimone, Deng, & Gage, 2011.

80. The iCASA thinking framework was first developed and elaborated in Koutstaal, 2012.

81. Figure 1.10 is adapted and revised from Koutstaal, 2012.

82. Figure 1.11 is adapted from Koutstaal, 2012.

PART 2

1. The example of folding and levels of abstraction in Figure 2.1 is adapted from Linsey, Markman, & Wood, 2012.
2. Hayes, Flower, Schriver, Stratman, & Carey, 1987.
3. Moore, 1955, p. 77.
4. Knuth, 2014, np.
5. The "think aloud" study of artists and nonartists is reported in Fayena-Tawil, Kozbelt, & Sitaras, 2011.
6. See, for example, Brainerd & Reyna, 1990, 2001; Brown, 1958; Reyna, 2012; Rosch, Mervis, Gray, Johnson, & Boyes-Braem, 1976; Winocur, Moscovitch, & Bontempi, 2010.
7. Conway, 2005; Conway 2009; Conway & Pleydell-Pearce, 2000; James, 1909/1978; Liberman & Trope, 2014; Renoult, Davidson, Palombo, Moscovitch, & Levine, 2012; Trope & Liberman, 2003, 2010.
8. The analogy from a ferryboat to a movable x-ray stand design is found in Kalogerakis, Lüthje, & Herstatt, 2010.
9. The philosopher and polymath C. S. Peirce pioneered the term "abduction" to describe forms of "hunch-like" inferential thinking that shade from perception to concepts; Peirce, 1901/1935.
10. Doyle, 1902/2006.
11. For the checkerboard problem experiment see Kaplan & Simon, 1990.
12. Kaplan & Simon, 1990, p. 413, original emphasis.
13. Weick, Sutcliffe, & Obstfeld, 2005, pp. 410 and 412.
14. Goel, Vattam, Wiltgen, & Helms, 2012, p. 882.
15. Gerber, McKenna, Hirsch, & Yarnoff, 2010, p. 3.
16. We thank Shane Hoversten for pointing us to the read-eval-print loop analogy.
17. The parallel prototyping experiment is described in Dow, Glassco, Kass, Schwarz, Schwartz, & Klemmer, 2010.
18. Figure 2.5 is a schematic depiction of the method and results of Dow, Glassco, Kass, Schwarz, Schwartz, & Klemmer, 2010.
19. On the importance of juxtaposing contrasting cases see Schwartz & Bransford, 1998.
20. See Dow, Glassco, Kass, Schwarz, Schwartz, & Klemmer, 2010.
21. Jansson & Smith, 1991; Marsh, Landau, & Hicks, 1996; Marsh, Ward, & Landau, 1999; Perttula & Sipilä, 2007; S. M. Smith, Ward, & Schumacher, 1993.
22. Jansson & Smith, 1991.
23. Linsey, Tseng, Fu, Cagan, Wood, & Schunn, 2010.
24. Linsey, Tseng, Fu, Cagan, Wood, & Schunn, 2010.
25. The value of a "scrutiny-reduced" making-and-finding team environment was demonstrated in a field experiment conducted in a very large Chinese factory that produced mobile phones. The factory had a massive open floor plan where the workers on the production lines and the supervisors were continually and readily seen. In the study, four production lines were randomly chosen to be surrounded by a privacy curtain. Over the course of several months, the privacy curtains increased improvisation, encouraged "productive deviance," and lead to higher productivity and quality—in part because the increase in team

privacy allowed temporary, smaller issues to be solved locally and it promoted collective team knowledge. The privacy curtain study is described in Bernstein, 2012. On creativity friendly environments, and prototyping our thinking/making spaces, see, for example, Doorley & Witthoft, 2012; McCoy & Evans, 2002; Oksanen & Ståhle, 2013.

26. Heath & Anderson, 2010, in an essay examining the many ways our environments can support our will; the quotation is found at pp. 244–245.

27. Larkin & Simon, 1987.

28. Kirsh, 1995.

29. See Koutstaal, 2001, for a broader discussion of words as physical objects with visual and auditory "edges."

30. The Scrabble example is based on Kirsh, 2011; the quotation appears in Kirsh, 2011, p. 4.

31. On making-finding as "back talk" with materials, see Schon, 1983.

32. Jang & Schunn, 2012.

33. On the role of models and model-based reasoning in the generation of novel concepts in science and conceptual innovation, see Nersessian, 2008.

34. See Barsalou, 1999, 2003.

35. The driving versus washing a car example is part of a study by Borghi, Glenberg, & Kaschak, 2004.

36. Borghi, Glenberg, & Kaschak, 2004; Clement, 2009; Trickett, Trafton, & Schunn, 2009; Vukovic & Williams, 2014; see also Barsalou, 1999.

37. See, for example, B. T. Christensen & Schunn, 2009; Foxley, 2010; Youmans, 2011.

38. On how our current use of an object may make it more difficult to see alternative possible uses, see Ye, Cardwell, & Mark, 2009.

39. See German & Defeyter, 2000; Ye, Cardwell, & Mark, 2009.

40. On five-year-olds' versus seven-year-olds' thinking of alternative uses of common objects, see Defeyter & German, 2003; German & Johnson, 2002.

41. Gilhooly, Fioratou, Anthony, & Wynn, 2007; see also Barsalou, 1999.

42. See Chrysikou, 2006; Wen, Butler, & Koutstaal, 2013. On the relation between our ability to move flexibly between different levels of abstraction in memory and on-the-spot novel problem solving, see Aizpurua & Koutstaal, 2010.

43. The term and concept of affordances was developed by the psychologist James J. Gibson, 1977, 1979/1986. The psychologist Donald A. Norman extensively applied the concept of affordances specifically to the design of everyday objects, and emphasized the continuing value of perceived affordances. As he noted, "Affordances specify the range of possible activities, but affordances are of little use if they are not visible to the users. Hence, the art of the designer is to ensure that the desired, relevant actions are readily perceivable. . . . Personally, I believe that our reliance on abstract representations and actions is a mistake and that people would be better served if we would return to control through physical objects, to real knobs, sliders, buttons, to simpler, more concrete objects and actions." D. A. Norman, 1999, pp. 41–42; see also D. A. Norman, 1988.

44. See Gero & Kannengiesser, 2012; Maier & Fadel, 2009.

45. See Guindon, 1990; Wetzel, Anderson, Gini, & Koutstaal, in preparation

46. The quotation of the painter and sculptor appears in Silbey, 2011, p. 2108.

47. See, for example, Beilock, & Goldin-Meadow, 2010; Broaders, Cook, Mitchell, & Goldin-Meadow, 2007; Schwartz & Black, 1996. For a discussion of gestures as "representational actors" within thinking see Koutstaal, 2012, pp. 154–161.

48. See Alibali & Goldin-Meadow, 1993; Alibali, Spencer, Knox, & Kita, 2011; Roth, 2000.

49. On the pervasive role of metaphor in how we think and act, see, for example, the seminal work of Lakoff & Johnson, 1980a,b; and Schon, 1963. For a recent experimental demonstration of how even apparently incidental metaphors can structure the direction of our thinking, see Thibodeau & Boroditsky, 2011. The quotation from William James occurs in 1890/1981, p. 233.

50. Vattam, Helms, & Goel, 2010; compare with the time-keeping design scenario we worked through in Part 1.

51. Kalogerakis, Lüthje, & Herstatt, 2010.

52. See Chan, Fu, Schunn, Cagan, Wood, & Kotovsky, 2011; B. T. Christensen & Schunn, 2007; Dahl & Moreau, 2002; Saner & Schunn, 1999; see also Fu, Chan, Cagan, Kotovsky, Schunn, & Wood, 2013.

53. See Kalogerakis, Lüthje, & Herstatt, 2010.

54. See Dunbar, 1995; Kalogerakis, Lüthje, & Herstatt, 2010.

55. Ball, Ormerod, & Morley, 2004.

56. Gassman & Zeschky, 2008.

57. See Benkler, 2006; Boudreau, Lacetera, & Lakhani, 2011; Boudreau & Lakhani, 2015; Jeppesen & Lakhani, 2010; Lakhani, Boudreau, Loh, Backstrom, Baldwin, Lonstein, … Guinan, 2013; Lakhani, Jeppesen, Lohse, & Panetta, 2007; Terwiesch & Xu, 2008.

58. On biologically inspired design, see, for example, Goel, Vattam, Wiltgen, & Helms, 2012; Vattam, Helms, & Goel, 2010; Vincent & Mann, 2002.

59. Nakrani & Tovey, 2004; Nakrani & Tovey, 2007.

60. See, for example, Alvarado-Iniesta, Garcia-Alcaraz, Rodriguez-Borbon, & Maldonado, 2013; Todorovic & Petrovic, 2013.

61. Werfel, Petersen, & Nagpal, 2014.

62. Werfel, Petersen, & Nagpal, 2014, p. 755.

63. We drew the examples of changing our abstraction levels and seeking "champion adaptors" from Helms, Vattam, & Goel, 2009.

64. I. Chiu & Shu, 2012.

65. Goel, Vattam, Wiltgen, & Helms, 2012; Mak & Shu, 2008; Shu, Ueda, Chiu, & Cheong, 2011; Wilson, Rosen, Nelson, & Yen, 2010; for overview, see Hayes, Goel, Tumer, Agogino, & Regli, 2011.

66. The concept of mental time travel, toward the past or the future, and the important related concept of episodic memory, was first developed by Endel Tulving. See, for example, Suddendorf & Corballis, 1997; Suddendorf & Redshaw, 2013; Tulving, 1983.

67. For overview and theoretical background, see Brainerd & Reyna, 1990; Parkinson, Liu, & Wheatley, 2014; Reyna & Brainerd, 1995; Trope & Liberman, 2003; 2010; Vallacher & Wegner, 1987; 1989; Watkins, 2011.

68. Atance & O'Neill, 2001; Christian, Miles, Fung, Best, & Macrae, 2013; Irish & Piguet, 2013; S. B. Klein, 2013; Renoult, Davidson, Palombo, Moscovitch, & Levine, 2012.

69. See, for example, Greenberg & Verfaellie, 2010; Schacter, Addis, & Buckner, 2007; Schacter, Addis, Hassabis, Martin, Spreng, & Szpunar, 2012; Szpunar, 2010.

70. Figure 2.9 is broadly schematically based on Conway, 2005; see also Renoult, Davidson, Palombo, Moscovitch, & Levine, 2012.

71. See, for example, Irish & Piguet, 2013; Raes, Hermans, Williams, Demyttenaere, Sabbe, Pieters, & Eelen, 2005; Rasmussen & Berntsen, 2010; Stöber, 1998; Stöber, Tepperwien, & Staak, 2000; Van Daele, Van den Bergh, Van Aundenhove, Raes, & Hermans, 2013; Williams, Barnhofer, Crane, Hermans, Raes, Watkins, & Dagleish, 2007.

72. The concept of action identification is developed in Vallacher & Wegner, 1987, 1989; for recent discussion see Watkins, 2011.

73. The ideas in Table 2.1 are based on Goldstone & Son, 2005. For a more recent practice-focused discussion on the value of varying our level of abstractness versus concreteness in various interpersonal and managerial settings, particularly through changing our "psychological distance," see Hamilton, 2015.

74. Meyer & Marion, 2010, p. 27.

75. Leveson, 2011, p. 61.

76. See, for example, Amalberti, Auroy, Berwick, & Barach, 2005; Espin, Lingard, Baker, & Regehr, 2006; Leveson, 2011; Tucker & Edmondson, 2003.

77. Fuster, 2006, 2009; Fuster & Bressler, 2012; see also Madl, Baars, & Franklin, 2011.

78. See, for example, Barsalou, 1999; Binder & Desai, 2011.

79. See, for example, Binder, & Desai, 2011; O'Craven & Kanwisher, 2000; Patterson, Nestor, & Rogers, 2007; Pulvermüller, 2013; Wheeler, Peterson, & Buckner, 2000.

80. Figure 2.10 is adapted from Patterson, Nestor, & Rogers, 2007, and Binder & Desai, 2011.

81. Figure 2.11 is schematically adapted from Fuster, 2006.

82. See, especially, Badre, 2008; Badre & D'Esposito, 2007; Badre, Kayser, & D'Esposito, 2010; Koechlin, Ody, & Kouneiher, 2003.

83. On abstraction and relational and analogical processing in anterior frontal regions see, for example, Green, Kraemer, Fugelsang, Gray, & Dunbar, 2012; Ramnani & Owen, 2004; Vartanian, 2012; Wendelken, Nakhabenko, Donohue, Carter, & Bunge, 2008. Findings from our own and other labs suggest that gradients of increasing abstraction likewise may be found in the temporal lobes with, for example, more abstract conceptual or semantic representations occurring in comparatively more anterior, relative to posterior, regions within the temporal lobes. See, for instance, Binney, Parker, & Lambon Ralph, 2012.

84. See, for example, Garoff, Slotnick, & Schacter, 2005; Koutstaal, Wagner, Rotte, Maril, Buckner, & Schacter, 2001; Marsolek, 1999; Simons, Koutstaal, Prince, Wagner, & Schacter, 2003.

85. On laterality differences in coarse- versus fine-grained semantic processing see Beeman, 1998; Beeman, Friedman, Grafman, Perez, Diamond, & Lindsay, 1994; Ben-Artzi, Faust, & Moeller, 2009; Seger, Desmond, Glover, & Gabrieli, 2000; Stringaris, Medford, Giora, Giampietro, Brammer, & David 2006; Yang, 2014; the example of "sourness" provided here is from Zeev-Wolf, Goldstein, Levkovitz & Faust, 2014. More generally, for a recent review on the joint contributions of left and right cerebral hemispheres to creative cognition in all its manifestations see Zaidel, 2013.

86. Smith, 2010, p. 3.

87. See, for example, Conway, 2005; Dickson & Moberly, 2013; Stöber, 1998; Stöber, Tepperwein, & Staak, 2000; Williams, Barnhofer, Crane, Hermans, Raes, Watkins, & Dagleish, 2007.

88. Addis, Wong, & Schacter, 2007; Marien, Aarts, & Custers, 2012; Schacter, Addis, & Buckner, 2007; Woolley, 2009.

89. Viola, 2007, p. 5.

90. Rodrik, 2009, p. 40.

91. Riley v. California, 2014, 134 S. Ct. 2473, at pp. 2488-2489.

92. Kirsh, 1995, p. 49.

PART 3

1. On degrees of cognitive control as a continuum see Bugg & Crump, 2012; Cleeremans & Jiménez, 2002; Dunwoody, Haarbauer, Mahan, Marino, & Tang, 2000; Dux, Roseboom, & Olivers, 2013; Hammond, Hamm, Grassia, & Pearson, 1987; Koutstaal, 2012, pp. 15-26; Zabelina & Robinson, 2010.

2. Block & Kremen, 1996; Nijstad, De Dreu, Rietzschel, & Baas, 2010; see also Mieg, Bedenk, Braun, & Neyer, 2012.

3. For the "expected value of control" account, see Shenhav, Botvinick, & Cohen, 2013. For broader conceptual perspectives on factors influencing cognitive control, see Job, Dweck, & Walton, 2010; Leary, Adams, & Tate, 2006.

4. For overview, see Koutstaal, 2012, pp. 190-214; Zabelina, Robinson, & Anicha, 2007; Zimbardo & Boyd, 1999.

5. Tangney, Baumeister, & Boone, 2004.

6. See, for example, Berman, Jonides, & Kaplan, 2008; Block & Kremen, 1996; Zimbardo & Boyd, 1999.

7. See, for example, Bocanegra & Hommel, 2014; Olivers & Nieuwenhuis, 2006; Su, Bowman, & Barnard, 2011; Taatgen, Juvina, Schipper, Borst, & Martens, 2009.

8. Bocanegra & Hommel, 2014, p. 1249.

9. Anderson, 1983; Collins & Loftus, 1975; Neely, 1977; Yaniv & Meyer, 1987.

10. Martindale & Dailey, 1996.

11. Kvavilashvili & Mandler, 2004; Mandler, 1994.

12. Basadur, 1995; Basadur, Graen, & Green, 1982; Ellamil, Dobson, Beeman, & Christoff, 2012; Gabora, 2010.

13. Groves, Vance, Choi, & Mendez, 2008.

14. Smallwood, Brown, Baird, & Schooler, 2012.

15. Vartanian, Martindale, & Kwiatkowski, 2007, p. 1471, emphasis added.

16. Zabelina & Beeman, 2013, p. 7. See also Zabelina & Robinson, 2010. For a recent review and discussion of the role of shifting between comparatively more generative and comparatively more evaluative modes of processing in creative thinking, and varied dual process models as applied to creativity, see Sowden, Pringle, & Gabora, 2015.

17. Fuster, 2006, 2009; Schon & Wiggins, 1992.

18. Gollwitzer, 1999; Gollwitzer & Sheeran, 2006.

19. Wieber, Thürmer, & Gollwitzer, 2012. For a recent set of suggestions on how to use if-then thinking in teams, see Halvorson, 2014.

20. On "strategic automatization," see Gollwitzer & Schall, 1998, and Gallo, Keil, McCulloch, Rockstroh, & Gollwitzer, 2009. On implementation intentions broadly, see, for example, Brandstätter, Lengfelder, & Gollwitzer, 2001; Gollwitzer, 1999; Seifert & Patalano, 2001.

21. See, for example, Oettingen, 2012; Oettingen, Pak, & Schnetter, 2001.

22. Kvavilashvili & Mandler, 2004; Mandler, 1994.

23. See, for example, Baird, Smallwood, Mrazek, Kam, Franklin, & Schooler, 2012; Sio & Ormerod, 2009.

24. On the tip of the tongue experience, see R. Brown & McNeill, 1966; Maril, Wagner, & Schacter, 2001.

25. See, for example, May, 1999; May & Hasher, 1998.

26. Wieth & Zacks, 2011.

27. On a proposed application of times in between to professional work settings, see Elsbach & Hargadon, 2006.

28. Carver, 2004.

29. Bolte, Goschke, & Kuhl, 2003; Subramaniam, Kounios, Parrish, & Jung-Beeman, 2009.

30. See, for example, Gilhooly, Georgiou, & Devery, 2013; Sio & Ormerod, 2009; Wallas, 1926.

31. On the role of sleep in facilitating abstraction, see Oudiette, Antony, Creery, & Paller, 2013; Stickgold & Walker, 2013; Wagner, Gals, Haider, Verleger, & Born, 2004.

32. Eaglestone, Ford, Brown, & Moore, 2007, p. 454.

33. Killingsworth & Gilbert, 2010.

34. Smallwood & Andrews-Hanna, 2013.

35. See, for example, Baird, Smallwood, & Schooler, 2011; Finnbogadóttir & Berntsen, 2013; Klein, Robertson, Delton, & Lax, 2012; Schacter, Addis, & Buckner, 2007.

36. Munro, 1982, p. 224.

37. The salt-and-pepper design heuristics study is reported in Yilmaz, Seifert, & Gonzalez, 2010.

38. Yilmaz, Seifert, & Gonzalez, 2010, p. 338.

39. Yilmaz & Seifert, 2009.

40. Yilmaz, Seifert, & Gonzalez, 2010.

41. The notion of see-move-see is developed in Schon, 1983; Schon & Wiggins, 1992.

42. Yilmaz & Seifert, 2009.

43. The portable solar cooker design study is found in Daly, Yilmaz, Christian, Seifert, & Gonzalez, 2012.

44. Figure 3.4 is schematically based on Yilmaz and Seifert, 2009.

45. Abbott, 2004.

46. Fullbright, 2014, np.

47. Schon & Wiggins, 1992, p. 135.

48. Vallacher & Wegner, 1987; Vallacher & Wegner, 1989; Watkins, 2011.

49. On the concept of deliberate practice, see Ericsson, 2008; Ericsson, Krampe, & Tesch-Römer, 1993.

50. For research and discussion of recognition-primed decision making see, for example, Fadde, 2006; 2009; G. A. Klein, 1993, 2008.

51. Moulton, Regehr, Lingard, Merritt, & MacRae, 2010.

52. Moulton, Regehr, Lingard, Merritt, & MacRae, 2010, p. 1577, emphasis added.

53. The characterization of the preconditions for flow states is found in Nakamura & Csíkszentmihályi, 2002, p. 90.

54. For seminal research and discussion of flow states see Csíkszentmihályi, 1990; 1996; Keller & Bless, 2008; Nakamura & Csíkszentmihályi, 2002.

55. Baumann & Scheffer, 2011.

56. Hefferon & Ollis, 2006; J. J. Martin & Cutler, 2002; Wrigley & Emmerson, 2013.

57. de Manzano, Theorell, Harmat, & Ullén, 2010.

58. For a pioneering characterization of absorption as "total" attention, "involving a *full commitment of available perceptual, motoric, imaginative and ideational resources*," see Tellegen & Atkinson, 1974, p. 274 (original emphasis). On the ways that short-term meditation may improve our attention and also alter the interaction of the central and autonomic nervous system, see Tang, Ma, Wang, Fan, Feng, Lu, . . . Posner, 2007; Tang, Ma, Fan, Feng, Wang, Feng, . . . Fan, 2009.

59. On the importance of keeping track of our goals and subgoals, and precisely where we are in the sequential steps of a multistep complex task, see Altmann, & Trafton, 2002; on the interconnected brain regions and changing ensembles of neurons that help to encode, maintain, and then deactivate subgoals as we move through a multistep procedure, see Duncan, 2010. For the essay writing study see Foroughi, Werner, Nelson, & Boehm-Davis, 2014. We thank Ben Denkinger for prompting us to elaborate on the various forms of "task switching."

60. König & Waller, 2010.

61. On our goals and mental processing in the background of our awareness, see Ellwood, Pallier, Snyder, & Gallate, 2009; Gallate, Wong, Ellwood, Roring, & Snyder, 2012; Klinger, 2013.

62. Beeftink, van Eerde, & Rutte, 2008.

63. Madjar & Oldham, 2009.

64. Ivanovski & Malhi, 2007; Jha, Krompinger, & Baime, 2007; see Horan, 2009, for review.

65. Tang, Ma, Fan, Feng, Wang, Fen, . . . Fan, 2009; Tang, Ma, Wang, Fan, Feng, Lu, . . . Posner, 2007. See also Grant, Duerden, Courtemanche, Cherkasova, Duncan, & Rainville, 2013.

66. Colzato, Ozturk, & Hommel, 2012.

67. Ostafin & Kassman, 2012.

68. Wenk-Sormaz, 2005, p. 53.

69. Luchins, 1942.

70. Greenberg, Reiner, & Meiran, 2012.

71. Greenberg, Reiner, & Meiran, 2012.

72. Schwartz, Chase, & Bransford, 2012.

73. Genco, Johnson, Hölttä-Otto, & Seepersad, 2011, 2012.

74. Genco, Johnson, Hölttä-Otto, & Seepersad, 2012, p. 75.

75. Gaver, Beaver, & Benford, 2003; Sengers & Gaver, 2006; Yamamoto & Nakakoji, 2005.

76. See, for example, Kouprie & Visser, 2009; Postma, Zwartkruis-Pelgrim, Daemen, & Du, 2012.

77. See, for example, Osborn, 1957; Paulus, Kohn, & Arditti, 2011; R. I. Sutton & Hargadon, 1996.

78. See, for example, Schröer, Kain, & Lindemann, 2010.

79. See, for example, Otto & Wood, 2001; Shah, 1998; Shah, Vargas-Hernandez, Summers, & Kulkarni, 2001.

80. See, for example, Geschka, 1983.

81. See, for example, DeRosa, Smith, & Hantula, 2007.

82. Altshuller, 2000; Stratton & Mann, 2003; Wang, Chang, & Kao, 2010; see Daly, Yilmaz, Christian, Seifert, & Gonzalez, 2012; Hernandez, Shah, & Smith, 2010, VanGundy, 1988 for additional techniques and discussion.

83. Anderson, 1983; Collins & Loftus, 1975.

84. Sutton & Hargadon, 1996.

85. Diehl & Stroebe, 1987; Mullen, Johnson, & Salas, 1991; Stroebe, Nijstad, & Rietzschel, 2010.

86. Sutton & Hargadon, 1996; see also Hinsz, Tindale, & Vollrath, 1997.

87. DeRosa, Smith, & Hantula, 2007.

88. Paulus, Kohn, Arditti, & Korde, 2013.

89. Gero, Jiang, & Williams, 2013; see also Genco, Johnson, Hölttä-Otto, & Seepersad, 2012; Weaver, Kuhr, Wang, Crawford, Wood, Jensen, & Linsey, 2009; Wodehouse & Ion, 2012; for a systematic comparison of some of the methods see Chulvi, Sonseca, Mulet, & Chakrabarti, 2012; Linsey, Clauss, Kurtoglu, Murphy, Wood, & Markman, 2011.

90. Gaver, Beaver, & Benford, 2003; Yamamoto & Nakakoji, 2005.

91. Kouprie & Visser, 2009; Postma, Zwartkruis-Pelgrim, Daemen, & Du, 2012.

92. Goldenberg, Larson, & Wiley, 2013.

93. Bonnardel, 2000.

94. Cross, 1997.

95. Dorst & Cross, 2001, p. 434.

96. Ellamil, Dobson, Beeman, & Christoff, 2012.

97. Fayena-Tawil, Kozbelt, & Sitaras, 2011.

98. Fayena-Tawil, Kozbelt, & Sitaras, 2011.

99. See, for example, Dodson, Johnson, & Schooler, 1997; Schooler, 2002.

100. The reflective verbalization questions in the outdoor garden grill study are from Wetztein & Hacker, 2004.

101. Wetztein & Hacker, 2004.

102. Chris Bertoni quoted in Sutton, 2013, p. 214.

103. Shirouzu, Miyake, & Masukawa, 2002. For a recent review of how teams can take advantage of reflective verbalization to counteract common

team information-processing failures see Schippers, Edmondson, & West, 2014.

104. Winkelmann & Hacker, 2011.
105. Gill Clarke quoted in deLahunta, Clarke, & Barnard, 2012, p. 247.
106. Beaty & Silvia, 2012; Gilhooly, Fioratou, Anthony, & Wynn, 2007.
107. Ward, Patterson, Sifonis, Dodds, & Saunders, 2002.
108. See, for example, De Dreu, Baas, & Nijstad, 2008; Nijstad, De Dreu, Rietzschel, & Baas, 2010. For evidence on the importance of short-term attentional *perseveration* in real world creativity see Zabelina & Beeman, 2013.
109. The study of cellists is reported in De Dreu, Nijstad, Baas, Wolsink, & Roskes, 2012.
110. Tangney, Baumeister, & Boone, 2004.
111. Caspi, 2000; Mischel, Shoda, & Peake, 1988; Mischel, Shoda, & Rodriguez, 1989; Shoda, Mischel, & Peake, 1990.
112. Zabelina & Robinson, 2010; Zabelina, Robinson, & Anicha, 2007; Zimbardo & Boyd, 1999; see also Grant & Schwartz, 2011; Webster, 2011.
113. See, for example, Hockey, 2011; Kool & Botvinick, 2013; Kool, McGuire, Wang, & Botvinick, 2013; Kurzban, Duckworth, Kable, & Myers, 2013. For the account of the dorsal anterior cingulate cortex as important in computing the expected value of control, see Shenhav, Botvinick, & Cohen, 2013.
114. See, for example Berman, Jonides, & Kaplan, 2008; for a broader review, see Russell, Guerry, Balvanera, Gould, Basurto . . . Tam, 2013.
115. See, for example, Job, Dweck, & Walton, 2010; Muraven, Gagné, & Rosman, 2008.
116. L. Martin & Schwartz, 2009.
117. L. Martin & Schwartz, 2009, p. 374.
118. See, for example, Clark, 2001, 2008; Eccles, 2006; Patel, Chapman, Luo, Woodruff, & Arora, 2012; Marian, Dexter, Tucker, & Todd, 2012.
119. Wood & Neal, 2007; Wood, Tam, & Witt, 2005.
120. See, for example, Desimone & Duncan, 1995; Duncan, 2010; Miller & Cohen, 2001.
121. Howard-Jones, Blakemore, Samuel, Summers, & Claxton, 2005.
122. Bengtsson, Csíkszentmihályi, & Ullén, 2007.
123. Kounios, Fleck, Green, Payne, Stevenson, Bowden, & Jung-Beeman, 2008; Subramaniam, Kounios, Parrish, & Jung-Beeman, 2009.
124. Geake & Hansen, 2005.
125. Ellamil, Dobson, Beeman, & Christoff, 2012.
126. Bengtsson, Csíkszentmihályi, & Ullén, 2007, p. 837.
127. Buckner, Andrews-Hanna, & Schacter, 2008, p. 2; see also Limb & Braun, 2008.
128. Craig, 2009; Damasio, 1996; Su, Bowman, & Barnard, 2011. Visceral responses might include "gut reactions," autonomic responses include changes in heart rate or breathing, and hedonic responses relate to whether a particular experience elicits sensations of liking or disliking.
129. Sridharan, Levitin, & Menon, 2008, p. 12573.
130. M. A. Eckert, Menon, Walczak, Ahlstrom, Denslow, Horwitz, & Dubno, 2009.

131. Christoff, 2012; Ellamil, Dobson, Beeman, & Christoff, 2012; Spreng, Stevens, Chamberlain, Gilmore, & Schacter, 2010. See also Dixon, Fox, & Christoff, 2014.
132. The schematic depiction shown in Figure 3.8 is based on Bressler and Menon, 2010.
133. Ellamil, Dobson, Beeman, & Christoff, 2012, p. 1791.
134. Cabeza & Moscovitch, 2013, p. 52.
135. Craig, 2009, p. 67.
136. Mayer, 2011, p. 461.
137. Craig, 2009.
138. Cools & D'Esposito, 2011. For a discussion of the three broad classes of mechanisms that contribute to flexible cognitive control, including broadcast neuromodulation, large-scale brain network interactions (involving direct communication and topological reconfiguration), and the recruitment of specific brain computational hubs, see Braver, Krug, Chiew, Kool, Westbrook, Clement . . . Somerville, 2014.
139. See, for example, Leber, Turk-Browne, & Chun, 2008.
140. McGinley, 2012, np.
141. Ondaatje, 2002, p. 37.
142. Gillian Welch interviewed in Hogan, 2011, np.
143. William Eggleston quoted in O'Hagan, 2004, np.
144. Rauschenberg, 1981, np.
145. John Kruse, of 3M User experience and product design, in a personal e-mail communication, September 2014.
146. Pinker, 2014, p. 76.
147. J. Norman, 2014, p. 53.

PART 4

1. The perception-action cycle and see-move-see have been described from neuroscience, design, and art historical perspectives; see Fuster, 2006, 2009; Schon & Wiggins, 1992; Shiff, 1986.
2. The playground design study is from Atman, Chimka, Bursic, & Nachtmann, 1999.
3. The think aloud protocols shown in Figure 4.2 are modified and adapted from Atman, Chimka, Bursic, & Nachtmann, 1999.
4. Atman, Chimka, Bursic, & Nachtmann, 1999, pp. 146–147.
5. Dobson, 2013, p. 140.
6. The definition of creativity as "novel generation fitted to the constraints of a particular task" is found in Green, Kraemer, Fugelsang, Gray, & Dunbar, 2012, p. 264. On the co-evolution of constraints see Dorst & Cross, 2001; see also Bonnardel, 2000; Simon, 1973.
7. Stokes, 2001, 2007, 2009, 2014.
8. This characterization of the successive constraints that Claude Monet set himself is found in Stokes, 2001; the quotation is from Stokes, 2001, p. 357.
9. Stokes, 2001, p. 357.
10. The six possible classification dimensions of constraints are provided in Onarheim, 2012.

11. The four interrelated origins of constraints are described in Eckert, Stacey, Wyatt, & Garthwaite, 2012.

12. Ive, 2014, np.

13. The intensive case study of the engineering design company, and how the engineers spoke of and treated constraints, is from Onarheim, 2012.

14. The Tate Modern art museum landscape redesign is described in Foxley, 2010.

15. Foxley, 2010, p. 295.

16. Foxley, 2010, p. 298. One contemporary ceramicist, Michelle Erickson, deliberately searched the shores of the Thames, including near Tate Modern, as a source of inspiration and meaning for her studio work. She said of her "mudlarking" expeditions, "I found everything from late 16th-century borderware to 19th-century willow pattern but the finds I kept were things that I recognized parallels to from American archeological contexts." See M. Erickson, 2012, np.

17. Hackman, 2011, p. 73, original emphasis.

18. Woolley, 2009.

19. Eckert, Stacey, Wyatt, & Garthwaite, 2012.

20. Onarheim, 2012, p. 329.

21. Rosso, 2014.

22. See, for example, Baer & Oldham, 2006.

23. The Dutch construction industry example is drawn from Pries & Dorée, 2005. The example, and quotation, relating the genesis of *Star Wars* is found in Fishman, 2015, p. 1336.

24. The novel noun combinations are from Connell & Lynott, 2013.

25. Clark & Clark, 1979; Connell & Lynott, 2013; Kaschak & Glenberg, 2000.

26. The lemonade stand experiment described in the next several paragraphs is from Ederer & Manso, 2013.

27. The study on the shorter- versus longer-term research support structures for scientists discussed in the next several paragraphs is from Azoulay, Graff Zivin, & Manso, 2011.

28. Lerner & Wulf, 2007.

29. Hemel & Ouellette, 2013, p. 382.

30. See, for example, Cohen, McClure, & Yu, 2007; Daw, O'Doherty, Dayan, Seymour, & Dolan, 2006; Laursen, 2012; March 1991.

31. Adler & Chen, 2011; Gibson & Birkinshaw, 2004.

32. See Gupta, Smith, & Shalley, 2006.

33. Amabile, Hill, Hennessey, & Tighe, 1994; Walker, Greene, & Mansell, 2006.

34. Gagné & Deci, 2005.

35. Adler & Chen, 2011.

36. Eisenberger & Armeli, 1997.

37. Kasof, Chen, Himsel, & Greenberger, 2007.

38. Boice, 1983.

39. See, for example, Byron & Khazanchi, 2012; Deci, Koestner, & Ryan, 1999; Gagné & Deci, 2005. See Bénabou & Tirole, 2003, for a formal analysis of the circumstances under which "explicit incentive schemes may sometimes backfire, especially in the long run, by undermining agents' confidence in

their own abilities or in the value of the rewarded task." Bénabou & Tirole, 2003, p. 516.

40. See, for example, Adler & Chen, 2011.

41. Burroughs, Dahl, Moreau, Chattopadhyay, & Gorn, 2011.

42. Birdi, Leach, & Magadley, 2012.

43. See, for example, Ford, 1996; Neuringer, 2004; Stokes, 2001.

44. The discussion of praise for children's intelligence versus children's effort is based on the research of Carol Dweck and colleagues, in Dweck & Leggett, 1988; Mueller & Dweck, 1998.

45. Yeager & Dweck, 2012.

46. For evidence that reinforcing variability can lead to increased exploration and innovative responding in children, undergraduate students, and animal species ranging from laboratory rats to trained porpoises, see Neuringer, 2002; 2004; A. Weiss & Neuringer, 2012; on learning to vary and the sources and role of behavioral variation in innovation also see Koutstaal, 2012, pp. 220–233.

47. Klahr & Chen, 2011; Siegler, 2007.

48. Rittle-Johnson, Star, & Durkin, 2012.

49. Bornstein, Hahn, & Suwalsky, 2013.

50. Bornstein, Hahn, & Suwalsky, 2013, p. 9.

51. Canham, Wiley, & Mayer, 2012.

52. Neuringer, 2004, p. 904.

53. On mindfulness, see Langer & Moldoveanu, 2000.

54. The study with the orchestral musicians is from Langer, Russell, & Eisenkraft, 2009.

55. Langer, Russell, & Eisenkraft, 2009, p. 129.

56. Langer, Russell, & Eisenkraft, 2009, p. 132.

57. Stokes, 2008, p. 224; see also Ross & Neuringer, 2002; Stokes, 2007.

58. Yokochi & Okada, 2005, p. 250.

59. Tharp, 2003.

60. Tharp, 2003, p. 101, parentheses in the original.

61. On the impetus for change and the rich informational guidance provided by experiments and prototyping in social, economic, and political contexts see, for example, Gerken, 2014; Rodrik, 2009; Trencher, Bai, Evans, McCormick, & Yarime, 2014. On experimenting with our tools, such as virtual worlds and their potential role in organizational learning, see Dodgson, Gann, & Phillips, 2013; on experimenting with our search tools themselves, including visual-user interfaces that allow for making and finding, see Ruotsalo, Jacucci, Myllymäki, & Kaski, 2015.

62. The continuum shown in Figure 4.5 is based on Berliner, 1994, and Weick, 1998.

63. See, for example, Goel, Vattam, Wiltgen, & Helms, 2012; Ritter, Damian, Simonton, Van Baaren, Strick, Derks, & Dijksterhuis, 2012; Weick, 1998.

64. Miner, Bassoff, & Moorman, 2001.

65. Miner, Bassoff, & Moorman, 2001, p. 311.

66. Moorman & Miner, 1998.

67. Brews & Hunt, 1999.

68. Doll & Deng, 2011, p. 28.

69. Doll & Deng, 2011, p. 29.
70. Miner, Bassoff, & Moorman, 2001.
71. Vera & Crossan, 2005.
72. March, 1976, p. 77.
73. Mainemelis, Boyatzis, & Kolb, 2002.
74. Hecker, 2012, p. 431. See also Gino, Argote, Miron-Spektor, & Todorova, 2010.
75. Amabile & Kramer, 2011.
76. On the importance and experience of prototyping see Gerber & Carroll, 2012; see also Dow, Glassco, Kass, Schwarz, Schwartz, & Klemmer, 2010.
77. Yamamoto & Nakakoji, 2005.
78. Glynn, 1994.
79. Mesmer-Magnus, Glew, & Viswesvaran, 2012.
80. Humke & Schaefer, 1996; Kozbelt & Nishioka, 2010; N. Murray, Sujan, Hirt, & Sujan, 1990.
81. Dodgson, Gann, & Phillips, 2013.
82. James, 1890/1981, p. 239.
83. Cools & D'Esposito, 2011.
84. Cools, 2008 p. 382.
85. Cools, 2008.
86. Cools & D'Esposito, 2011; see also Akbari Chermahini & Hommel, 2010; Akbari Chermahini & Hommel, 2012.
87. On the effects of relatively momentary changes in our affect on cognitive performance see, for example, Baumann & Kuhl, 2005; Dreisbach & Goschke 2004; Subramaniam, Kounios, Parrish, & Jung-Beeman, 2009.
88. Ashby, Isen, & Turken, 1999.
89. For discussion of the modulatory role of dopamine in cognitive control see, for example, Braver, Barch, & Cohen, 1999; J. D. Cohen, Braver, & Brown, 2002.
90. D'Ardenne, Eshel, Luka, Lenartowicz, Nystrom, & Cohen, 2012; also see Badre, 2012; Frank, Loughry, & O'Reilly, 2001; Kriete, Noelle, Cohen, & O'Reilly, 2013.
91. See, for example, Cohen, McClure, & Yu, 2007.
92. See, for example, Carson, Peterson, & Higgins, 2003; McCrae, 1987.
93. Ziegler, Danay, Heene, Asendorpf, & Bühner, 2012.
94. DeYoung, 2013, p. 8, emphasis added.
95. Vera & Crossan, 2005, p. 203.
96. deLahunta, Clarke, & Barnard, 2012, p. 248, emphasis added.
97. Jocelyne Prince, in Dobson, 2013, p. 146.
98. Olson, 2013, np.

PART 5

1. For the study on student moving-in routines, see Feldman, 2000.
2. For the online customer service database study, see Orlikowski, 1996.
3. Orliowski, 1996, pp. 88–89.
4. The importance of striving in the modification of routines is noted by Feldman, 2000.
5. Feldman, 2000, p. 613.
6. Obstfeld, 2012.

7. Miner, Bassoff, & Moorman, 2001.

8. Orlikowski, 1996, p. 67.

9. Tsoukas & Robert Chi, 2002, p. 567.

10. For the direct versus indirect team experience experiments with origami that we discuss here and in the following several pages, see Gino, Argote, Miron-Spektor, & Todorova, 2010.

11. On transactive memory, see Argote & Ren, 2012; Gino, Argote, Miron-Spektor, & Todorova, 2010; Ren & Argote, 2011.

12. Gino, Argote, Miron-Spektor, & Todorova, 2010; see also Lewis, Belliveau, Herndon, & Keller, 2007.

13. For the Japanese soy sauce company case (the "Tornado" program) see Cooper & Markus, 1995.

14. Cooper & Markus, 1995, np.

15. For the detailed study of the phases of the innovation process in 10 different organizations, see Akbar & Tzokas, 2013.

16. The diagram shown in Figure 5.1 is based on the results reported in Akbar & Tzokas, 2013.

17. For the survey study on firm innovativeness, see Akgün, Keskin, & Byrne, 2012.

18. For the importance of a firm's procedural and emotional memory to innovation, see Akgün, Keskin, & Byrne, 2012.

19. Wang & Wang, 2012.

20. For characterization of the innovation approaches of 44 US design firms, see Meyer & Marion, 2010. For a recent description by Tom Kelley & David Kelley of the design practices at IDEO and the Stanford d.school, see T. Kelley & D. Kelley, 2013.

21. Levitt, List, & Syverson, 2013.

22. Levitt, List, & Syverson, 2013, p. 645.

23. MacCormack, Baldwin, & Rusnak, 2012.

24. MacCormack, Baldwin, & Rusnak, 2012, pp. 1317–1318.

25. For the study on the computerized design search tool, "Sweeper," see Howard, Culley, & Dekoninck, 2011; Howard, Dekoninck, & Culley, 2010.

26. Howard, Culley, & Dekoninck, 2011, p. 579.

27. See, for example, Collins & Koechlin, 2012; Oberauer, 2009; Siegler, 2007.

28. For the team process for developing shared mental models, see DeFranco, Neill, & Clariana, 2011.

29. Consoli, 2014, p. 883, reviewing M. Mazzucato's, 2013, *The Entrepreneurial State: Debunking Public vs. Private Sector Myths.*

30. Cohen & Levinthal, 1990.

31. Todorova & Durisin, 2007.

32. Wegner, 1986, p. 197. See also, Cohen & Levinthal, 1990.

33. For the example of rotationally based learning at IKEA, see Parkin, 2014; the quotation regarding General Electric is from Miller, Fern, & Cardinal, 2007, p. 308.

34. Cohen & Levinthal, 1990; Henderson & Newell, 2011. For an analysis of the value of longer-term collaborative and trust-based relationships in automobile design and manufacturing, see Helper & Henderson, 2014.

35. For the patent data study showing the combined benefits of in-house research and external collaboration, see Fabrizio, 2009.

36. For a discussion of business and organizational clusters, see Porter, 1998.

37. For the study of the Chilean wine producers and absorptive capacity, see Giuliani & Bell, 2005.

38. For the follow-up study of the wine producers, see Giuliani, 2013.

39. See O'Leary & Cummings, 2007.

40. The schematic diagram in Figure 5.3 is broadly based on Giuliani & Bell, 2005 and Giuliani, 2013.

41. For the study on the effects of distance on software development teams, see Magni, Maruping, Hoegl, & Proserpio, 2013.

42. Vera & Crossan, 2005, p. 206; see also Weick & Roberts, 1993.

43. See Dougherty & Takacs, 2004; Weick & Roberts, 1993.

44. The concept of heedfulness in thinking was developed by the philosopher Gilbert Ryle, in Ryle, 1949.

45. Dougherty & Takacs, 2004, p. 583.

46. On situational awareness, see Endsley, 1995.

47. For reviews, see Baard, Rench, & Kozlowski, 2014; Burke, Stagl, Salas, Pierce, & Kendall, 2006.

48. For the study of the film crews described in the next several paragraphs, see Bechky & Okhuysen, 2011.

49. On the process of bricolage, see Baker & Nelson, 2005; the quotation is from Baker & Nelson, p. 333.

50. Bechky & Okhuysen, 2011, p. 241.

51. On openness to experience see, for example, DeYoung, 2013; Koutstaal, 2012, pp. 269–278; McCrae, 1987.

52. For the computerized military aircraft simulation study on adaptability to change and openness to experience, see LePine, Colquitt, & Erez, 2000.

53. LePine, Colquitt, & Erez, 2000.

54. For the three-member team version of the computerized military aircraft simulation study, see LePine, 2003.

55. LePine, 2003; see also Schilpzand, Herold, & Shalley, 2011.

56. Bradley, Klotz, Postlethwaite, & Brown, 2013.

57. On the role of intentional unlearning in successful change, see Akgün, Byrne, Lynn, & Keskin, 2007.

58. For the study of large-scale organizational learning and unlearning discussed in the next several paragraphs, see Becker, 2010.

59. For the study of intentional unlearning and organizational change in the Spanish hotel industry, discussed here and in the following paragraph, see Cegarra-Navarro, Martinez-Martinez, Gutiérrez, & Leal-Rodríguez, 2013.

60. The diagram in Figure 5.4 is adapted from Becker, 2010.

61. Cegarra-Navarro, Martinez-Martinez, Gutiérrez, & Leal-Rodríguez, 2013; see also Wang, Lu, Zhao, Gong, & Li, 2013.

62. See, for example, De Dreu, Nijstad, Bechtoldt, & Baas, 2011; McCrae, 1987.

63. For the study on multicultural experience within student pairs, and the possibility of achieving "superadditive" levels of creativity, see Tadmor, Satterstrom, Jang, & Polzer, 2012.

64. Mitchell, Nicholas, & Boyle, 2009.

65. See, for example, Barrett & Sexton, 2006; Bourgeois, 1981; Mallidou, Cummings, Ginsburg, Chuang, Kang, Norton, & Estabrooks, 2011.

66. For first-order versus second-order problem solving in the context of hospitals, see Tucker & Edmondson, 2003.
67. Bourgeois, 1981, p. 30.
68. Nohria & Gulati, 1996.
69. Danneels, 2008.
70. Our discussion, in the next several pages, of the exploration-exploitation challenges facing nonprofit professional theaters is based on Voss, Sirdeshmukh, & Voss, 2008; Voss & Voss, 2013.
71. Voss, Sirdeshmukh, & Voss, 2008, p. 155.
72. Voss, Sirdeshmukh, & Voss, 2008, p. 155, original emphasis.
73. The results described here are from Voss, Sirdeshmukh, & Voss, 2008.
74. Voss & Voss, 2013.
75. Voss & Voss, 2013, p. 1470.
76. Compare Henderson & Clark, 1990; Voss & Voss, 2013.
77. For the study of the process and learning of the NASA science and engineering teams, described in this section, see Paletz, Kim, Schunn, Tollinger, & Vera, 2013; Paletz, Schunn, & Kim, 2013.
78. Paletz, Schunn, & Kim, 2013, p. 5.
79. See, for example, Squyres, Arvidson, Bell, Brückner, Cabrol, Calvin, . . . Yen, 2004.
80. Paletz, Kim, Schunn, Tollinger, & Vera, 2013.
81. On the concept of adaptive expertise, see Hatano & Inagaki, 1984.
82. Paletz, Kim, Schunn, Tollinger, & Vera, 2013, p. 421.
83. Raisch, Birkinshaw, Probst, & Tushman, 2009; Tushman & O'Reilly, 1996; for a recent overview and discussion on organizational ambidexterity, see O'Reilly & Tushman, 2013.
84. On the concept of an optimal adaptability corridor, see Schwartz, Bransford, & Sears, 2005; McKenna, 2007.
85. The diagram in Figure 5.5 is adapted from Schwartz, Bransford, & Sears, 2005, and McKenna, 2007.
86. Ohly, Sonnentag, & Pluntke, 2006; see also Mylopoulos & Regehr, 2009. For initial experimental evidence on how organizations "that endorse a culture of growth and development may encourage people to pursue learning goals" may, in turn, "not only equip people to deal with setbacks but may also result in mastery-oriented behaviors such as seeking opportunities for challenge and learning," see Murphy & Dweck, 2010, p. 294.
87. Li, Maggitti, Smith, Tesluk, & Katila, 2013, p. 893.
88. See, for example, Lin & Li, 2013.
89. See, for example, Bogers, Afuah, & Bastian, 2010; Lettl, Herstatt, & Gemuenden, 2006.
90. Baldwin & Von Hippel, 2011.
91. See, for example, Lettl, Herstatt, & Gemuenden, 2006.
92. Our discussion of the search processes of the Japanese manufacturer and retailer Muji is based on Nishikawa, Schreier, & Ogawa, 2013.
93. Nishikawa, Schreier, & Ogawa, 2013, p. 163.
94. Audia & Goncalo, 2007; Battilana & Casciaro, 2012; Rosenkopf & Almeida, 2003.

95. Jeppesen & Lakhani, 2010.
96. For the widely broadcasted search for the big data genetic sequencing problem, see Lakhani, Boudreau, Loh, Backstrom, Baldwin, Lonstein, ... Guinan, 2013.
97. Lakhani, Boudreau, Loh, Backstrom, Baldwin, Lonstein, ... Guinan, 2013, p. 110.
98. Lakhani, Boudreau, Loh, Backstrom, Baldwin, Lonstein, ... Guinan, 2013, p. 111.
99. March, 1991.
100. See, for example, Rosenkopf & Nerkar, 2001.
101. See, for example, Katila, 2002.
102. Katila & Chen, 2008, p. 596.
103. Katila & Chen, 2008, p. 605.
104. Katila & Chen, 2008, p. 619.
105. On the benefits of mental contrasting in goal pursuit and change see, for example, Oettingen, 2012; Sevincer & Oettingen, 2013.
106. Taylor, Pham, Rivkin, & Armor, 1998, p. 432.
107. Kappes, Wendt, Reinelt, & Oettingen, 2013.
108. Zhang & Fishbach, 2010.
109. Rasmussen & Berntsen, 2013.
110. Oettingen, Marquardt, & Gollwitzer, 2012.
111. Meleady, Hopthrow, & Crisp, 2013.
112. Liberman & Trope, 2014; Mann, de Ridder, & Fujita, 2013.
113. Armor, Massey, & Sackett, 2008.
114. See, for example, Carver, Scheier, & Segerstrom, 2010.
115. On optimism and our preparedness for the immediate future, see Sweeny, Carroll, & Shepperd, 2006.
116. Sweeny & Krizan, 2013.
117. Rego, Sousa, Marques, & Cunha, 2012.
118. Schacter, Addis, Hassabis, Martin, Spreng, & Szpunar, 2012; Spreng, Stevens, Chamberlain, Gilmore, & Schacter, 2010.
119. Ellamil, Dobson, Beeman, & Christoff, 2012.
120. D'Argembeau, Lardi, & Van der Linden, 2012; D'Argembeau & Van der Linden, 2012.
121. D'Argembeau, Stawarczyk, Majerus, Collette, Van der Linden, Feyers, ... & Salmon, 2010.
122. On the role of the default-mode network in autobiographical memory, future-related thinking, and imaginatively taking the perspectives of others, see Andrews-Hanna, 2012; Spreng & Grady, 2010.
123. Suddendorf & Redshaw, 2013, p. 136.
124. Suddendorf & Redshaw, 2013, p. 136.
125. Katila & Chen, 2008, p. 595.
126. Bonvillian, 2013, p. 1173.
127. The two quotations are from, respectively, Jennings, 2008, pp. 7–8, and Bell & Van Hecke, 2014, np.
128. Faust, 2011, np.
129. The thoughts on precedent are those of Schauer, 1987, pp. 572–573.
130. Davies, 1991, p. 89.

131. Chadha, 2013, np.
132. Sotomayor & Greenhouse, 2014, np.

PART 6

1. P. Smith, 2010, p. 3.
2. Conway, Meares, & Standart, 2004; Conway & Pleydell-Pearce, 2000.
3. On the distinction between experience-near and experience-far events, see, for example, Conway, 2005, 2009; Renoult, Davidson, Palombo, Moscovitch, & Levine, 2012.
4. D'Argembeau & Van der Linden, 2012, p. 1204; see also D'Argembeau, Renaud, & Van der Linden, 2011.
5. Rudenstine, 2001, p. 364.
6. Ravasi & Phillips, 2011, p. 116; our discussion in the following paragraphs of organizational change at Bang & Olufsen is based on Ravasi & Phillips, 2011.
7. Ravasi & Phillips, 2011, p. 119.
8. Ravasi & Phillips, 2011, p. 122.
9. Ravasi & Phillips, 2011, p. 120, original emphasis.
10. Sharma, 2013, p. 236.
11. See, for example, Brandstätter, Lengfelder, & Gollwitzer, 2001; Gollwitzer, Heckhausen, & Steller, 1990.
12. On Community Supported Agriculture see, for example, C. Brown & Miller, 2008; Hunt, Geiger-Oneto, & Varca, 2012. Under Advance Market Commitments (AMC), "the reward to the company is not paid simply for development of a product that meets a set of technical specifications but, rather, is tied to actual adoption and use of that product . . . Basing AMC payments in part on this measure of ex post use provides incentives for companies to focus their R&D efforts on products that actually would be used rather than on a product that somehow fits a set of predecided technical specifications but is not a good fit with what developing countries need or want." Kremer & Williams, 2010, p. 8.
13. See, for example, Balsamo, 2011; Kafai, Peppler, & Chapman, 2009.
14. See, for example, McGrane, 2012.
15. Kokonas, 2014.
16. These new variations on traditional corporate forms are more explicit and direct in promoting social, environmental, or public goals. Yet this is not to say that traditional for-profit firms don't or can't pursue social purposes or cannot rely on other means to promote social, environmental, or public goals, through, for instance, national and global corporate philanthropy, environmentally sensitive manufacturing processes, community development, and so on. For a review of some of the new corporate structures, see Clark & Babson, 2012; Cummings, 2012; Esposito, 2013; and Plerhoples, 2014. On the need for continuing innovation and experimentation in national and global corporate social responsibility, see Pitts, 2009.
17. For the fMRI study discussed in this research highlight, see Most, Chun, Johnson, & Kiehl, 2006.
18. The quotations on the meaning-manageability tradeoff in the specificity with which we conceive our personal projects are found in Little, 2015, p. 97, and

Little, 2014, p. 338, respectively. We thank Chip Pitts for pointing us to Brian R. Little's work. See also Ülkümen & Cheema, 2013.

19. Oettingen, 2012, pp. 55–56.
20. Sonnentag & Volmer, 2010, p. 116; see also Pinto & Prescott, 1988; West & Anderson, 1996.
21. Winkelmann & Hacker, 2011.
22. Hackman, 2011, p. 73.
23. See, for example, Carson & Carson, 1993; Chua & Iyengar, 2008; Ford, 1996; Harrington, 1975; Litchfield, 2008; Shalley, 1991.
24. On how explicit cues to be creative can benefit our creative performance, see Green, Cohen, Kim, & Gray, 2012; see also Prabhakaran, Green, & Gray, 2014.
25. Litchfield, Fan, & Brown, 2011.
26. Pearce & Ensley, 2004, p. 273; see also Pirola-Merlo & Mann, 2004.
27. See Watkins, 2011 for the need for flexible regulation of goal or action identification across changing circumstances.
28. Our discussion here of Aravind Eye Hospital is based on Ebrahim & Rangan, 2014.
29. Ebrahim & Rangan, 2014, p. 129.
30. Ebrahim & Rangan, 2014, p. 129.
31. Goldstone, Roberts, & Gureckis, 2008; Hackman, Kosslyn, & Woolley, 2008; Woolley, Chabris, Pentland, Hashmi, & Malone, 2010; Woolley, Hackman, Jerde, Chabris, Bennett, & Kosslyn, 2007.
32. Woolley, Gerbasi, Chabris, Kosslyn, & Hackman, 2008.
33. Gerber, McKenna, Hirsch, & Yarnoff, 2010.
34. Köpetz, Faber, Fishbach, & Kruglanski, 2011; see also Kruglanski, Shah, Fishbach, Friedman, Chun, & Sleeth-Keppler, 2002.
35. Kiviniemi, Snyder, & Omoto, 2002.
36. Kiviniemi, Snyder, & Omoto, 2002; Linville, 1987.
37. Snyder, 2009, p. 235; see also Omoto & Snyder, 2002.
38. Voss, Cable, & Voss, 2006.
39. March, 1976, p. 78, original italics.
40. For empirical findings on the distinction between conceptual artists and experimental artists, see Galenson, 2006, 2010.
41. Galenson, 2006, 2010.
42. Kapur, 2008; Kapur & Bielaczyc, 2012.
43. Hirst, 2013, p. 46.
44. See, for example, Eitam & Higgins, 2010; Hedberg & Higgins, 2011.
45. See, for example, Einstein, McDaniel, Richardson, Guynn, & Cunfer, 1995; Ellis & Milne, 1996; Gilbert, Gollwitzer, Cohen, Oettingen, & Burgess, 2009; Gollwitzer, & Brandstätter, 1997; Sheeran, Webb, & Gollwitzer, 2005.
46. Marsh, Hicks, & Cook, 2006.
47. See, for example Carver, 2003, 2004; Louro, Pieters, & Zeelenberg, 2007.
48. Fredrickson, 2001, 2004.
49. Nesse, 2004, p. 1339.
50. See, for example, Carver, 2003; Eaglestone, Ford, Brown, & Moore, 2007.

51. Duncan, 2010; Duncan, Parr, Woolgar, Thompson, Bright, Cox, Bishop, & Nimmo-Smith, 2008; Heath & Staudenmayer, 2000; Kane & Engle, 2002.

52. Altmann, & Trafton, 2002; Dodhia & Dismukes, 2009.

53. Catmull, 2014, p. x.

54. Byron & Khazanchi, 2012.

55. Baas, De Dreu, & Nijstad, 2008.

56. Ericsson, 2008; Ericsson, Krampe, & Tesch-Römer, 1993, Kahneman & Klein, 2009; Klein, 2008; Osbeck, 1999.

57. Our discussion of the rapid feedback approach for baseball players is based on Fadde, 2006, 2009.

58. Erickson, Li, Kim, Deshpande, Sahu, Chao, Sukaviriya, & Naphade, 2013.

59. Barber, Bagsby, Grawitch, & Buerck, 2011; see also Pennebaker, Gosling, & Ferrell, 2013.

60. Meyer & Marion, 2010.

61. Our discussion in the next several paragraphs of The Nature Conservancy's efforts to assess their goal progress is based on Sawhill & Williamson, 2001.

62. On the need for remindings and environmental support in remaining constant to our ideals, see Koutstaal, 1995. On the role of hospital-employed patient advocates see, for example, Heaphy, 2013. A contemporary legal scholar argues for the need for "designing more tailored or 'bespoke' processes and institutions for the necessary processes of recognizing, taking responsibility for, and apologizing for past wrongs, while at the same time, focusing on more complex remedies for moving from the past to the future, including compensation, apologies, and affirmative action to improve and repair the lives of those who suffer from the legacies of great harm." See Menkel-Meadow, 2014, p. 622.

63. Agarwal & Helfat, 2009, p. 282.

64. Raffaelli, 2013.

65. Bandura, 1997, p. 131.

66. Our discussion in the next several paragraphs of the "City Hospital" case study is based on Valentine & Edmondson, 2015.

67. Valentine & Edmondson, 2015, p. 412.

68. Our discussion, in the next few paragraphs, of the experimental initiative for cotton growers in rural India is based on Cole & Fernando, 2012.

69. See Patel, Chittamuru, Jain, Dave, & Parikh, 2010.

70. The study of the collaborative efforts of researchers using the Large Hadron Collider Computing Grid is found in Zheng, Venters, & Cornford, 2011.

71. Yumer & Kara, 2012.

72. Yumer & Kara, 2012.

73. See, for example, Brainerd & Reyna, 1990, 2001; Winocur, Moscovitch, & Bontempi, 2010.

74. See, for example, Schwartz & Bransford, 1998.

75. Our discussion of patterns of online course-related information exchange among university students is based on Vaquero & Cebrian, 2013.

76. Figure 6.2 is adapted from Vaquero & Cebrian, 2013.

77. The study of developing computerized aids to the complex task of train scheduling, that we discuss in the next several paragraphs, is found in Van Wezel & Jorna, 2009.
78. Jorna, Van Wezel, & Bos, 2012.
79. De Snoo, Van Wezel, & Jorna, 2011, p. 188.
80. Our discussion over the next few pages of the diverse modes of communication in creating a new dance piece is based on Kirsh, Muntanyola, Jao, Lew, & Sugihara, 2009.
81. Kirsh, Muntanyola, Jao, Lew, & Sugihara, 2009, p. 190.
82. Figure 6.3 is adapted from Kirsh, Muntanyola, Jao, Lew, & Sugihara, 2009.
83. Kirsh, Muntanyola, Jao, Lew, & Sugihara, 2009, p. 192.
84. Kirsh, Muntanyola, Jao, Lew, & Sugihara, 2009, p. 192.
85. See, for example, Bertsch, Pesta, Wiscott, & McDaniel, 2007.
86. The quotation on the value of "tinkering" in the policy design process is found in Ostrom, 2012, p. 1401. On encouraging diverse action at multiple scales, using multiple methods, and multiple decisionmaking units in order to reduce global greenhouse gas emissions, see Ostrom, 2009. See also Rodrik, 2009.
87. Rodrik, 2009, p. 43.
88. Munro, 1982, p. 224.
89. Hackman, 2011, p. 70.
90. Henderson & Gibbons, 2013, p. 697.
91. March, 1976, p. 80.
92. Amabile & Flanagan, 2014, p. 15, original emphasis.

A CONCEPTS GUIDE

1. Stokes, 2009, p. 174.
2. Chiu & Shu, 2012, p. 274, original emphasis.
3. Buckner, Andrews-Hanna, & Schacter, 2008, p. 2.
4. The quotation characterizes Donald Schon's philosophy of design, and is from Waks, 2001, p. 44; the italics are in the original. The three key properties of design are from Lei, Taura & Numata, 1996, pp. 268–269.
5. Jansson & Smith, 1991, p. 4.
6. Yilmaz, Seifert, Gonzalez, 2010 p. 337.
7. Genco, Johnson, Höltta-Otto, & Seepersad, 2011, p. 2.
8. Dougherty & Takacs, 2004, pp. 571 and 575.
9. See, for example, R. Brown & McNeill, 1966; Tulving & Pearlstone, 1966.
10. See, for example, Nee & Jonides, 2014.
11. Wen, Butler, & Koutstaal, 2013, p. 98.
12. Simon, 1973, p. 187.
13. Webb, Sheeran, & Armitage, 2006, p. 335.
14. Segal, 2004, p. 147.
15. See Koutstaal, 2012.
16. Burton, Lydon, D'Alessandro, & Koestner, 2006, p. 751.
17. See, for example, Fuster, 2006.

18. Wetzstein & Hacker, 2004, p. 146.
19. Bressler & Menon, 2010, p. 285.
20. Weick, Sutcliffe, & Obstfeld, 2005, pp. 411–412.
21. Gino, Argote, Miron-Spektor, & Todorova, 2010, p. 103.
22. Kozlowski & Ilgen, 2006, p. 85.

REFERENCES

Abbott, A. (2004). *Methods of discovery: Heuristics for the social sciences.* New York: W. W. Norton.

Abraham, A. (2014). Creative thinking as orchestrated by semantic processing vs. cognitive control brain networks. *Frontiers in Human Neuroscience, 8,* Article 95, 1–8.

Addis, D. R., Wong, A. T., & Schacter, D. L. (2007). Remembering the past and imagining the future: Common and distinct neural substrates during event construction and elaboration. *Neuropsychologia, 45,* 1363–1377.

Adler, P. S., & Chen, C. X. (2011). Combining creativity and control: Understanding individual motivation in large-scale collaborative creativity. *Accounting, Organizations and Society, 36,* 63–85.

Agarwal, R., & Helfat, C. E. (2009). Strategic renewal of organizations. *Organization Science, 20,* 281–293.

Aimone, J. B., Deng, W., & Gage, F. H. (2011). Resolving new memories: A critical look at the dentate gyrus, adult neurogenesis, and pattern separation. *Neuron, 70,* 589–596.

Aizpurua, A., & Koutstaal, W. (2010). Aging and flexible remembering: Contributions of conceptual span, fluid intelligence, and frontal functioning. *Psychology and Aging, 25,* 193–207.

Akbar, H., & Tzokas, N. (2013). An exploration of new product development's front-end knowledge conceptualization process in discontinuous innovations. *British Journal of Management, 24,* 245–263.

Akbari Chermahini, S., & Hommel, B. (2010). The b(link) between creativity and dopamine: Spontaneous eye blink rates predict and dissociate divergent and convergent thinking. *Cognition, 115,* 458–465.

Akbari Chermahini, S., & Hommel, B. (2012). More creative through positive mood? Not everyone! *Frontiers in Human Neuroscience, 6,* Article 319, 1–7.

Akgün, A. E., Byrne, J. C., Lynn, G. S., & Keskin, H. (2007). Organizational unlearning as changes in beliefs and routines in organizations. *Journal of Organizational Change Management, 20,* 794–812.

Akgün, A. E., Keskin, H., & Byrne, J. (2012). The role of organizational emotional memory on declarative and procedural memory and firm innovativeness. *Journal of Product Innovation Management, 29,* 432–451.

Alibali, M. W., & Goldin-Meadow, S. (1993). Gesture-speech mismatch and mechanisms of learning: What the hands reveal about a child's state of mind. *Cognitive Psychology, 25,* 468–523.

Alibali, M. W., Spencer, R. C., Knox, L., & Kita, S. (2011). Spontaneous gestures influence strategy choices in problem solving. *Psychological Science, 22,* 1138–1144.

Altmann, E. M., & Trafton, J. G. (2002). Memory for goals: An activation-based model. *Cognitive Science, 26,* 39–83.

Altshuller, G. S. (2000). *The innovation algorithm: TRIZ, systematic innovation and technical creativity.* Worcester, MA: Technical Innovation Center.

Alvarado-Iniesta, A., Garcia-Alcaraz, J. L, Rodriguez-Borbon, M. I., & Maldonado, A. (2013). Optimization of the material flow in a manufacturing plant by use of artificial bee colony algorithm. *Expert Systems with Applications, 40,* 4785–4790.

Amabile, T. M., Barsade, S. G., Mueller, J. S., & Staw, B. M. (2005). Affect and creativity at work. *Administrative Science Quarterly, 50,* 367–403.

Amabile, T. M., & Flanagan, K. (2014). *Making progress at IDEO.* HBS No. 9-814-123. Boston, MA: Harvard Business School Publishing.

Amabile, T. M., Hill, K. G., Hennessey, B. A., & Tighe, E. M. (1994). The work preference inventory: Assessing intrinsic and extrinsic motivational orientations. *Journal of Personality and Social Psychology, 66,* 950–967.

Amabile, T. M., & Kramer, S. (2011). *The progress principle: Using small wins to ignite joy, engagement, and creativity at work.* Boston: Harvard Business Review Press.

Amalberti, R., Auroy, Y., Berwick, D., & Barach, P. (2005). Five system barriers to achieving ultrasafe health care. *Annals of Internal Medicine, 142,* 756–764.

Anderson, J. R. (1983). A spreading activation theory of memory. *Journal of Verbal Learning and Verbal Behavior, 22,* 261–295.

Andrews-Hanna, J. R. (2012). The brain's default network and its adaptive role in internal mentation. *The Neuroscientist, 18,* 251–270.

Argote, L., & Ren, Y. (2012). Transactive memory systems: A microfoundation of dynamic capabilities. *Journal of Management Studies, 49,* 1375–1382.

Armor, D. A., Massey, C., & Sackett, A. M. (2008). Prescribed optimism: Is it right to be wrong about the future? *Psychological Science, 19,* 329–331.

Ashby, F. G., Isen, A. M., & Turken, A. U. (1999). A neuropsychological theory of positive affect and its influence on cognition. *Psychological Review, 106,* 529–550.

Atance, C. M., & O'Neill, D. K. (2001). Episodic future thinking. *Trends in Cognitive Sciences, 5,* 533–539.

Atman, C. J., Chimka, J. R., Bursic, K. M., & Nachtmann, H. L. (1999). A comparison of freshman and senior engineering design processes. *Design Studies, 20,* 131–152.

Atman, C. J., Yasuhara, K., Adams, R. S., Barker, T. J., Turns, J., & Rhone, E. (2008). Breadth in problem scoping: A comparison of freshman and senior engineering students. *International Journal of Engineering Education, 24,* 234–245.

Audia, P. G., & Goncalo, J. A. (2007). Past success and creativity over time: A study of inventors in the hard disk drive industry. *Management Science, 53,* 1–15.

Azoulay, P., Graff Zivin, J. S., & Manso, G. (2011). Incentives and creativity: Evidence from the academic life sciences. *RAND Journal of Economics, 42*, 527–554.

Baard, S. K., Rench, T. A., & Kozlowski, S. W. J. (2014). Performance adaptation: A theoretical integration and review. *Journal of Management, 40*, 48–99.

Baas, M., De Dreu, C. K. W., & Nijstad, B. A. (2008). A meta-analysis of 25 years of mood-creativity research: Hedonic tone, activation, or regulatory focus? *Psychological Bulletin, 134*, 779–806.

Baas, M., De Dreu, C. K. W., & Nijstad, B. A. (2011). When prevention promotes creativity: The role of mood, regulatory focus, and regulatory closure. *Journal of Personality and Social Psychology, 100*, 794–809.

Badre, D. (2008). Cognitive control, hierarchy, and the rostro-caudal organization of the frontal lobes. *Trends in Cognitive Sciences, 12*, 193–200.

Badre, D. (2012). Opening the gate to working memory. *Proceedings of the National Academy of Sciences, USA, 109*, 19878–19879.

Badre, D., & D'Esposito, M. (2007). Functional magnetic resonance imaging evidence for a hierarchical organization of the prefrontal cortex. *Journal of Cognitive Neuroscience, 19*, 2082–2099.

Badre, D., Kayser, A. S., & D'Esposito, M. (2010). Frontal cortex and the discovery of abstract action rules. *Neuron, 66*, 315–326.

Baer, M., & Oldham, G. R. (2006). The curvilinear relation between experienced creative time pressure and creativity: Moderating effects of openness to experience and support for creativity. *Journal of Applied Psychology, 91*, 963–970.

Baird, B., Smallwood, J., Mrazek, M. D., Kam, J.W.Y., Franklin, M. S., & Schooler, J. W. (2012). Inspired by distraction: Mind wandering facilitates creative incubation. *Psychological Science, 23*, 1117–1122.

Baird, B., Smallwood, J., & Schooler, J. W. (2011). Back to the future: Autobiographical planning and the functionality of mind-wandering. *Consciousness and Cognition, 20*, 1604–1611.

Baker, T., & Nelson, R. E. (2005). Creating something from nothing: Resource construction through entrepreneurial bricolage. *Administrative Science Quarterly, 50*, 329–366.

Baldwin, C., & Von Hippel, E. (2011). Modeling a paradigm shift: From producer innovation to user and open collaborative innovation. *Organization Science, 22*, 1399–1417.

Ball, L. J., Ormerod, T. C., & Morley, N. J. (2004). Spontaneous analogising in engineering design: A comparative analysis of experts and novices. *Design Studies, 25*, 495–508.

Balsamo, A. (2011). *Designing culture: The technological imagination at work.* Durham, NC: Duke University Press.

Bandura, A. (1997). *Self-efficacy: The exercise of control.* New York: W. H. Freeman.

Barber, L. K., Bagsby, P. G., Grawitch, M. J., & Buerck, J. P. (2011). Facilitating self-regulated learning with technology: Evidence for student motivation and exam improvement. *Teaching of Psychology, 38*, 303–308.

Barrett, P., & Sexton, M. (2006). Innovation in small, project-based construction firms. *British Journal of Management, 17*, 331–346.

Barsalou, L. W. (1999). Perceptual symbol systems. *Behavioral and Brain Sciences, 22*, 577–660.

Barsalou, L. W. (2003). Situated simulation in the human conceptual system. *Language and Cognitive Processes, 18*, 513–562.

Basadur, M. (1995). The optimal ideation-evaluation ratios. *Creativity Research Journal, 8*, 63–75.

Basadur, M., Graen, G. B., & Green, S. G. (1982). Training in creative problem solving: Effects on ideation and problem finding and solving in an industrial research organization. *Organizational Behavior and Human Performance, 30*, 41–70.

Battilana, J., & Casciaro, T. (2012). Change agents, networks, and institutions: A contingency theory of organizational change. *Academy of Management Journal, 55*, 381–398.

Baumann, N., & Kuhl, J. (2002). Intuition, affect, and personality: Unconscious coherence judgments and self-regulation of negative affect. *Journal of Personality and Social Psychology, 83*, 1213–1223.

Baumann, N., & Kuhl, J. (2005). Positive affect and flexibility: Overcoming the precedence of global over local processing of visual information. *Motivation and Emotion, 29*, 123–134.

Baumann, N., & Scheffer, D. (2011). Seeking flow in the achievement domain: The achievement flow motive behind flow experience. *Motivation and Emotion, 35*, 267–284.

Beaty, R. E., & Silvia, P. J. (2012). Why do ideas get more creative across time? An executive interpretation of the serial order effect in divergent thinking tasks. *Psychology of Aesthetics, Creativity, and the Arts, 6*, 309–319.

Bechara, A., Damasio, H., & Damasio, A. R. (2000). Emotion, decision making and the orbitofrontal cortex. *Cerebral Cortex, 10*, 295–307.

Bechky, B. A., & Okhuysen, G. A. (2011). Expecting the unexpected? How SWAT officers and film crews handle surprises. *Academy of Management Journal, 54*, 239–261.

Becker, K. (2010). Facilitating unlearning during implementation of new technology. *Journal of Organizational Change Management, 23*, 251–268.

Beeftink, F., van Eerde, W., & Rutte, C. G. (2008). The effect of interruptions and breaks on insight and impasses: Do you need a break right now? *Creativity Research Journal, 20*, 358–364.

Beeman, M. J. (1998). Coarse semantic coding and discourse comprehension. In M. Beeman & C. Chiarello (Eds.), *Right hemisphere language comprehension: Perspectives from cognitive neuroscience* (pp. 255–284). Mahwah, NJ: Erlbaum.

Beeman, M. J., Friedman, R. B., Grafman, J., Perez, E., Diamond, S., & Lindsay, M. B. (1994). Summation priming and coarse semantic coding in the right hemisphere. *Journal of Cognitive Neuroscience, 6*, 26–45.

Beilock, S. L., & Goldin-Meadow, S. (2010). Gesture changes thought by grounding it in action. *Psychological Science, 21*, 1605–1610.

Bell, J., & Van Hecke, W. (2014). Design Explosions, Issue #1: Mapping on iOS. Retrieved December 7, 2014, from https://medium.com/design-explosion/design-explosions-mapping-on-ios-ad4ec6ba5c59

Bénabou, R., & Tirole, J. (2003). Intrinsic and extrinsic motivation. *Review of Economic Studies, 70,* 489–520.

Ben-Artzi, E., Faust, M., & Moeller, E. (2009). Hemispheric asymmetries in discourse processing: Evidence from false memories for lists and texts. *Neuropsychologia, 47,* 430–438.

Benedek, M., Könen, T., & Neubauer, A. C. (2012). Associative abilities underlying creativity. *Psychology of Aesthetics, Creativity, and the Arts, 6,* 273–281.

Bengtsson, S. L., Csíkszentmihályi, M., & Ullén, F. (2007). Cortical regions involved in the generation of musical structures during improvisation in pianists. *Journal of Cognitive Neuroscience, 19,* 830–842.

Benkler, Y. (2006). *The wealth of networks: How social production transforms markets and freedom.* New Haven, CT: Yale University Press.

Berliner, P. F. (1994). *Thinking in jazz: The infinite art of improvisation.* Chicago: University of Chicago Press.

Berman, M. G., Jonides, J., & Kaplan, S. (2008). The cognitive benefits of interacting with nature. *Psychological Science, 19,* 1207–1212.

Bernstein, E. S. (2012). The transparency paradox: A role for privacy in organizational learning and operational control. *Administrative Science Quarterly, 57,* 181–216.

Bertsch, S., Pesta, B. J., Wiscott, R., & McDaniel, M. A. (2007). The generation effect: A meta-analytic review. *Memory & Cognition, 35,* 201–210.

Binder, J., & Desai, R. H. (2011). The neurobiology of semantic memory. *Trends in Cognitive Sciences, 15,* 527–536.

Binnewies, C., & Wörnlein, S. C. (2011). What makes a creative day? A diary study on the interplay between affect, job stressors, and job control. *Journal of Organizational Behavior, 32,* 589–607.

Binney, R. J., Parker, G. J. M., & Lambon Ralph, M. A. (2012). Convergent connectivity and graded specialization in the rostral human temporal lobe as revealed by diffusion-weighted imaging probabilistic tractography. *Journal of Cognitive Neuroscience, 24,* 1998–2014.

Birdi, K., Leach, D., & Magadley, W. (2012). Evaluating the impact of TRIZ creativity training: An organizational field study. *R&D Management, 42,* 315–326.

Bittner, J. V., & Heidemeier, H. (2013). Competitive mindsets, creativity, and the role of regulatory focus. *Thinking Skills and Creativity, 9,* 59–68.

Bledow, R., Rosing, K., & Frese, M. (2013). A dynamic perspective on affect and creativity. *Academy of Management Journal, 56,* 432–450.

Block, J., & Kremen, A. M. (1996). IQ and ego-resiliency: Conceptual and empirical connections and separateness. *Journal of Personality and Social Psychology, 70,* 349–361.

Bocanegra, B. R., & Hommel, B. (2014). When cognitive control is not adaptive. *Psychological Science, 25,* 1249–1255.

Bogers, M., Afuah, A., & Bastian, B. (2010). Users as innovators: A review, critique, and future research directions. *Journal of Management, 36,* 857–875.

Boice, R. (1983). Contingency management in writing and the appearance of creative ideas: Implications for the treatment of writing blocks. *Behaviour Research and Therapy, 21,* 537–543.

Bolte, A., Goschke, T., & Kuhl, J. (2003). Emotion and intuition: Effects of positive and negative mood on implicit judgments of semantic coherence. *Psychological Science, 14,* 416–421.

Bonnardel, N. (2000). Towards understanding and supporting creativity in design: Analogies in a constrained cognitive environment. *Knowledge-Based Systems, 13,* 505–513.

Bonnardel, N. & Moscardini, L. (2012). Toward a situated cognition approach to design: Effect of emotional context on designers' ideas. *European Conference on Cognitive Ergonomics (ECCE'12),* 15–21.

Bonvillian, W. B. (2013). Advanced manufacturing policies and paradigms for innovation. *Science, 342,* 1173–1175.

Borghi, A. M., Glenberg, A. M., & Kaschak, M. P. (2004). Putting words in perspective. *Memory & Cognition, 32,* 863–873.

Bornstein, M. H., Hahn, C-S., & Suwalsky, J. T. D. (2013). Physically developed and exploratory young infants contribute to their own long-term academic achievement. *Psychological Science, 24,* 1906–1917.

Boudreau, K. J., Lacetera, N., & Lakhani, K. R. (2011). Incentives and problem uncertainty in innovation contests: An empirical analysis. *Management Science, 57,* 843–863.

Boudreau, K. J., & Lakhani, K. R. (2015). 'Open' disclosure of innovations, incentives and follow-on reuse: Theory on processes of cumulative innovation and a field experiment in computational biology. *Research Policy, 44,* 4–19.

Bourgeois, L. J. III (1981). On the measurement of organizational slack. *Academy of Management Review, 6,* 29–39.

Bowden, E. M., & Jung-Beeman, M. (2003). Aha!—Insight experience correlates with solution activation in the right hemisphere. *Psychonomic Bulletin and Review, 10,* 730–737.

Bradley, B. H., Klotz, A. C., Postlethwaite, B. E., & Brown, K. G. (2013). Ready to rumble: How team personality composition and task conflict interact to improve performance. *Journal of Applied Psychology, 98,* 385–392.

Brainerd, C. J., & Reyna, V. F. (1990). Gist is the grist: Fuzzy-trace theory and the new intuitionism. *Developmental Review, 10,* 3–47.

Brainerd, C. J., & Reyna, V. F. (2001). Fuzzy-trace theory: Dual processes in memory, reasoning, and cognitive neuroscience. *Advances in Child Development and Behavior, 28,* 41–100.

Brandstätter, V., Lengfelder, A., & Gollwitzer, P. M. (2001). Implementation intentions and efficient action initiation. *Journal of Personality and Social Psychology, 81,* 946–960.

Braver, T. S., Barch, D. M., & Cohen, J. D. (1999). Cognition and control in schizophrenia: A computational model of dopamine and prefrontal function. *Biological Psychiatry, 46,* 312–328.

Braver, T. S., Krug, M. K., Chiew, K. S., Kool, W., Westbrook, J. A., Clement, N. J., . . . Somerville, L. H. (2014). Mechanisms of motivation-cognition interaction: Challenges and opportunities. *Cognitive, Affective, and Behavioral Neuroscience, 14,* 443–472.

Bressler, S. L., & Menon, V. (2010). Large-scale brain networks in cognition: Emerging methods and principles. *Trends in Cognitive Sciences, 14*, 277–290.

Brews, P. J., & Hunt, M. R. (1999). Learning to plan and planning to learn: Resolving the planning school/learning school debate. *Strategic Management Journal, 20*, 889–913.

Broaders, S. C., Cook, S. W., Mitchell, Z., & Goldin-Meadow, S. (2007). Making children gesture brings out implicit knowledge and leads to learning. *Journal of Experimental Psychology: General, 136*, 539–550.

Brooks, A. W. (2013). Get excited: Reappraising pre-performance anxiety as excitement. *Journal of Experimental Psychology: General, 143*, 1144–1158.

Brown, C., & Miller, S. (2008). The impacts of local markets: A review of research on farmers markets and community supported agriculture (CSA). *American Journal of Agricultural Economics, 90*, 1296–1302.

Brown, R. (1958). How shall a thing be called? *Psychological Review, 65*, 14–21.

Brown, R., & McNeill, D. (1966). The "tip-of-the-tongue" phenomenon. *Journal of Verbal and Verbal Behavior, 5*, 325–337.

Buckner, R. L., Andrews-Hanna, J. R., & Schacter, D. L. (2008). The brain's default network: Anatomy, function, and relevance to disease. *Annals of the New York Academy of Sciences, 1124*, 1–38.

Bugg, J. M., & Crump, M. J. C. (2012). In support of a distinction between voluntary and stimulus-driven control: A review of the literature on proportion congruent effects. *Frontiers in Psychology, 3*, Article 367, 1–16.

Burke, C. S., Stagl, K. C., Salas, E., Pierce, L., & Kendall, D. (2006). Understanding team adaptation: A conceptual analysis and model. *Journal of Applied Psychology, 91*, 1189–1207.

Burroughs, J. E., Dahl, D. W., Moreau, C. P., Chattopadhyay, A., & Gorn, G. J. (2011). Facilitating and rewarding creativity during new product development. *Journal of Marketing, 75*, 53–67.

Burton, K. D., Lydon, J. E., D'Alessandro, D. U., & Koestner, R. (2006). The differential effects of intrinsic and identified motivation on well-being and performance: Prospective, experimental, and implicit approaches to self-determination theory. *Journal of Personality and Social Psychology, 91*, 750–762.

Byron, K., & Khazanchi, S. (2012). Rewards and creative performance: A meta-analytic test of theoretically derived hypotheses. *Psychological Bulletin, 138*, 809–830.

Cabeza, R., & Moscovitch, M. (2013). Memory systems, processing modes, and components: Functional neuroimaging evidence. *Perspectives on Psychological Science, 8*, 49–55.

Canham, M. S., Wiley, J., & Mayer, R. E. (2012). When diversity in training improves dyadic problem solving. *Applied Cognitive Psychology, 26*, 421–430.

Carnevale, P. J., & Isen, A. M. (1986). The influence of positive affect and visual access on the discovery of integrative solutions in bilateral negotiation. *Organizational Behavior and Human Decision Processes, 37*, 1–13.

Carson, P. P., & Carson, K. D. (1993). Managing creativity enhancement through goal-setting and feedback. *Journal of Creative Behavior, 27*, 36–43.

Carson, S., Peterson, J. B., & Higgins, D. (2003). Decreased latent inhibition is asso-ciated with increased creative achievement in high-functioning individuals. *Journal of Personality and Social Psychology, 85*, 499–506.

Carver, C. S. (2003). Pleasure as a sign you can attend to something else: Placing positive feelings within a general model of affect. *Cognition and Emotion, 17*, 241–261.

Carver, C. S. (2004). Negative affects deriving from the behavioral approach system. *Emotion, 4*, 3–22.

Carver, C. S., Scheier, M. F., & Segerstrom, S. C. (2010). Optimism. *Clinical Psychology Review, 30*, 879–889.

Caspi, A. (2000). The child is father of the man: Personality continuities from child-hood to adulthood. *Journal of Personality and Social Psychology, 78*, 158–172.

Catmull, E. E. (2014). *Creativity, Inc.: Overcoming the unseen forces that stand in the way of true inspiration* (with Amy Wallace). New York: Random House.

Cegarra-Navarro, J-G., Martinez-Martinez, A., Gutiérrez, J. O., & Leal-Rodríguez, A. L. (2013). Environmental knowledge, unlearning, and performance in hospi-tality companies. *Management Decision, 51*, 341–360.

Chadha, G. (2013, December 23). University education: How to get into film-making. *The Daily Telegraph*, London. Retrieved April 8, 2015, from http://www.telegraph.co.uk/education/10520812/University-education-how-to-get-into-filmmaking.html

Chan, J., Fu, K., Schunn, C., Cagan, J., Wood, K., & Kotovsky, K. (2011). On the benefits and pitfalls of analogies for innovative design: Ideation performance based on analogical distance, commonness, and modality of examples. *Journal of Mechanical Design, 133*, Article 061004, 1–11.

Chermahini, S. A., & Hommel, B. (2012). Creative mood swings: Divergent and convergent thinking affect mood in opposite ways. *Psychological Research, 76*, 634–640.

Chiu, I., & Shu, L. H. (2012). Investigating effects of oppositely related semantic stimuli on design concept creativity. *Journal of Engineering Design, 23*, 271–296.

Christensen, B. T., & Schunn, C. D. (2007). The relationship of analogical distance to analogical function and preinventive structure: The case of engineering design. *Memory & Cognition, 35*, 29–38.

Christensen, B. T., & Schunn, C. D. (2009). The role and impact of mental simulation in design. *Applied Cognitive Psychology, 23*, 327–344.

Christian, B. M., Miles, L. K., Fung, F.H.K., Best, S., & Macrae, C. N. (2013). The shape of things to come: Exploring goal-directed prospection. *Consciousness and Cognition, 22*, 471–478.

Christoff, K. (2012). Undirected thought: Neural determinants and correlates. *Brain Research, 1428*, 51–59.

Chrysikou, E. G. (2006). When shoes become hammers: Goal-derived categoriza-tion training enhances problem-solving performance. *Journal of Experimental Psychology: Learning, Memory, and Cognition, 32*, 935–942.

Chua, Y.-J., & Iyengar, S. S. (2008). Creativity as a matter of choice: Prior experience and task instruction as boundary conditions for the positive effect of choice on creativity. *Journal of Creative Behavior, 42*, 164–180.

Chulvi, V., Sonseca, Á., Mulet, E., & Chakrabarti, A. (2012). Assessment of the relationships among design methods, design activities, and creativity. *Journal of Mechanical Design, 134,* Article 111004, 1–11.

Clark, A. (2001). Reasons, robots and the extended mind. *Mind and Language, 16,* 121–145.

Clark, A. (2008). *Supersizing the mind: Embodiment, action, and cognitive extension.* New York: Oxford University Press.

Clark, E. V., & Clark, H. A. (1979). When nouns surface as verbs. *Language, 55,* 767–811.

Clark, W. H., & Babson E. K. (2012). How benefit corporations are redefining the purpose of business corporations. *William Mitchell Law Review, 38,* 817–851.

Cleeremans, A., & Jiménez, L. (2002). Implicit learning and consciousness: A graded, dynamic perspective. In R. M. French and A. Cleeremans, Eds., *Implicit learning and consciousness* (pp. 1–40). New York: Taylor & Francis.

Clement, J. J. (2009). The role of imagistic simulation in scientific thought experiments. *Topics in Cognitive Science, 1,* 686–710.

Cohen, J. D., Braver, T. S., & Brown, J. W. (2002). Computational perspectives on dopamine function in prefrontal cortex. *Current Opinion in Neurobiology, 12,* 223–229.

Cohen, J. D., McClure, S. M., & Yu, A. J. (2007). Should I stay or should I go? How the human brain manages the trade-off between exploitation and exploration. *Philosophical Transactions of the Royal Society, B, 362,* 933–942.

Cohen, L. (1992/2003). Leonard Cohen, in P. Zollo (Ed.), *Songwriters on songwriting* (pp. 329–349). Cambridge, MA: Da Capo Press.

Cohen, W. M., & Levinthal, D. A. (1990). Absorptive capacity: A new perspective on learning and innovation. *Administrative Science Quarterly, 35,* 128–152.

Cole, S. A., & Fernando, A. N. (2012, November 21). The value of advice: Evidence from mobile phone-based agricultural extension. *Harvard Business School Working Paper* 13-047, 1–31.

Collins, A., & Koechlin, E. (2012). Reasoning, learning, and creativity: Frontal lobe function and human decision-making. *PLoS Biology, 10,* Article e1001293, 1–16.

Collins, A. M., & Loftus, E. F. (1975). A spreading-activation theory of semantic processing. *Psychological Review, 82,* 407–428.

Colzato, L. S., Ozturk, A., & Hommel, B. (2012). Meditate to create: The impact of focused-attention and open-monitoring training on convergent and divergent thinking. *Frontiers in Psychology, 3,* Article 116, 1–5.

Colzato, L. S., Van den Wildenberg, W. P. M., & Hommel, B. (2013). Increasing self-other integration through divergent thinking. *Psychonomic Bulletin & Review, 20,* 1011–1016.

Connell, L., & Lynott, D. (2013). Flexible and fast: Linguistic shortcut affects both shallow and deep conceptual processing. *Psychonomic Bulletin & Review, 20,* 542–550.

Consoli, D. (2014). Innovation: Myths and prospects. *Science, 345,* 883.

Conway, M. A. (2005). Memory and the self. *Journal of Memory and Language, 53,* 594–628.

Conway, M. A. (2009). Episodic memories. *Neuropsychologia, 47,* 2305–2313.

Conway, M. A., Meares, K., & Standart, S. (2004). Images and goals. *Memory, 12,* 525–531.

Conway, M. A., & Pleydell-Pearce, C. W. (2000). The construction of autobiographical memories in the self-memory system. *Psychological Review, 107,* 261–288.

Cools, R. (2008). Role of dopamine in the motivational and cognitive control of behaviour. *Neuroscientist, 14,* 381–395.

Cools, R., & D'Esposito, M. (2011). Inverted U-shaped dopamine actions on human working memory and cognitive control. *Biological Psychiatry, 69,* e113–e125.

Cooper, R., & Markus, M. L. (1995). Human reengineering. *Sloan Management Review, 36,* 39–50.

Cowan, N. (2001). The magical number 4 in short-term memory: A reconsideration of mental storage capacity. *Behavioral and Brain Sciences, 24,* 87–114; discussion 114–185.

Craig, A. D. (2009). How do you feel—now? The anterior insula and human awareness. *Nature Reviews Neuroscience, 10,* 59–70.

Crane, C., Winder, R., Hargus, E., Amarasinghe, M., & Barnhoffer, T. (2012). Effects of mindfulness-based cognitive therapy on specificity of life goals. *Cognitive Therapy & Research, 36,* 182–189.

Cross, N. (1997). Descriptive models of creative design: Application to an example. *Design Studies, 18,* 427–455.

Crump, J. (2013). On photography and influence: James Welling in conversation with Eva Respini. In *James Welling: Monograph* (pp. 119–124). New York: Aperture.

Csíkszentmihályi, M. (1990). *Flow: The psychology of optimal experience.* New York: HarperCollins.

Csíkszentmihályi, M. (1996). *Creativity: Flow and the psychology of discovery and invention.* New York: HarperCollins.

Cummings, B. (2012). Benefit corporations: How to enforce a mandate to promote the public interest. *Columbia Law Review, 112,* 578–672.

Curlik, D. M., & Shors, T. J. (2013). Training your brain: Do mental and physical (MAP) training enhance cognition through the process of neurogenesis in the hippocampus? *Neuropharmacology, 64,* 506–514.

Curtis, D. E., & Resnik, J. (1987). Images of justice. *Yale Law Journal, 96,* 1727–1772.

Dahl, D. W., & Moreau, P. (2002). The influence and value of analogical thinking during new product ideation. *Journal of Marketing Research, 39,* 47–60.

Daly, S. R., Yilmaz, S., Christian, J. L., Seifert, C. M., & Gonzalez, R. (2012). Design heuristics in engineering concept generation. *Journal of Engineering Education, 101,* 601–629.

Damasio, A. R. (1996). The somatic marker hypothesis and the possible functions of the prefrontal cortex. *Philosophical Transactions of the Royal Society of London, B, 351,* 1413–1420.

Danneels, E. (2008). Organizational antecedents of second-order competences. *Strategic Management Journal, 29,* 519–543.

D'Ardenne, K. D., Eshel, N., Luka, J., Lenartowicz, A., Nystrom, L. E., & Cohen, J. D. (2012). Role of prefrontal cortex and the midbrain dopamine system in working memory updating. *Proceedings of the National Academy of Sciences, USA, 109,* 19900–19909.

D'Argembeau, A., Lardi, C., & Van der Linden, M. (2012). Self-defining future projections: Exploring the identity function of thinking about the future. *Memory,* *20*, 110–120.

D'Argembeau, A., Renaud, O., & Van der Linden, M. (2011). Frequency, characteristics and functions of future-oriented thoughts in daily life. *Applied Cognitive Psychology, 25*, 96–103.

D'Argembeau, A., Stawarczyk, D., Majerus, S., Collette, F., Van der Linden, M., Feyers, D., . . . Salmon, E. (2010). The neural basis of personal goal processing when envisioning future events. *Journal of Cognitive Neuroscience, 22*, 1701–1713.

D'Argembeau, A., & Van der Linden, M. (2012). Predicting the phenomenology of episodic future thoughts. *Consciousness and Cognition, 21*, 1198–1206.

Davies, R. (1991). *The Tanner lectures on human values* (Vol. 13). Salt Lake City: University of Utah Press.

Davis, M. A. (2009). Understanding the relationship between mood and creativity: A meta-analysis. *Organizational Behavior and Human Decision Processes, 108*, 25–38.

Daw, N. D., O'Doherty, J. P., Dayan, P., Seymour, B., & Dolan, R. J. (2006). Cortical substrates for exploratory decisions in humans. *Nature, 441*, 876–879.

DeChurch, L. A., & Mesmer-Magnus, J. R. (2010a). Measuring shared team mental models: A meta-analysis. *Group Dynamics: Theory, Research, and Practice, 14*, 1–14.

DeChurch, L. A., & Mesmer-Magnus, J. R. (2010b). The cognitive underpinnings of effective teamwork: A meta-analysis. *Journal of Applied Psychology, 95*, 32–53.

Deci, E. L., Koestner, R., & Ryan, R. M. (1999). A meta-analytic review of experiments examining the effects of extrinsic rewards on intrinsic motivation. *Psychological Bulletin, 125*, 627–668.

De Dreu, C.K.W., Baas, M., & Nijstad, B. A. (2008). Hedonic tone and activation level in the mood-creativity link: Toward a dual pathway to creativity model. *Journal of Personality and Social Psychology, 94*, 739–756.

De Dreu, C. K. W., Nijstad, B. A., Baas, M., Wolsink, I., & Roskes, M. (2012). Working memory benefits creative insight, musical improvisation, and original ideation through maintained task-focused attention. *Personality and Social Psychology Bulletin, 38*, 656–669.

De Dreu, C. K. W., Nijstad, B. A., Bechtoldt, M. N., & Baas, M. (2011). Group creativity and innovation: A motivated information processing perspective. *Psychology of Aesthetics, Creativity, and the Arts, 5*, 81–89.

Defeyter, M. A., & German, T. P. (2003). Acquiring an understanding of design: Evidence from children's insight problem solving. *Cognition, 89*, 133–155.

DeFranco, J. F., Neill, C. J., & Clariana, R. B. (2011). A cognitive collaborative model to improve performance in engineering teams: A study of team outcomes and mental model sharing. *Systems Engineering, 14*, 267–278.

Dehaene, S., & Changeux, J.-P. (2011). Experimental and theoretical approaches to conscious processes. *Neuron, 70*, 200–227.

Dehaene, S., & Naccache, L. (2001). Towards a cognitive neuroscience of consciousness: Basic evidence and a workspace framework. *Cognition, 79*, 1–37.

deLahunta, S., Clarke, G., & Barnard, P. (2012). A conversation about choreographic thinking tools. *Journal of Dance & Somatic Practices, 3,* 243–259.

de Manzano, Ö., Theorell, T., Harmat, L., & Ullén, F. (2010). The psychophysiology of flow during piano playing. *Emotion, 10,* 301–311.

DeRosa, D. M., Smith, C. L., & Hantula, D. A. (2007). The medium matters: Mining the long-promised merit of group interaction in creative idea generation tasks in a meta-analysis of the electronic group brainstorming literature. *Computers in Human Behavior, 23,* 1549–1581.

Desai, R. H., Conant, L. L., Binder, J. R., Park, H., & Seidenberg, M. S. (2013). A piece of the action: Modulation of sensory-motor regions by action idioms and metaphors. *NeuroImage, 83,* 862–869.

Desimone, R., & Duncan, J. (1995). Neural mechanisms of selective visual attention. *Annual Review of Neuroscience, 18,* 193–222.

De Snoo, C., Van Wezel, W., & Jorna, R. J. (2011). An empirical investigation of scheduling performance criteria. *Journal of Operations Management, 29,* 181–193.

Desroches, A. S., Newman, R. L., & Joanisse, M. F. (2009). Investigating the time course of spoken word recognition: Electrophysiological evidence for the influences of phonological similarity. *Journal of Cognitive Neuroscience, 21,* 1893–1906.

DeYoung, C. G. (2013). The neuromodulator of exploration: A unifying theory of the role of dopamine in personality. *Frontiers in Human Neuroscience, 7,* Article 762, 1–26.

Dickson, J. M., & Moberly, N. J. (2013). Reduced specificity of personal goals and explanations for goal attainment in major depression. *PLoS ONE, 8,* Article e64512, 1–8.

Diehl, M., & Stroebe, W. (1987). Productivity loss in brainstorming groups: Toward the solution of a riddle. *Journal of Personality and Social Psychology, 53,* 497–509.

Dixon, M. L., Fox, K. C. R., & Christoff, K. (2014). A framework for understanding the relationship between externally and internally directed cognition. *Neuropsychologia, 62,* 321–330.

Dobson, K. (2013). Conversation: Materials. In R. Somerson & M. L. Hermano (Eds.), *The art of critical making: Rhode Island School of Design on creative practice* (pp. 138–163). Hoboken, NJ: Wiley.

Dodgson, M., Gann, D. M., & Phillips, N. (2013). Organizational learning and the technology of foolishness: The case of virtual worlds at IBM. *Organization Science, 24,* 1358–1376.

Dodhia, R. M., & Dismukes, R. K. (2009). Interruptions create prospective memory tasks. *Applied Cognitive Psychology, 23,* 73–89.

Dodson, C. S., Johnson, M. K., & Schooler, J. W. (1997). The verbal overshadowing effect: Why descriptions impair face recognition. *Memory & Cognition, 25,* 129–139.

Dolcos, F., Iordan, A. D., & Dolcos, S. (2011). Neural correlates of emotion-cognition interactions: A review of evidence from brain imaging investigations. *Journal of Cognitive Psychology, 23,* 669–694.

Doll, W. J., & Deng, X. (2011). Antecedents of improvisation in IT-enabled engineering work. *Journal of Organizational and End User Computing, 23,* 26–47.

Doorley, S., & Witthoft, S. (2012). *Make space: How to set the stage for creative collaboration.* Hoboken, NJ: Wiley.

Dorst, K., & Cross, N. (2001). Creativity in the design process: Co-evolution of problem–solution. *Design Studies, 22,* 425–437.

Dougherty, D., & Takacs, C. H. (2004). Team play: Heedful interrelating as the boundary for innovation. *Long Range Planning, 37,* 569–590.

Dow, S. P., Glassco, A., Kass, J., Schwarz, M., Schwartz, D. L., & Klemmer, S. R. (2010). Parallel prototyping leads to better design results, more divergence, and increased self-efficacy. *ACM Transactions on Computer-Human Interaction, 17,* Article 18, 1–24.

Doyle, A. C. (1902/2006). The Hound of the Baskervilles. In L. S. Klinger (Ed.), *The new annotated Sherlock Holmes: The novels* (Vol. 3, pp. 383–627). New York: W. W. Norton.

Draganski, B., Gaser, C., Busch, V., Schuierer, G., Bogdahn, U., & May, A. (2004). Changes in grey matter induced by training. *Nature, 427,* 311–312.

Dreisbach, G., & Goschke, T. (2004). How positive affect modulates cognitive control: Reduced perseveration at the cost of increased distractibility. *Journal of Experimental Psychology: Learning, Memory, and Cognition, 30,* 343–353.

Dunbar, K. (1995). How scientists really reason: Scientific reasoning in real world laboratories. In R. J. Sternberg & J. E. Davidson (Eds.), *The nature of insight* (pp. 365–395). Cambridge, MA: MIT Press.

Duncan, J. (2010). The multiple-demand (MD) system of the primate brain: Mental programs for intelligent behavior. *Trends in Cognitive Sciences, 14,* 172–179.

Duncan, J., Parr, A., Woolgar, A., Thompson, R., Bright, P., Cox, S., Bishop, S., & Nimmo-Smith, I. (2008). Goal neglect and Spearman's *g:* Competing parts of a complex task. *Journal of Experimental Psychology: General, 137,* 131–148.

Dunwoody, P. T., Haarbauer, E., Mahan, R. P., Marino, C., & Tang, C. C. (2000). Cognitive adaptation and its consequences: A test of cognitive continuum theory. *Journal of Behavioral Decision Making, 13,* 35–54.

Dux, P. E., Roseboom, W., & Olivers, C. N. L. (2013). Attentional tuning resets after failures of perceptual awareness. *PLoS ONE, 8,* Article e60623, 1–6.

Dweck, C. S., & Leggett, E. L. (1988). A social-cognitive approach to motivation and personality. *Psychological Review, 95,* 256–273.

Eaglestone, B., Ford, N., Brown, G. J., & Moore, A. (2007). Information systems and creativity: An empirical study. *Journal of Documentation, 63,* 443–464.

Ebrahim, A., & Rangan, V. K. (2014). What impact? A framework for measuring the scale and scope of social performance. *California Management Review, 56,* 118–141.

Eccles, D. W. (2006). Thinking outside of the box: The role of environmental adaptation in the acquisition of skilled and expert performance. *Journal of Sports Sciences, 24,* 1103–1114.

Eckert, C. M., Stacey, M., Wyatt, D., & Garthwaite, P. (2012). Change as little as possible: Creativity in design by modification. *Journal of Engineering Design, 23,* 337–360.

Eckert, M. A., Menon, V., Walczak, A., Ahlstrom, J., Denslow, S., Horwitz, A., & Dubno, J. R. (2009). At the heart of the ventral attention system: The right anterior insula. *Human Brain Mapping, 30,* 2530–2541.

Ederer, F., & Manso, G. (2013). Is pay for performance detrimental to innovation? *Management Science, 59,* 1496–1513.

Einstein, G. O., McDaniel, M. A., Richardson, S. L., Guynn, M. J., & Cunfer, A. R. (1995). Aging and prospective memory: Examining the influences of self-initiated retrieval processes. *Journal of Experimental Psychology: Learning, Memory, and Cognition, 21,* 996–1007.

Eisenberger, R., & Armeli, S. (1997). Can salient reward increase creative performance without reducing intrinsic creative interest? *Journal of Personality and Social Psychology, 72,* 652–665.

Eitam, B., & Higgins, E. T. (2010). Motivation in mental accessibility: Relevance of a representation (ROAR) as a new framework. *Social and Personality Psychology Compass, 3,* 1–17.

Ellamil, M., Dobson, C., Beeman, M., & Christoff, K. (2012). Evaluative and generative modes of thought during the creative process. *NeuroImage, 59,* 1783–1794.

Ellis, J. & Milne, A. (1996). Retrieval cue specificity and the realization of delayed intentions. *Quarterly Journal of Experimental Psychology, 49A,* 862–887.

Ellwood, S., Pallier, G., Snyder, A., & Gallate, J. (2009). The incubation effect: Hatching a solution? *Creativity Research Journal, 21,* 6–14.

Elsbach, K. D., & Hargadon, A. B. (2006). Enhancing creativity through "mindless" work: A framework for workday design. *Organization Science, 17,* 470–483.

Endsley, M. R. (1995). Toward a theory of situation awareness in dynamic systems. *Human Factors, 37,* 32–64.

Erickson, M. (2012, October 10). "Mudlark." Retrieved November 22, 2014 from http://michelleericksonceramics.blogspot.com/2012/10/mudlark.html

Erickson, T., Li, M., Kim, Y., Deshpande, A., Sahu, S., Chao, T., . . . Naphade, M. (2013). The Dubuque electricity portal: Evaluation of a city-scale residential electricity consumption feedback system. *Proceedings of the SIGCHI Conference on Human Factors in Computing Systems (CHI '13),* 1203–1212.

Ericsson, K. A. (2008). Deliberate practice and acquisition of expert performance: A general overview. *Academic Emergency Medicine, 15,* 988–994.

Ericsson, K. A., Krampe, R. T., & Tesch-Römer, C. (1993). The role of deliberate practice in the acquisition of expert performance. *Psychological Review, 100,* 363–406.

Ernst, A., Alkass, K., Bernard, S., Salehpour, M., Perl, S., Tisdale, J., . . . Frisén, J. (2014). Neurogenesis in the striatum of the adult human brain. *Cell, 156,* 1072–1083.

Espin, S., Lingard, L., Baker, G. R., & Regehr, G. (2006). Persistence of unsafe practice in everyday work: An exploration of organizational and psychological factors constraining safety in the operating room. *Quality and Safety in Health Care, 15,* 165–170.

Esposito, R. T. (2013). The social enterprise revolution in corporate law: A primer on emerging corporate entities in Europe and the United States and the case for the benefit corporation. *William & Mary Business Law Review, 4,* 639–714.

Estrada, C. A., Isen, A. M., & Young, M. J. (1997). Positive affect facilitates integration of information and decreases anchoring in reasoning among physicians. *Organizational Behavior and Human Decision Processes, 72,* 117–135.

Fabrizio, K. R. (2009). Absorptive capacity and the search for innovation. *Research Policy, 38*, 255–267.

Fadde, P. J. (2006). Interactive video training of perceptual decision-making in the sport of baseball. *Technology, Instruction, Cognition and Learning, 4*, 265–285.

Fadde, P. J. (2009). Instructional design for advanced learners: Training recognition skills to hasten expertise. *Educational Technology and Research Development, 57*, 359–376.

Faust, D. G. (2011, December 26). Women in leadership: Drew Gilpin Faust, *Nightly Business Report.* Retrieved April 8, 2015, from http://wp.nbr.com/transcripts/women-in-leadership-drew-gilpin-faust-20111226

Fayena-Tawil, Kozbelt, A., & Sitaras, L. (2011). Think global, act local: A protocol analysis comparison of artists' and nonartists' cognitions, metacognitions, and evaluations while drawing. *Psychology of Aesthetics, Creativity, and the Arts, 5*, 135–145.

Feldman, M. S. (2000). Organizational routines as a source of continuous change. *Organization Science, 11*, 611–629.

Finnbogadóttir, H., & Berntsen, D. (2013). Involuntary future projections are as frequent as involuntary memories, but more positive. *Consciousness and Cognition, 22*, 272–280.

Fishman, J. P. (2015). Creating around copyright. *Harvard Law Review, 128*, 1333–1404.

Fong, C. T. (2006). The effects of emotional ambivalence on creativity. *Academy of Management Journal, 49*, 1016–1030.

Ford, C. M. (1996). A theory of individual creative action in multiple social domains. *Academy of Management Review, 21*, 1112–1142.

Forgas, J. P., & Eich, E. (2012). Affective influences on cognition: Mood congruence, mood dependence, and mood effects on processing strategies. In A. F. Healy & R. W. Proctor (Eds.), *Handbook of Psychology* (pp. 61–82). New York: Wiley.

Forgas, J. P., & George, J. M. (2001). Affective influences on judgments and behavior in organizations: An information processing perspective. *Organizational Behavior and Human Decision Processes, 86*, 3–34.

Foroughi, C. K., Werner, N. E., Nelson, E. T., & Boehm-Davis, D. A. (2014). Do interruptions affect quality of work? *Human Factors, 56*, 1262–1271.

Foxley, A. (2010). *Distance and engagement: Walking, thinking and making landscape.* Baden, Switzerland: Lars Müller Publishers.

Frank, M. J., Loughry, B., & O'Reilly, R. C. (2001). Interactions between frontal cortex and basal ganglia in working memory: A computational model. *Cognitive, Affective, & Behavioral Neuroscience, 1*, 137–160.

Fredrickson, B. L. (2001). The role of positive emotions in positive psychology: The broaden-and-build theory of positive emotions. *American Psychologist, 56*, 218–226.

Fredrickson, B. L. (2004). The broaden-and-build theory of positive emotions. *Philosophical Transactions of the Royal Society of London, B, 359*, 1367–1377.

Fu, K., Chan, J., Cagan, J., Kotovsky, K., Schunn, C., & Wood, K. (2013). The meaning of "near" and "far": The impact of structuring design databases and the effect of distance of analogy on design output. *Journal of Mechanical Design, 135*, Article 021007, 1–12.

Fullbright, J. (2014, June 2). Songwriters on songwriting: John Fullbright. (Interview with Kim Ruehl). *The Bluegrass Situation.* Retrieved April 8, 2015, from www.thebluegrasssituation.com/read/songwriters-songwriting-john-fullbright

Furr, N. R., Cavarretta, F., & Garg, S. (2012). Who changes course? The role of domain knowledge and novel framing in making technology changes. *Strategic Entrepreneurship Journal, 6*, 236–256.

Fuster, J. (2006). The cognit: A network model of cortical representation. *International Journal of Psychophysiology, 60*, 125–132.

Fuster, J. (2009). Cortex and memory: Emergence of a new paradigm. *Journal of Cognitive Neuroscience, 21*, 2047–2072.

Fuster, J., & Bressler, S. L. (2012). Cognit activation: A mechanism for enabling temporal integration in working memory. *Trends in Cognitive Sciences, 16*, 207–218.

Gabora, L. (2010). Revenge of the "neurds": Characterizing creative thought in terms of the structure and dynamics of memory. *Creativity Research Journal, 22*, 1–13.

Gagné, M., & Deci, E. L. (2005). Self-determination theory and work motivation. *Journal of Organizational Behavior, 26*, 331–362.

Galenson, D. W. (2006). *Old masters and young geniuses: The two life cycles of artistic creativity.* Princeton, NJ: Princeton University Press.

Galenson, D. W. (2010). Understanding creativity. *Journal of Applied Economics, 13*, 351–362.

Gallate, J., Wong, C., Ellwood, S., Roring, R. W., & Snyder, A. (2012). Creative people use nonconscious processes to their advantage. *Creativity Research Journal, 24*, 146–151.

Gallo, I. S., Keil, A., McCulloch, K. C., Rockstroh, B., & Gollwitzer, P. M. (2009). Strategic automation of emotion regulation. *Journal of Personality and Social Psychology, 96*, 11–31.

Garoff, R. J., Slotnick, S. D., & Schacter, D. L. (2005). The neural origins of specific and general memory: The role of fusiform cortex. *Neuropsychologia, 43*, 847–859.

Gassman, O., & Zeschky, M. (2008). Opening up the solution space: The role of analogical thinking for breakthrough product innovation. *Creativity and Innovation Management, 17*, 97–106.

Gaver, W. W., Beaver, J., & Benford, S. (2003). Ambiguity as a resource for design. *Proceedings of the SIGCHI Conference on Human Factors in Computing Systems (CHI '03)*, 233–240.

Geake, J. G., & Hansen, P. C. (2005). Neural correlates of intelligence as revealed by fMRI of fluid analogies. *NeuroImage, 26*, 555–564.

Genco, N., Johnson, D., Hölttä-Otto, K., & Seepersad, C. C. (2011). A study of the effectiveness of empathic experience design as a creativity technique. *Proceedings of the ASME 2011 International Design Engineering Technical Conferences & Computers and Information in Engineering Conference*, Washington, DC. Article DETC2011-021711, 1–9.

Genco, N., Johnson, D., Hölttä-Otto, K., & Seepersad, C. C. (2012). An experimental investigation of the innovation capabilities of undergraduate engineering students. *Journal of Engineering Education, 101,* 60–81.

George, J. M. (2011). Dual tuning: A minimum condition for understanding affect in organizations? *Organizational Psychology Review, 1,* 147–164.

George, J. M., & Zhou, J. (2007). Dual tuning in a supportive context: Joint contributions of positive mood, negative mood, and supervisory behaviors to employee creativity. *Academy of Management Journal, 50,* 605–622.

Gerber, E., & Carroll, M. (2012). The psychological experience of prototyping. *Design Studies, 33,* 64–84.

Gerber, E., McKenna, A., Hirsch, P., & Yarnoff, C. (2010). Learning to waste and wasting to learn? How to use cradle to cradle principles to improve the teaching of design. *International Journal of Engineering Education, 26,* 314–323.

Gerken, H. K. (2014). Federalism as the new nationalism: An overview. *Yale Law Journal, 123,* 1889–1918.

German, T. P., & Defeyter, M. A. (2000). Immunity to functional fixedness in young children. *Psychonomic Bulletin & Review, 7,* 707–712.

German, T. P., & Johnson, S. C. (2002). Function and the origins of the design stance. *Journal of Cognition and Development, 3,* 279–300.

Gero, J., Jiang, H., & Williams, C. B. (2013). Design cognition differences when using structured and unstructured concept generation creativity techniques. *International Journal of Design Creativity and Innovation, 1,* 196–214.

Gero, J. S., & Kannengiesser, U. (2012). Representational affordances in design, with examples from analogy making and optimization. *Research in Engineering Design, 23,* 235–249.

Geschka, H. (1983). Creativity techniques in product-planning and development: A view from West Germany. *R&D Management, 13,* 169–183.

Gibson, C. B., & Birkinshaw, J. (2004). The antecedents, consequences, and mediating role of organizational ambidexterity. *Academy of Management Journal, 47,* 209–226.

Gibson, J. (1977). The theory of affordances. In Shaw, R., & Bransford, J. (Eds.), *Perceiving, acting and knowing* (pp. 67–82). New York: Wiley.

Gibson, J. J. (1979/1986). *The ecological approach to visual perception.* Hillsdale, NJ: Erlbaum.

Gilbert, S. J., Gollwitzer, P. M., Cohen, A-L., Oettingen, G., & Burgess, P. W. (2009). Separable brain systems supporting cued versus self-initiated realization of delayed intentions. *Journal of Experimental Psychology: Learning, Memory, and Cognition, 35,* 905–915.

Gilhooly, K. J., Fioratou, E., Anthony, S. H., & Wynn, V. (2007). Divergent thinking: Strategies and executive involvement in generating novel uses for familiar objects. *British Journal of Psychology, 98,* 611–625.

Gilhooly, K. J., Georgiou, G., & Devery, U. (2013). Incubation and creativity: Do something different. *Thinking and Reasoning, 19,* 137–149.

Gino, F., Argote, L., Miron-Spektor, E., & Todorova, G. (2010). First, get your feet wet: The effects of learning from direct and indirect experience on team creativity. *Organizational Behavior and Human Decision Processes, 111,* 102–115.

Giuliani, E. (2013). Network dynamics in regional clusters: Evidence from Chile. *Research Policy, 42*, 1406–1419.

Giuliani, E., & Bell, M. (2005). The micro-determinants of meso-level learning and innovation: Evidence from a Chilean wine cluster. *Research Policy, 34*, 47–68.

Glynn, M. A. (1994). Effects of work task cues and play task cues on information processing, judgment, and motivation. *Journal of Applied Psychology, 79*, 34–45.

Goel, A. K., Vattam, S., Wiltgen, B., & Helms, M. (2012). Cognitive, collaborative, conceptual and creative—Four characteristics of the next generation of knowledge-based CAD systems: A study in biologically inspired design. *Computer-Aided Design, 44*, 879–900.

Goldenberg, O., Larson, J. R., & Wiley, J. (2013). Goal instructions, response format, and idea generation in groups. *Small Group Research, 44*, 227–256.

Goldstone, R. L., Roberts, M. E., & Gureckis, T. M. (2008). Emergent processes in group behavior. *Current Directions in Psychological Science, 17*, 10–15.

Goldstone, R. L., & Son, J. Y. (2005). The transfer of scientific principles using concrete and idealized simulations. *Journal of the Learning Sciences, 14*, 69–110.

Gollwitzer, P. M. (1999). Implementation intentions: Strong effects of simple plans. *American Psychologist, 54*, 493–503.

Gollwitzer, P. M., & Brandstätter, V. (1997). Implementation intentions and effective goal pursuit. *Journal of Personality and Social Psychology, 73*, 186–199.

Gollwitzer, P. M., Heckhausen, H., & Steller, B. (1990). Deliberative and implemental mind-sets: Cognitive tuning toward congruous thoughts and information. *Journal of Personality and Social Psychology, 59*, 1119–1127.

Gollwitzer, P. M., & Schaal, B. (1998). Metacognition in action: The importance of implementation intentions. *Personality and Social Psychology Review, 2*, 124–136.

Gollwitzer, P. M., & Sheeran, P. (2006). Implementation intentions and goal achievement: A meta-analysis of effects and processes. *Advances in Experimental Social Psychology, 38*, 69–119.

Grant, A. M., & Schwartz, B. (2011). Too much of a good thing: The challenge and opportunity of the inverted U. *Perspectives on Psychological Science, 6*, 61–76.

Grant, J. A., Duerden, E. G., Courtemanche, J., Cherkasova, M., Duncan, G. H., & Rainville, P. (2013). Cortical thickness, mental absorption and meditative practice: Possible implications for disorders of attention. *Biological Psychology, 92*, 275–281.

Green, A. E., Cohen, M. S., Kim, J. U., & Gray, J. R. (2012). An explicit cue improves creative analogical reasoning. *Intelligence, 40*, 598–603.

Green, A. E., Kraemer, D. J. M., Fugelsang, J. A., Gray, J. R., & Dunbar, K. N. (2012). Neural correlates of creativity in analogical reasoning. *Journal of Experimental Psychology: Learning, Memory, and Cognition, 38*, 264–272.

Greenberg, D. L., & Verfaellie, M. (2010). Interdependence of episodic and semantic memory: Evidence from neuropsychology. *Journal of the International Neuropsychological Society, 16*, 748–753.

Greenberg, J., Reiner, K., & Meiran, N. (2012). "Mind the trap": Mindfulness reduces cognitive rigidity. *PLoS ONE, 7*, Article e36206, 1–8.

Groves, K. S., Vance, C. M., Choi, D. Y., & Mendez, J. L. (2008). An examination of the nonlinear thinking style profile stereotype of successful entrepreneurs. *Journal of Enterprising Culture, 16*, 133–159.

Guilford, J. P. (1960). Basic conceptual problems in the psychology of thinking. *Annals of the New York Academy of Sciences, 91*, 6–21.

Guindon, R. (1990). Designing the design process: Exploiting opportunistic thoughts. *Human-Computer Interaction, 5*, 305–344.

Gupta, A. K., Smith, K. G., & Shalley, C. E. (2006). The interplay between exploration and exploitation. *Academy of Management Journal, 49*, 693–706.

Hackman, J. R. (2002). *Leading teams: Setting the stage for great performances.* Boston: Harvard Business School Press.

Hackman, J. R. (2011). *Collaborative intelligence: Using teams to solve hard problems.* San Francisco: Berrett-Koehler.

Hackman, J. R. (2012). From causes to conditions in group research. *Journal of Organizational Behavior, 33*, 428–444.

Hackman, J. R., Kosslyn, S. M., & Woolley, A. W. (2008, March). The design and leadership of intelligence analysis teams. *The group brain project*, Department of Psychology, Harvard University, Technical Report No. 11, 1–93.

Halvorson, H. G. (2014, May). Get your team to do what it says it's going to do. *Harvard Business Review, 92*, 82–87.

Hamilton, R. (2015, March). Bridging psychological distance. *Harvard Business Review, 93*, 116–119.

Hammond, K. R., Hamm, R. M., Grassia, J., & Pearson, T. (1987). Direct comparison of the efficacy of intuitive and analytical cognition in expert judgment. *IEEE Transactions on Systems, Man, and Cybernetics, 17*, 753–770.

Harmon-Jones, E., Gable, P. A., & Price, T. F. (2013). Does negative affect always narrow and positive affect always broaden the mind? Considering the influence of motivational intensity on cognitive scope. *Current Directions in Psychological Science, 22*, 301–307.

Harrington, D. M. (1975). Effects of explicit instructions to "be creative" on the psychological meaning of divergent thinking test scores. *Journal of Personality, 43*, 434–454.

Hatano, G., & Inagaki, K. (1984). Two courses of expertise. *Research and Clinical Center for Child Development Annual Report, 6*, 27–36.

Hayes, C. C., Goel, A. K., Tumer, I. Y., Agogino, A. M., & Regli, W. C. (2011). Intelligent support for product design: Looking backward, looking forward. *Journal of Computing and Information Science in Engineering, 11*, Article No. 021007, 1–9.

Hayes, J. R., Flower, L. S., Schriver, K. A., Stratman, J., & Carey, L. (1987). Cognitive processes in revision. In S. Rosenberg (Ed.), *Advances in psycholinguistics: Vol. II. Reading, writing, and language processing* (pp. 176–240). Cambridge, UK: Cambridge University Press.

Heaphy, E. D. (2013). Repairing breaches with rules: Maintaining institutions in the face of everyday disruptions. *Organization Science, 24*, 1291–1315.

Heath, C., & Staudenmayer, N. (2000). Coordination neglect: How lay theories of organizing complicate coordination in organizations. *Research in Organizational Behaviour, 22*, 155–193.

Heath, J., & Anderson J. (2010). Procrastination and the extended will. In C. Andreou & M. D. White (Eds), *The thief of time: Philosophical essays on procrastination* (pp. 233–252). New York: Oxford University Press.

Hecker, A. (2012). Knowledge beyond the individual? Making sense of a notion of collective knowledge in organization theory. *Organization Studies, 33*, 423–445.

Hedberg, P. H., & Higgins, E. T. (2011). What remains on your mind after you are done? Flexible regulation of knowledge accessibility. *Journal of Experimental Social Psychology, 47*, 882–890.

Hefferon, K. M., & Ollis, S. (2006). "Just clicks": An interpretive phenomenological analysis of professional dancers' experience of flow. *Research in Dance Education, 7*, 141–159.

Helms, M., Vattam, S., & Goel, A. (2009). Biologically inspired design: Process and products. *Design Studies, 30*, 606–622.

Helper, S., & Henderson, R. M. (2014). Management practices, relational contracts and the decline of General Motors. *Journal of Economic Perspectives, 28*, 49–72.

Hemel, D. J., & Ouellette, L. L. (2013). Beyond the patents-prizes debate. *Texas Law Review, 92*, 304–382.

Henderson, R. M., & Clark, K. B. (1990). Architectural innovation: The reconfiguration of existing product technologies and the failure of established firms. *Administrative Science Quarterly, 35*, 9–30.

Henderson, R. M., & Gibbons, R. (2013). What do managers do? Exploring persistent performance differences among seemingly similar enterprises. In R. Gibbons & J. Roberts (Eds.), *The handbook of organizational economics* (pp. 680–731). Princeton, NJ: Princeton University Press.

Henderson, R. M., & Newell, R. G. (Eds.) (2011). *Accelerating energy innovation: Insights from multiple sectors.* Chicago: University of Chicago Press.

Hernandez, N. V., Shah, J. J., & Smith, S. M. (2010). Understanding design ideation mechanisms through multilevel aligned empirical studies. *Design Studies, 31*, 382–410.

Higgins, E. T. (2000). Making a good decision: Value from fit. *American Psychologist, 5*, 217–230.

Hinsz, V. B., Tindale, R. S., & Vollrath, D. A. (1997). The emerging conceptualization of groups as information processors. *Psychological Bulletin, 121*, 43–64.

Hirst, L. (2013). Groundwork. In R. Somerson & M. L. Hermano (Eds.), *The art of critical making: Rhode Island School of Design on creative practice* (pp. 32–51). Hoboken, NJ: Wiley.

Hirt, E. R., Levine, G. M., McDonald, H. E., & Melton, R. J. (1997). The role of mood in quantitative and qualitative aspects of performance: Single or multiple mechanisms? *Journal of Experimental Social Psychology, 33*, 602–629.

Hockey, G. R. J. (2011). A motivational control theory of cognitive fatigue. In P. L. Ackerman (Ed.), *Cognitive fatigue: Multidisciplinary perspectives on current research and future applications* (pp. 167–187). Washington, DC: American Psychological Association.

Hogan, P. (2011, November 19). Gillian Welch: "A lot of the songs are done in one take. Maybe two." *The Observer.* Retrieved April 8, 2015, from http://www.the-guardian.com/music/2011/nov/20/gillian-welch-david-rawlings-interview

Horan, R. (2009). The neuropsychological connection between creativity and meditation. *Creativity Research Journal, 21*, 199–222.

Horga, G., & Maia, T. V. (2012). Conscious and unconscious processes in cognitive control: A theoretical perspective and novel empirical approach. *Frontiers in Human Neuroscience, 6*, Article 199, 1–7.

Howard, T. J., Culley, S., & Dekoninck, E. A. (2011). Reuse of ideas and concepts for creative stimuli in engineering design. *Journal of Engineering Design, 22*, 565–581.

Howard, T. J., Dekoninck, E. A., & Culley, S. (2010). The use of creative stimuli at early stages of industrial product innovation. *Research in Engineering Design, 21*, 263–274.

Howard-Jones, P. A., Blakemore, S-J., Samuel, E. A., Summers, I. R., & Claxton, G. (2005). Semantic divergence and creative story generation: An fMRI investigation. *Cognitive Brain Research, 25*, 240–250.

Humke, C., & Schaefer, C. E. (1996). Sense of humor and creativity. *Perceptual and Motor Skills, 82*, 544–546.

Hunkin, T. (2013). Making. Retrieved April 8, 2015, from www.timhunkin.com/a194_rubegoldberg-essay.htm

Hunt, D. M., Geiger-Oneto, S., & Varca, P. E. (2012). Satisfaction in the context of customer co-production: A behavioral involvement perspective. *Journal of Consumer Behaviour, 11*, 347–356.

Irish, M., & Piguet, O. (2013). The pivotal role of semantic memory in remembering the past and imagining the future. *Frontiers in Behavioral Neuroscience, 7*, Article 27, 1–11.

Isen, A. M., & Daubman, K. A. (1984). The influence of affect on categorization. *Journal of Personality and Social Psychology, 47*, 1206–1217.

Ivanovski, B., & Malhi, G. S. (2007). The psychological and neurophysiological concomitants of mindfulness forms of meditation. *Acta Neuropsychiatrica, 19*, 76–91.

Ive, J. (2014, June 16). In Chen, B. X., & Richtel, M., Jonathan Ive on Apple's design process and product philosophy. *The New York Times*. Retrieved April 8, 2015, from http://bits.blogs.nytimes.com/2014/06/16/jonathan-ive-on-apples-design-process-and-product-philosophy/

Jain, A., & Kogut, B. (2013). Memory and organizational evolvability in a neutral landscape. *Organization Science, 25*, 479–493.

James, W. (1890/1981). *The principles of psychology*, Vol. 1 (F. H. Burkhardt, F. Bowers, & I. K. Skrupskelis, Eds.). Cambridge, MA: Harvard University Press.

James, W. (1909/1978). *Pragmatism and the meaning of truth* (F. T. Bowers & I. K. Skrupskelis, Eds.). Cambridge, MA: Harvard University Press.

Jang, J., & Schunn, C. D. (2012). Physical design tools support and hinder innovative engineering design. *Journal of Mechanical Design, 134*, Article 041001, 1–9.

Jansson, D. G., & Smith, S. M. (1991). Design fixation. *Design Studies, 12*, 3–11.

Jennings, K. E. (2008, March). Adjusting the novelty thermostat: Courting creative success through judicious randomness. *Proceedings of the AAAI Spring Symposium on Creative Intelligent Systems*, Stanford, CA.

Jeppesen, L. B., & Lakhani, K. R. (2010). Marginality and problem-solving effectiveness in broadcast search. *Organization Science, 21*, 1016–1033.

Jha, A. P., Krompinger, J., & Baime, M. J. (2007). Mindfulness training modifies subsystems of attention. *Cognitive, Affective, and Behavioral Neuroscience, 7*, 109–119.

Job, V., Dweck, C. S., & Walton, G. M. (2010). Ego depletion—Is it all in your head?: Implicit theories about will power affect self-regulation. *Psychological Science, 21*, 1686–1693.

Jorna, R. J., Van Wezel, W., & Bos, J. (2012). An analysis of the usability of a planning algorithm: An empirical study in the Netherlands Railways. In J. R. Wilson, A. Mills, T. Clarke, J. Rajan, & N. Dadashi (Eds.), *Rail human factors around the world: Impacts on and of people for successful rail operations*. Leiden, The Netherlands: CRC Press.

Kafai, Y. B., Peppler, K. A., & Chapman, R. N. (2009). *The computer clubhouse: Constructionism and creativity in youth communities*. New York: Teachers College Press.

Kahn, B. E., & Isen, A. M. (1993). The influence of positive affect on variety seeking among safe, enjoyable products. *Journal of Consumer Research, 20*, 257–270.

Kahneman, D. (2003). A perspective on judgment and choice: Mapping bounded rationality. *American Psychologist, 58*, 697–720.

Kahneman, D., & Klein, G. (2009). Conditions for intuitive expertise: A failure to disagree. *American Psychologist, 64*, 515–526.

Kalogerakis, K., Lüthje, C., & Herstatt, C. (2010). Developing innovations based on analogies: Experience from design and engineering consultants. *Journal of Product Innovation Management, 27*, 418–436.

Kane, M. J., & Engle, R. W. (2002). The role of prefrontal cortex in working-memory capacity, executive attention, and general fluid intelligence: An individual-differences perspective. *Psychonomic Bulletin & Review, 9*, 637–671.

Kaplan, C. A., & Simon, H. A. (1990). In search of insight. *Cognitive Psychology, 22*, 374–419.

Kappes, A., Wendt, M., Reinelt, T., & Oettingen, G. (2013). Mental contrasting changes the meaning of reality. *Journal of Experimental Social Psychology, 49*, 797–810.

Kapur, M. (2008). Productive failure. *Cognition and Instruction, 26*, 379–424.

Kapur, M., & Bielaczyc, K. (2012). Designing for productive failure. *Journal of the Learning Sciences, 21*, 45–83.

Kaschak, M. P., & Glenberg, A. M. (2000). Constructing meaning: The role of affordances and grammatical constructions in sentence comprehension. *Journal of Memory and Language, 43*, 508–529.

Kasof, J., Chen, C., Himsel, A., & Greenberger, E. (2007). Values and creativity. *Creativity Research Journal, 19*, 105–122.

Katila, R. (2002). New product search over time: Past ideas in their prime? *Academy of Management Journal, 45*, 995–1010.

Katila, R., & Chen, E. L. (2008). Effects of search timing on innovation: The value of not being in sync with rivals. *Administrative Science Quarterly, 53*, 593–625.

Keller, J., & Bless, H. (2008). Flow and regulatory compatibility: An experimental approach to the flow model of intrinsic motivation. *Personality and Social Psychology Bulletin, 34*, 196–209.

Kelley, T., & Kelley, D. (2013). *Creative confidence: Unleashing the creative potential within us all.* New York: Crown.

Kempermann, G. (2008). The neurogenic reserve hypothesis: What is adult hippocampal neurogenesis good for? *Trends in Neurosciences, 31*, 163–169.

Keynes, R. (2009). Darwin's ways of working: The opportunity for education. *Journal of Biological Education, 43*, 101–103.

Killingsworth, M. A., & Gilbert, D. T. (2010). A wandering mind is an unhappy mind. *Science, 330*, 932.

Kirsh, D. (1995). The intelligent use of space. *Artificial Intelligence, 73*, 31–68.

Kirsh, D. (2011). Creative cognition in choreography. *Proceedings of the 2nd International Conference on Computational Creativity*, 1–6.

Kirsh, D., Muntanyola, D., Jao, R. J., Lew, A., & Sugihara, M. (2009). Choreographic methods for creating novel, high quality dance. *The 5th International Workshop on Design and Semantics of Form and Movement*, 188–195.

Kiviniemi, M. T., Synder, M., & Omoto, A. M. (2002). Too many of a good thing? The effects of multiple motivations on stress, cost, fulfillment, and satisfaction. *Personality and Social Psychology Bulletin, 28*, 732–743.

Klahr, D., & Chen, Z. (2011). Finding one's place in transfer space. *Child Development Perspectives, 5*, 196–204.

Klein, G. A. (1993). A recognition-primed decision (RPD) model of rapid decision making. In G. A. Klein, J. Orasanu, R. Calderwood, & C. E. Zsambok (Eds.), *Decision making in action: Models and methods* (pp. 138–147). Norwood, NJ: Ablex.

Klein, G. A. (2007, September). Performing a project premortem. *Harvard Business Review, 85*, 18–19.

Klein, G. A. (2008). Naturalistic decision making, *Human Factors, 50*, 456–460.

Klein, G. A., Moon, B., & Hoffman, R. R. (2006a). Making sense of sensemaking 1: Alternative perspectives. *Intelligent Systems, 21*, 70–73.

Klein, G. A., Moon, B., & Hoffman, R. R. (2006b). Making sense of sensemaking 2: A macrocognitive model. *Intelligent Systems, 21*, 88–92.

Klein, S. B. (2013). The complex act of projecting oneself into the future. *WIREs Cognitive Science, 4*, 63–79.

Klein, S. B., Robertson, T. E., Delton, A. W., & Lax, M. L. (2012). Familiarity and personal experience as mediators of recall when planning for future contingencies. *Journal of Experimental Psychology: Learning, Memory, and Cognition, 38*, 240–245.

Klinger, E. (2013). Goal commitments and the content of thoughts and dreams: Basic principles. *Frontiers in Psychology, 4*, Article 415, 1–17.

Knuth, D. (2014, June 5). People of ACM: Donald Knuth. *Association for Computing Machinery (ACM) Bulletin.*

Koechlin, E., Ody, C., & Kouneiher, F. (2003). The architecture of cognitive control in the human prefrontal cortex. *Science, 302*, 1181–1185.

Kokonas, N. (2014, June 4). Tickets for restaurants. Retrieved April 8, 2015, from website.alinearestaurant.com/site/2014/06/tickets-for-restaurants

König, C. J., & Waller, M. J. (2010). Time for reflection: A critical examination of polychronicity. *Human Performance, 23*, 173–190.

Kool, W., & Botvinick, M. M. (2013). A labor/leisure tradeoff in cognitive control. *Journal of Experimental Psychology: General, 143*, 131–141.

Kool, W., McGuire, J. T., Wang, G. J., & Botvinick, M. M. (2013). Neural and behavioral evidence for an intrinsic cost of self-control. *PLoS ONE, 8*, Article e72626, 1–6.

Köpetz, C., Faber, T., Fishbach, A., & Kruglanski, A. W. (2011). The multifinality constraints effect: How goal multiplicity narrows the means set to a focal end. *Journal of Personality and Social Psychology, 100*, 810–826.

Kounios, J., Fleck, J. I., Green, D. L., Payne, L., Stevenson, J. L., Bowden, E. M., & Jung-Beeman, M. (2008). The origins of insight in resting-state brain activity. *Neuropsychologia, 46*, 281–291.

Kouprie, M., & Visser, F. S. (2009). A framework for empathy in design: Stepping into and out of the user's life. *Journal of Engineering Design, 20*, 437–448.

Koutstaal, W. (1995). Situating ethics and memory. *American Philosophical Quarterly, 32*, 253–262.

Koutstaal, W. (2001). The edges of words. *Semiotica, 137*, 57–97.

Koutstaal, W. (2012). *The agile mind*. New York: Oxford University Press.

Koutstaal, W., Wagner, A. D., Rotte, M., Maril, A., Buckner, R. L., & Schacter, D. L. (2001). Perceptual specificity in visual object priming: Functional magnetic resonance imaging evidence for a laterality difference in fusiform cortex. *Neuropsychologia, 39*, 184–199.

Kozbelt, A., & Nishioka, K. (2010). Humor comprehension, humor production, and insight: An exploratory study. *Humor, 23*, 375–401.

Kozlowski, S.W.J., & Ilgen, D. R. (2006). Enhancing the effectiveness of work groups and teams. *Psychological Science in the Public Interest, 7*, 77–124.

Kremer, M. & Williams, H. (2010). Incentivizing innovation: Adding to the tool kit. In J. Lerner & S. Stern (Eds.), *Innovation policy and the economy, Vol. 10* (pp. 1–17). Chicago, IL: University of Chicago Press.

Kriete, T., Noelle, D. C., Cohen, J. D., & O'Reilly, R. C. (2013). Indirection and symbol-like processing in the prefrontal cortex and basal ganglia. *Proceedings of the National Academy of Sciences, USA, 110*, 16390–16395.

Kruglanski, A. W., Shah, J. Y., Fishbach, A., Friedman, R., Chun, W. Y., & Sleeth-Keppler, D. (2002). A theory of goal systems. *Advances in Experimental Social Psychology, 34*, 331–378.

Kurzban, R., Duckworth, A., Kable, J. W., & Myers, J. (2013). An opportunity cost model of subjective effort and task performance. *Behavioral and Brain Sciences, 36*, 661–679.

Kvavilashvili, L., & Mandler, G. (2004). Out of one's mind: A study of involuntary semantic memories. *Cognitive Psychology, 48*, 47–94.

Lakhani, K. R., Boudreau, K. J., Loh, P-R., Backstrom, L., Baldwin, C., Lonstein, E., . . . Guinan, E. C. (2013). Prize-based contests can provide solutions to computational biology problems. *Nature Biotechnology, 31*, 108–111.

Lakhani, K. R., Jeppesen, L. B., Lohse, P. A., & Panetta, J. A. (2007). The value of openness in scientific problem solving. *Harvard Business School Working Paper No. 07-050*, 1–57.

Lakoff, G., & Johnson, M. (1980a). The metaphorical structure of the human conceptual system. *Cognitive Science, 4*, 195–208.

Lakoff, G., & Johnson, M. (1980b). Conceptual metaphor in everyday language. *Journal of Philosophy, 77*, 453–486.

Langer, E. J., & Moldoveanu, M. (2000). The construct of mindfulness. *Journal of Social Issues, 56*, 1–9.

Langer, E. J., Russell, T., & Eisenkraft, N. (2009). Orchestral performance and the footprint of mindfulness. *Psychology of Music, 37*, 125–136.

Larkin, J. H., & Simon, H. A. (1987). Why a diagram is (sometimes) worth ten thousand words. *Cognitive Science, 11*, 65–99.

Laursen, K. (2012). Keep searching and you'll find: What do we know about variety creation through firms' search activities for innovation? *Industrial and Corporation Change, 21*, 1181–1220.

Leary, M. R., Adams, C. E., & Tate, E. B. (2006). Hypo-egoic self-regulation: Exercising self-control by diminishing the influence of the self. *Journal of Personality, 74*, 1803–1831.

Leber, A. B., Turk-Browne, N. B., & Chun, M. M. (2008). Neural predictors of moment-to-moment fluctuations in cognitive flexibility. *Proceedings of the National Academy of Sciences, USA, 105*, 13592–13597.

Lee, C. S., & Therriault, D. J. (2013). The cognitive underpinnings of creative thought: A latent variable analysis exploring the roles of intelligence and working memory in three creative processes. *Intelligence, 41*, 306–320.

Lei, B., Taura, T., & Numata, J. (1996). Representing the collaborative design process: A product model-oriented approach. In J. S. Gero & F. Sudweeks (Eds.), *Advances in formal design methods for CAD* (pp. 267–285). London: Chapman & Hall.

LePine, J. A. (2003). Team adaptation and postchange performance: Effects of team composition in terms of members' cognitive ability and personality. *Journal of Applied Psychology, 88*, 27–39.

LePine, J. A., Colquitt, J. A., & Erez, A. (2000). Adaptability to changing task contexts: Effects of general cognitive ability, conscientiousness, and openness to experience. *Personnel Psychology, 53*, 563–593.

Lerner, J., & Wulf, J. (2007). Innovation and incentives: Evidence from corporate R&D. *Review of Economics and Statistics, 89*, 634–644.

Lettl, C., Herstatt, C., & Gemuenden, H. G. (2006). Users' contributions to radical innovation: Evidence from four cases in the field of medical equipment technology. *R&D Management, 36*, 251–272.

Leung, A. K., & Chiu, C. (2010). Multicultural experience, idea receptiveness, and creativity. *Journal of Cross-Cultural Psychology, 41*, 723–741.

Leveson, N. G. (2011). Applying systems thinking to analyze and learn from events. *Safety Science, 49*, 55–64.

Levitt, S. D., List, J. A., & Syverson, C. (2013). Toward an understanding of learning by doing: Evidence from an automobile assembly plant. *Journal of Political Economy, 121,* 643–681.

Lewis, C., & Lovatt, P. J. (2013). Breaking away from set patterns of thinking: Improvisation and divergent thinking. *Thinking Skills and Creativity, 9,* 46–58.

Lewis, K., Belliveau, M., Herndon, B., & Keller, J. (2007). Group cognition, membership change, and performance: Investigating the benefits and detriments of collective knowledge. *Organizational Behavior and Human Decision Processes, 103,* 159–178.

Li, Q., Maggitti, P. G., Smith, K. G., Tesluk, P. E., & Katila, R. (2013). Top management attention to innovation: The role of search selection and intensity in new product introductions. *Academy of Management Journal, 56,* 893–916.

Liberman, N., & Trope, Y. (2014). Traversing psychological distance. *Trends in Cognitive Sciences, 18,* 364–369.

Limb, C. J., & Braun, A. R. (2008). Neural substrates of spontaneous musical performance: An fMRI study of jazz improvisation. *PLoS ONE, 3,* Article e1679, 1–9.

Lin, C-J., & Li, C-R. (2013). The effect of boundary-spanning search on breakthrough innovations of new technology ventures. *Industry and Innovation, 20,* 93–113.

Linsey, J. S., Clauss, E. F., Kurtoglu, T., Murphy, J. T., Wood, K. L., & Markman, A. B. (2011). An experimental study of group idea generation techniques: Understanding the roles of idea representation and viewing methods. *Journal of Mechanical Design, 133,* Article 031008, 1–15.

Linsey, J. S., Markman, A. B., & Wood, K. L. (2012). Design by analogy: A study of the WordTree method for problem re-representation. *Journal of Mechanical Design, 134,* Article 041009, 1–12.

Linsey, J. S., Tseng, I., Fu, K., Cagan, J., Wood, K. L., & Schunn, C. (2010). A study of design fixation, its mitigation and perception in engineering design faculty. *Journal of Mechanical Design, 132,* Article 041003, 1–12.

Linville, P. W. (1987). Self-complexity as a cognitive buffer against stress-related illness and depression. *Journal of Personality and Social Psychology, 52,* 663–676.

Litchfield, R. C. (2008). Brainstorming reconsidered: A goal-based view. *Academy of Management Review, 33,* 649–668.

Litchfield, R. C., Fan, J., & Brown, V. R. (2011). Directing idea generation using brainstorming with specific novelty goals. *Motivation and Emotion, 35,* 135–143.

Little, B. R. (2014). Well-doing: Personal projects and the quality of lives. *Theory and Research in Education, 12,* 329–346.

Little, B. R. (2015). The integrative challenge in personality science: Personal projects as units of analysis. *Journal of Research in Personality, 56,* 93–101.

Louro, M. J., Pieters, R., & Zeelenberg, M. (2007). Dynamics of multiple-goal pursuit. *Journal of Personality and Social Psychology, 93,* 174–193.

Luchins, A. S. (1942). Mechanization in problem solving: The effect of Einstellung. *Psychological Monographs, 54* (No. 248), 1–95.

MacCormack, A., Baldwin, C., & Rusnak, J. (2012). Exploring the duality between product and organizational architectures: A test of the "mirroring" hypothesis. *Research Policy, 41*, 1309–1324.

Mackey, A. P., Singley, A. T. M., & Bunge, S. A. (2013). Intensive reasoning training alters patterns of brain connectivity at rest. *Journal of Neuroscience, 33*, 4796–4803.

Mackey, A. P., Whitaker, K. J., & Bunge, S. A. (2012). Experience-dependent plasticity in white matter microstructure: Reasoning training alters structural connectivity. *Frontiers in Neuroanatomy, 6*, Article 32, 1–9.

Madjar, N., & Oldham, G. R. (2009). Task rotation and polychronicity: Effects on individuals' creativity. *Human Performance, 19*, 117–131.

Madl, T., Baars, B. J., & Franklin, S. (2011). The timing of the cognitive cycle. *PLoS ONE, 6*, Article e14803, 1–16.

Magni, M., Maruping, L. M., Hoegl, M., & Proserpio, L. (2013). Managing the unexpected across space: Improvisation, dispersion, and performance in NPD teams. *Journal of Product Innovation Management, 30*, 1009–1026.

Maia, T. V., & Cleeremans, A. (2005). Consciousness: Converging insights from connectionist modeling and neuroscience. *Trends in Cognitive Sciences, 9*, 395–404.

Maier, J. R. A., & Fadel, G. M. (2009). Affordance based design: A relational theory for design. *Research in Engineering Design, 20*, 13–27.

Mainemelis, C., Boyatzis, R. E., & Kolb, D. A. (2002). Learning styles and adaptive flexibility: Testing experiential learning theory. *Management Learning, 33*, 5–33.

Mak, T. W., & Shu, L. H. (2008). Using descriptions of biological phenomena for idea generation. *Research in Engineering Design, 19*, 21–28.

Mallidou, A. A., Cummings, J. G., Ginsburg, L. R., Chuang, Y-T., Kang, S., Norton, P. G., & Estabrooks, C. A. (2011). Staff, space, and time as dimensions of organizational slack: A psychometric assessment. *Health Care Management Review, 36*, 252–264.

Mandler, G. (1994). Hypermnesia, incubation, and mind popping: On remembering without really trying. *Attention and Performance, 15*, 3–33.

Mann, T., de Ridder, D., & Fujita, K. (2013). Self-regulation of health behavior: Social psychological approaches to goal setting and goal striving. *Health Psychology, 32*, 487–498.

March, J. G. (1976). The technology of foolishness. In J. G. March & J. P. Olsen (Eds.), *Ambiguity and choice in organizations* (pp. 69–81). Bergen, Norway: Universitetsforlaget.

March, J. G. (1991). Exploration and exploitation in organizational learning. *Organization Science, 2*, 71–87.

Marian, A. A., Dexter, F., Tucker, P., & Todd, M. M. (2012). Comparison of alphabetical versus categorical display format for medication order entry in a simulated touch screen anesthesia information management system: An experiment in clinician-computer interaction in anesthesia. *BMC Medical Informatics and Decision Making, 12*, Article 46, 1–7.

Marien, H., Aarts, H., & Custers, R. (2012). Being flexible or rigid in goal-directed behavior: When positive affect implicitly motivates the pursuit of goals or means. *Journal of Experimental Social Psychology, 48,* 277–283.

Maril, A., Wagner, A. D., & Schacter, D. L. (2001). On the tip of the tongue: An event-related fMRI study of semantic retrieval failure and cognitive control. *Neuron, 31,* 653–660.

Marsh, R. L., Hicks, J. L., & Bink, M. L. (1998). Activation of completed, uncompleted, and partially completed intentions. *Journal of Experimental Psychology: Learning, Memory, and Cognition, 24,* 350–361.

Marsh, R. L., Hicks, J. L., & Cook, G. I. (2006). Task interference from prospective memories covaries with contextual associations of fulfilling them. *Memory & Cognition, 34,* 1037–1045.

Marsh, R. L., Landau, J. D., & Hicks, J. L. (1996). How examples may (and may not) constrain creativity. *Memory & Cognition, 24,* 669–680.

Marsh, R. L., Ward, T. B., & Landau, J. D. (1999). The inadvertent use of prior knowledge in a generative cognitive task. *Memory & Cognition, 27,* 94–105.

Marsolek, C. J. (1999). Dissociable neural subsystems underlie abstract and specific object recognition. *Psychological Science, 10,* 111–118.

Martin, J. J., & Cutler, K. (2002). An exploratory study of flow and motivation in theater actors. *Journal of Applied Sport Psychology, 14,* 344–352.

Martin, L., & Schwartz, D. L. (2009). Prospective adaptation in the use of external representations. *Cognition and Instruction, 27,* 370–400.

Martindale, C., & Dailey, A. (1996). Creativity, primary process cognition and personality. *Personality and Individual Differences, 20,* 409–414.

May, C. P. (1999). Synchrony effects in cognition: The costs and a benefit. *Psychonomic Bulletin & Review, 6,* 142–147.

May, C. P., & Hasher, L. (1998). Synchrony effects in inhibitory control over thought and action. *Journal of Experimental Psychology: Human Perception and Performance, 24,* 363–379.

Mayer, E. A. (2011). Gut feelings: The emerging biology of gut-brain communication. *Nature Reviews Neuroscience, 12,* 453–466.

McClelland, J. L., Botvinick, M. M., Noelle, D. C., Plaut, D. C., Rogers, T. T., Seidenberg, M. S., & Smith, L. B. (2010). Letting structure emerge: Connectionist and dynamical systems approaches to cognition. *Trends in Cognitive Sciences, 14,* 348–356.

McCoy, J. M., & Evans, G. W. (2002). The potential role of the physical environment in fostering creativity. *Creativity Research Journal, 14,* 409–426.

McCrae, R. R. (1987). Creativity, divergent thinking, and openness to experience. *Journal of Personality and Social Psychology, 52,* 1258–1265.

McGinley, R. (2012, June 8). In a panel discussion of the DeYoung Museum's *Real to Real* exhibition, Playing the field: Photography and collecting today. Retrieved April 8, 2015, from https://www.youtube.com/watch?v=FgWAqUv2dCE

McGrane, S. (2012, May 8). An effort to bury a throwaway culture one repair at a time. *New York Times.* Retrieved April 8, 2015, from http://www.nytimes.com/2012/05/09/world/europe/amsterdam-tries-to-change-culture-with-repair-cafes.html?_r=0

McKenna, A. F. (2007). An investigation of adaptive expertise and transfer of design process knowledge. *Transactions of the ASME, 129,* 730–734.

Mednick, S. A. (1962). The associative basis of the creative process. *Psychological Review, 69,* 220–232.

Meleady, R., Hopthrow, T., & Crisp, R. J. (2013). Simulating social dilemmas: Promoting cooperative behavior through imagined group discussion. *Journal of Personality and Social Psychology, 104,* 839–853.

Menkel-Meadow, C. (2014). Unsettling the lawyers: Other forms of justice in Indigenous claims of expropriation, abuse, and injustice. *University of Toronto Law Journal, 64,* 620–639.

Mesmer-Magnus, J., Glew, D. J., & Viswesvaran, C. (2012). A meta-analysis of positive humor in the workplace. *Journal of Managerial Psychology, 27,* 155–190.

Mesulam, M.-M. (1998). From sensation to cognition. *Brain, 121,* 1013–1052.

Meyer, M. H., & Marion, T. J. (2010). Innovating for effectiveness: Lessons from design firms. *Research Technology Management,* Sept.-Oct., 21–28.

Mieg, H. A., Bedenk, S. J., Braun, A., & Neyer, F. J. (2012). How emotional stability and openness to experience support invention: A study with German independent inventors. *Creativity Research Journal, 24,* 200–207.

Miller, D. J., Fern, M. J., & Cardinal, L. B. (2007). The use of knowledge for technological innovation within diversified firms. *Academy of Management Journal, 50,* 308–326.

Miller, E. K., & Cohen, J. D. (2001). An integrative theory of prefrontal cortex function. *Annual Review of Neuroscience, 24,* 167–202.

Miner, A. S., Bassoff, P., & Moorman, C. (2001). Organizational improvisation and learning: A field study. *Administrative Science Quarterly, 46,* 304–337.

Mischel, W., Shoda, Y., & Peake, P. K. (1988). The nature of adolescent competencies predicted by preschool delay of gratification. *Journal of Personality and Social Psychology, 54,* 687–696.

Mischel, W., Shoda, Y., & Rodriguez, M. L. (1989). Delay of gratification. *Science, 244,* 933–938.

Mitchell, R., Nicholas, S., & Boyle, B. (2009). The role of openness to cognitive diversity and group processes in knowledge creation. *Small Group Research, 40,* 535–554.

Moore, H. (1955). Notes on sculpture. In B. Ghiselin (Ed.), *The creative process.* New York: Mentor.

Moorman, C., & Miner, A. S. (1998). Organizational improvisation and organizational memory. *Academy of Management Review, 23,* 698–723.

Moss, J., Kotovsky, K., & Cagan, J. (2007). The influence of open goals on the acquisition of problem-relevant information. *Journal of Experimental Psychology: Learning, Memory, and Cognition, 33,* 876–891.

Most, S. B., Chun, M. M., Johnson, M. R., & Kiehl, K. A. (2006). Attentional modulation of the amygdala varies with personality. *NeuroImage, 31,* 934–944.

Moulton, C-A., Regehr, G., Lingard, L., Merritt, C., & MacRae, H. (2010). Slowing down to stay out of trouble in the operating room: Remaining attentive in automaticity. *Academic Medicine, 85,* 1571–1577.

Mueller, C. M., & Dweck, C. S. (1998). Praise for intelligence can undermine children's motivation and performance. *Journal of Personality and Social Psychology, 75*, 33–52.

Mullen, B., Johnson, C., & Salas, E. (1991). Productivity loss in brainstorming groups: A meta-analytic integration. *Basic and Applied Social Psychology, 12*, 3–23.

Munro, A. (1982). What is real? In J. Metcalf (Ed.), *Making it new: Contemporary Canadian stories* (pp. 223–226). Toronto: Methuen.

Munro, A., & Awano, L. D. (2006). An interview with Alice Munro. *Virginia Quarterly Review*. Retrieved April 8, 2015, from http://www.vqronline.org/web-exclusive/interview-alice-munro

Muraven, M., Gagné, M., & Rosman, H. (2008). Helpful self-control: Autonomy support, vitality, and depletion. *Journal of Experimental Social Psychology, 44*, 573–585.

Murphy, M. C., & Dweck, C. S. (2010). A culture of genius: How an organization's lay theory shapes people's cognition, affect, and behavior. *Personality and Social Psychology Bulletin, 36*, 283–296.

Murray, N., Sujan, H., Hirt, E. R., & Sujan, M. (1990). The influence of mood on categorization: A cognitive flexibility interpretation. *Journal of Personality and Social Psychology, 59*, 411–425.

Mylopoulos, M., & Regehr, G. (2009). How student models of expertise and innovation impact the development of adaptive expertise in medicine. *Medical Education, 43*, 127–132.

Nakamura, J., & Csíkszentmihályi, M. (2002). The concept of flow. In C. R. Snyder, & S. J. Lopez (Eds.), *Handbook of positive psychology* (pp. 89–105). Oxford, UK: Oxford University Press.

Nakrani, S., & Tovey, C. (2004). On honey bees and dynamic server allocation in Internet hosting centers. *Adaptive Behavior, 12*, 223–240.

Nakrani, S., & Tovey, C. (2007). From honeybees to Internet servers: Biomimicry for distributed management of Internet hosting centers. *Bioinspiration and Biomimetics, 2*, S182–S197.

Nee, D. E., & Jonides, J. (2014). Trisecting representational states in short-term memory. *Frontiers in Human Neuroscience, 7*, Article 796, 1–16.

Neely, J. H. (1977). Semantic priming and retrieval from lexical memory: Roles of inhibitionless spreading activation and limited-capacity attention. *Journal of Experimental Psychology: General, 106*, 226–254.

Nersessian, N. J. (2008). *Creating scientific concepts*. Cambridge, MA: MIT Press.

Nesse, R. M. (2004). Natural selection and the elusiveness of happiness. *Philosophical Transactions of the Royal Society of London, B, 359*, 1333–1347.

Neuringer, A. (2002). Operant variability: Evidence, functions, and theory. *Psychonomic Bulletin & Review, 9*, 672–705.

Neuringer, A. (2004). Reinforced variability in animals and people: Implications for adaptive action. *American Psychologist, 59*, 891–906.

Nijstad, B. A., De Dreu, C. K. W., Rietzschel, E. F., & Baas, M. (2010). The dual pathway to creativity model: Creative ideation as a function of flexibility and persistence. *European Review of Social Psychology, 21*, 34–77.

Nishikawa, H., Schreier, M., & Ogawa, S. (2013). User-generated versus designer-generated products: A performance assessment at Muji. *International Journal of Research in Marketing, 30,* 160–167.

Nohria, N., & Gulati, R. (1996). Is slack good or bad for innovation? *Academy of Management Journal, 39,* 1245–1264.

Norman, D. A. (1988). *The psychology of everyday things.* New York: Basic Books.

Norman, D. A. (1999). Affordance, conventions, and design. *Interactions, 6,* 38–42.

Norman, J. (2014). *Stand up straight and sing!* Boston: Houghton Mifflin Harcourt.

Oberauer, K. (2009). Design for a working memory. *Psychology of Learning and Motivation, 51,* 45–100.

Obstfeld, D. (2012). Creative projects: A less routine approach toward getting new things done. *Organization Science, 23,* 1571–1592.

O'Craven, K. M., & Kanwisher, N. (2000). Mental imagery of faces and places activates corresponding stimulus-specific brain regions. *Journal of Cognitive Neuroscience, 12,* 1013–1023.

Oettingen, G. (2012). Future thought and behaviour change. *European Review of Social Psychology, 23,* 1–63.

Oettingen, G., Marquardt, M. K., & Gollwitzer, P. M. (2012). Mental contrasting turns positive feedback on creative potential into successful performance. *Journal of Experimental Social Psychology, 48,* 990–996.

Oettingen, G., Pak, H., & Schnetter, K. (2001). Self-regulation of goal setting: Turning free fantasies about the future into binding goals. *Journal of Personality and Social Psychology, 80,* 736–753.

O'Hagan, S. (2004, July 24). Out of the ordinary [interview with William Eggleston], *The Observer.* Retrieved April 8, 2015, from http://www.theguardian.com/artanddesign/2004/jul/25/photography1

Ohly, S., Sonnentag, S., & Pluntke, F. (2006). Routinization, work characteristics and their relationships with creative and proactive behaviors. *Journal of Organizational Behavior, 27,* 257–279.

Oksanen, K., & Ståhle, P. (2013). Physical environment as a source for innovation: Investigating the attributes of innovative space. *Journal of Knowledge Management, 17,* 815–827.

Okuda, S. M., Runco, M. A., & Berger, D. E. (1991). Creativity and the finding and solving of real-world problems. *Journal of Psychoeducational Assessment, 9,* 45–53.

O'Leary, M. B., & Cummings, J. N. (2007). The spatial, temporal, and configurational characteristics of geographic dispersion in teams. *MIS Quarterly, 31,* 433–452.

Olivers, C.N.L., & Nieuwenhuis, S. (2006). The beneficial effects of additional task load, positive affect, and instruction on the attentional blink. *Journal of Experimental Psychology: Human Perception and Performance, 32,* 364–379.

Olson, A. (2013, March 14). Studio talk with Dianna Molzan and Alex Olson, Walker Art Center. Retrieved April 8, 2015, from http://www.walkerart.org/channel/2013/studio-talk-with-dianna-molzan-and-alex-olson

Olsson, H. & Poom, L. (2005). Visual memory needs categories. *Proceedings of the National Academy of Sciences, USA, 102,* 8776–8780.

Omoto, A. M., & Snyder, M. (2002). Considerations of community: The context and process of volunteerism. *American Behavioral Scientist, 45,* 846–867.

Onarheim, B. (2012). Creativity from constraints in engineering design: Lessons learned at Coloplast. *Journal of Engineering Design, 23,* 323–336.

Ondaatje, M. (2002). In *The conversations: Walter Murch and the art of editing film.* New York: Knopf.

Oppezzo, M., & Schwartz, D. L. (2014). Give your ideas some legs: The positive effect of walking on creative thinking. *Journal of Experimental Psychology: Learning, Memory, and Cognition, 40,* 1142–1152.

O'Reilly, C. A. III, & Tushman, M. L. (2013). Organizational ambidexterity: Past, present, and future. *Academy of Management Perspectives, 27,* 324–338.

Orlikowski, W. J. (1996). Improvising organizational transformation over time: A situated change perspective. *Information Systems Research, 7,* 63–92.

Osbeck, L. M. (1999). Conceptual problems in the development of a psychological notion of "intuition." *Journal for the Theory of Social Behaviour, 29,* 229–250.

Osborn, A. F. (1957). *Applied imagination: Principles and procedures of creative thinking* (rev. ed.). New York: Scribner.

Ostafin, B. D., & Kassman, K. T. (2012). Stepping out of history: Mindfulness improves insight problem solving. *Consciousness and Cognition, 21,* 1031–1036.

Ostrom, E. (2009). A polycentric approach for coping with climate change. *Policy Research Working Paper 5095.* Washington, D.C.: World Bank.

Ostrom, E. (2012). Why do we need to protect institutional diversity? *European Political Science, 11,* 128–147.

Otto, K. L., & Wood, K. N. (2001). *Product design: Techniques in reverse engineering and new product development.* Upper Saddle River, NJ: Prentice Hall.

Oudiette, D., Antony, J. W., Creery, J. D., & Paller, K. A. (2013). The role of memory reactivation during wakefulness and sleep in determining which memories endure. *Journal of Neuroscience, 33,* 6672–6678.

Paletz, S. B. F., Kim, K. H., Schunn, C. D., Tollinger, I., & Vera, A. (2013). Reuse and recycle: The development of adaptive expertise, routine expertise, and novelty in a large research team. *Applied Cognitive Psychology, 27,* 415–428.

Paletz, S. B. F., Schunn, C. D., & Kim, K. H. (2013). The interplay of conflict and analogy in multidisciplinary teams. *Cognition, 126,* 1–19.

Parkin, K. (2014). Building 3D with IKEA. *CGSociety.* Retrieved April 8, 2015, from www.cgsociety.org/index.php/CGSFeatures/CGSFeatureSpecial/building_3d_with_ikea

Parkinson, C., Liu, S., & Wheatley, T. (2014). A common cortical metric for spatial, temporal, and social distance. *Journal of Neuroscience, 34,* 1979–1987.

Patalano, A. L., & Seifert, C. M. (1997). Opportunistic planning: Being reminded of pending goals. *Cognitive Psychology, 34,* 1–36.

Patel, B. K., Chapman, C. G., Luo, N., Woodruff, J. N., & Arora, V. M. (2012). Impact of mobile tablet computers on internal medicine resident efficiency. *Archives of Internal Medicine, 172,* 436–438.

Patel, N., Chittamuru, D., Jain, A., Dave, P., & Parikh, T. S. (2010). Avaaj Otalo— A field study of an interactive voice forum for small farmers in rural India.

Proceedings of the ACM Conference on Human Factors in Computing Systems (CHI 2010).

Patterson, K., Nestor, P. J., & Rogers, T. T. (2007). Where do you know what you know? The representation of semantic knowledge in the human brain. *Nature Reviews Neuroscience, 8,* 976–987.

Paulus, P. B., Kohn, N. W., & Arditti, L. E. (2011). Effects of quantity and quality instructions on brainstorming. *Journal of Creative Behavior, 45,* 38–46.

Paulus, P. B., Kohn, N. W., Arditti, L. E., & Korde, R. M. (2013). Understanding the group size effect in electronic brainstorming. *Small Group Research, 44,* 332–352.

Pearce, C. L., & Ensley, M. D. (2004). A reciprocal and longitudinal investigation of the innovation process: The central role of shared vision in product and process innovation teams (PPITs). *Journal of Organizational Behavior, 25,* 259–278.

Peirce, C. S. (1901/1935). *Collected papers of Charles Sanders Peirce* (Vols. 5–6). Cambridge, MA: Harvard University Press.

Pennebaker, J. W., Gosling, S. D., & Ferrell, J. D. (2013). Daily online testing in large classes: Boosting college performance while reducing achievement gaps. *PLoS ONE, 8,* Article e79774, 1–6.

Perttula, M., & Sipilä, P. (2007). The idea exposure paradigm in design idea generation. *Journal of Engineering Design, 18,* 93–102.

Pessoa, L. (2008). On the relationship between emotion and cognition. *Nature Reviews Neuroscience, 9,* 148–158.

Pinker, S. (2014). *The sense of style: The thinking person's guide to writing in the 21st century.* New York: Viking.

Pinto, J. K., & Prescott, J. E. (1988). Variations in critical success factors over the stages in the project life cycle. *Journal of Management, 14,* 5–18.

Pirola-Merlo, A., & Mann, L. (2004). The relationship between individual creativity and team creativity: Aggregating across people and time. *Journal of Organizational Behavior, 25,* 235–257.

Pitts, J. W. III (2009). Corporate social responsibility: Current status and future evolution. *Rutgers Journal of Law & Public Policy, 6,* 334–434.

Plerhoples, A. E. (2014). Delaware public benefit corporations 90 days out: Who's opting in? *UC Davis Business Law Journal, 14,* 247–277.

Porter, M. E. (1998, November-December). Clusters and the new economics of competition. *Harvard Business Review, 76,* 77–90.

Postma, C. E., Zwartkruis-Pelgrim, E., Daemen, E., & Du, J. (2012). Challenges of doing empathic design: Experiences from industry. *International Journal of Design, 6,* 59–70.

Pourtois, G., Notebaert, W., & Verguts, T. (2012). Cognitive and affective control. *Frontiers in Psychology, 3,* Article 477, 1–2.

Prabhakaran, R., Green, A. E., & Gray, J. R. (2014). Thin slices of creativity: Using single-word utterances to assess creative cognition. *Behavior Research Methods, 46,* 641–659.

Pries, F., & Dorée, A. (2005). A century of innovation in the Dutch construction industry. *Construction Management and Economics, 23,* 561–564.

Pulvermüller, F. (2013). How neurons make meaning: Brain mechanisms for embodied and abstract-symbolic semantics. *Trends in Cognitive Sciences, 17*, 458–470.

Raes, F., Hermans, D., Williams, J.M.G., Demyttenaere, K., Sabbe, B., Pieters, G., & Eelen, P. (2005). Reduced specificity of autobiographical memory: A mediator between rumination and ineffective problem-solving in major depression? *Journal of Affective Disorders, 87*, 331–335.

Raffaelli, R. (2013). Mechanisms of technology re-emergence and identity change in a mature field: Swiss watchmaking. *Academy of Management Proceedings, 1*, Article 13784.

Raisch, S., Birkinshaw, J., Probst, G., & Tushman, M. L. (2009). Organizational ambidexterity: Balancing exploitation and exploration for sustained performance. *Organization Science, 20*, 685–695.

Ramnani, N., & Owen, A. M. (2004). Anterior prefrontal cortex: Insights into function from anatomy and neuroimaging. *Nature Reviews Neuroscience, 5*, 184–194.

Rasmussen, A. S., & Berntsen, D. (2010). Personality traits and autobiographical memory: Openness is positively related to the experience and usage of recollections. *Memory, 18*, 774–786.

Rasmussen, A. S., & Berntsen, D. (2013). The reality of the past versus the ideality of the future: Emotional valence and functional differences between past and future mental time travel. *Memory & Cognition, 41*, 187–200.

Rauschenberg, R. (1981). Interview with Robert Rauschenberg [with Alain Sayag]. *Robert Rauschenberg: Photographs.* New York: Pantheon.

Ravasi, D., & Phillips, N. (2011). Strategies of alignment: Organizational identity management and strategic change at Bang & Olufsen. *Strategic Organization, 9*, 103–135.

Rego, A., Sousa, F., Marques, C., & Cunha, M. P. (2012). Optimism predicting employees' creativity: The mediating role of positive affect and the positivity ratio. *European Journal of Work and Organizational Psychology, 21*, 244–270.

Ren, Y., & Argote, L. (2011). Transactive memory systems 1985–2010: An integrative framework of key dimensions, antecedents, and consequences. *Academy of Management Annals, 5*, 189–229.

Renoult, L., Davidson, P.S.R., Palombo, D. J., Moscovitch, M., & Levine, B. (2012). Personal semantics: At the crossroads of semantic and episodic memory. *Trends in Cognitive Sciences, 16*, 550–558.

Reyna, V. F. (2012). A new intuitionism: Meaning, memory, and development in fuzzy-trace theory. *Judgment and Decision Making, 7*, 332–359.

Reyna, V. F., & Brainerd, C. J. (1995). Fuzzy-trace theory and framing effects in choice: Gist extraction, truncation, and conversion. *Journal of Behavioral Decision Making, 4*, 249–262.

Riley *v.* California, 2014, 134 S. Ct. 2473.

Ritter, S. M., Damian, R. I., Simonton, D. K., Van Baaren, R. B., Strick, M., Derks, J., & Dijksterhuis, A. (2012). Diversifying experiences enhance cognitive flexibility. *Journal of Experimental Social Psychology, 48*, 961–964.

Rittle-Johnson, B., Star, J. R., & Durkin, K. (2012). Developing procedural flexibility: Are novices prepared to learn from comparing procedures? *British Journal of Educational Psychology, 82*, 436–455.

Rodrik, D. (2009). The new development economics: We shall experiment, but how shall we learn? In J. Cohen & W. Easterly (Eds.), *What works in development? Thinking big and thinking small* (pp. 24–47). Washington DC: Brookings Institution Press.

Rosch, E., Mervis, C. B., Gray, W., Johnson, D., & Boyes-Braem, P. (1976). Basic objects in natural categories. *Cognitive Psychology, 8,* 382–439.

Rosenkopf, L., & Almeida, P. (2003). Overcoming local search through alliances and mobility. *Management Science, 49,* 751–766.

Rosenkopf, L., & Nerkar, A. (2001). Beyond local search: Boundary-spanning exploration, and impact in the optical disk industry. *Strategic Management Journal, 22,* 287–306.

Roskes, M., De Dreu, C.K.W., & Nijstad, B. A. (2012). Necessity is the mother of invention: Avoidance motivation stimulates creativity through cognitive effort. *Journal of Personality and Social Psychology, 103,* 242–256.

Ross, C., & Neuringer, A. (2002). Reinforcement of variations and repetitions along three independent response dimensions. *Behavioural Processes, 57,* 199–209.

Rosso, B. D. (2014). Creativity and constraints: Exploring the role of constraints in the creative processes of research and development teams. *Organization Studies, 35,* 551–585.

Roth, W. M. (2000). From gesture to scientific language. *Journal of Pragmatics, 32,* 1683–1714.

Rubin, D. (1995). *Memory in oral traditions: The cognitive psychology of epic, ballads, and counting-out rhymes.* New York: Oxford University Press.

Rudenstine, N. L. (2001). *Pointing our thoughts: Reflections on Harvard and higher education, 1991–2001.* Cambridge, MA: Harvard University Press.

Ruotsalo, T., Jacucci, G., Myllymäki, P., & Kaski, S. (2015, January). Interactive intent modeling: Information discovery beyond search. *Communications of the ACM, 58,* 86–92.

Russell, R., Guerry, A. D., Balvanera, P., Gould, R. K., Basurto, X., Chan, K.M.A., . . . Tam, J. (2013). Humans and nature: How knowing and experiencing nature affect well-being. *Annual Review of Environment and Resources, 38,* 473–502.

Ryle, G. (1949). *The concept of mind.* Chicago: University of Chicago Press.

Sakaki, M., & Niki, K. (2011). Effects of the brief viewing of emotional stimuli on understanding of insight solutions. *Cognitive, Affective, and Behavioral Neuroscience, 11,* 526–540.

Saner, L., & Schunn, C. D. (1999). Analogies out of the blue: When history seems to retell itself. *Proceedings of the 21st Annual Conference of the Cognitive Science Society.* Mahwah, NJ: Erlbaum.

Sawhill, J. C., & Williamson, D. (2001). Mission impossible? Measuring success in nonprofit organizations. *Nonprofit Management & Leadership, 11,* 371–386.

Schacter, D. L., Addis, D. R., & Buckner, R. L. (2007). Remembering the past to imagine the future: The prospective brain. *Nature Reviews Neuroscience, 8,* 657–661.

Schacter, D. L., Addis, D. R., Hassabis, D., Martin, V. C., Spreng, R. N., & Szpunar, K. K. (2012). The future of memory: Remembering, imagining, and the brain. *Neuron, 76,* 677–694.

Schauer, F. (1987). Precedent. *Stanford Law Review, 39,* 571–605.

Schilpzand, M. C., Herold, D. M., & Shalley, C. E. (2011). Members' openness to experience and teams' creative performance. *Small Group Research, 42,* 55–76.

Schippers, M. C., Edmondson, A. C., & West, M. A. (2014). Team reflexivity as an antidote to team information-processing failures. *Small Group Research, 45,* 731–769.

Scholz, J., Klein, M. C., Behrens, T.E.J., & Johansen-Berg, H. (2009). Training induces changes in white-matter architecture. *Nature Neuroscience, 11,* 1370–1371.

Schon, D. A. (1963). *Displacement of concepts.* London, UK: Tavistock.

Schon, D. A. (1983). *The reflective practitioner: How professionals think in action.* New York: Basic Books.

Schon, D. A., & Wiggins, G. (1992). Kinds of seeing and their functions in designing. *Design Studies, 13,* 135–156.

Schooler, J. W. (2002). Verbalization produces a transfer inappropriate processing shift. *Applied Cognitive Psychology, 16,* 989–997.

Schröer, B., Kain, A., & Lindemann, U. (2010). Supporting creativity in conceptual design: Method 635-extended. *Proceedings of the 11th International Design Conference (Design 2010)* (pp. 591–600). Dubrovnik, Croatia.

Schwartz, D. L., & Black, J. B. (1996). Shuttling between depictive models and abstract rules: Induction and fallback. *Cognitive Science, 20,* 457–497.

Schwartz, D. L., & Bransford, J. D. (1998). A time for telling. *Cognition and Instruction, 16,* 475–522.

Schwartz, D. L., Bransford, J. D., & Sears, D. (2005). Efficiency and innovation in transfer. In J. P. Mestre (Ed.), *Transfer of learning from a modern multidisciplinary perspective* (pp. 1–51). Greenwich, CT: Information Age Publishing.

Schwartz, D. L., Chase, C. C., & Bransford, J. D. (2012). Resisting overzealous transfer: Coordinating previously successful routines with needs for new learning. *Educational Psychologist, 47,* 204–214.

Schwarz, N., & Clore, G. L. (1983). Mood, misattribution, and judgments of well-being: Informative and directive functions of affective states. *Journal of Personality and Social Psychology, 45,* 513–523.

Segal, E. (2004). Incubation in insight problem solving. *Creativity Research Journal, 16,* 141–148.

Seger, C. A., Desmond, J. E., Glover, G. H., & Gabrieli, J.D.E. (2000). Functional magnetic resonance imaging evidence for right-hemisphere involvement in processing unusual semantic relationships. *Neuropsychology, 14,* 361–369.

Seifert, C. M., & Patalano, A. L. (2001). Opportunism in memory: Preparing for chance encounters. *Current Directions in Psychological Science, 10,* 198–201.

Sengers, P., & Gaver, B. (2006). Staying open to interpretation: Engaging multiple meanings in design and evaluation. *Proceedings of the 6th Conference on Designing Interactive Systems (DIS '06),* 99–108.

Sevincer, A. T., & Oettingen, G. (2013). Spontaneous mental contrasting and selective goal pursuit. *Personality and Social Psychology Bulletin, 39,* 1240–1254.

Shah, J. J. (1998). Experimental investigation of collaborative techniques for progressive idea generation. *Proceedings of the ASME Design Theory and Methodology Conference,* Atlanta, GA.

Shah, J. J., Vargas-Hernandez, N., Summers, J. D., & Kulkarni, S. (2001). Collaborative sketching (C-Sketch): An idea generation technique for engineering design. *Journal of Creative Behavior, 35*, 168–198.

Shalley, C. E. (1991). Effects of productivity goals, creativity goals, and personal discretion on individual creativity. *Journal of Applied Psychology, 76*, 179–185.

Sharma, P. (2013). Acting into the unknown. In R. Somerson & M. L. Hermano (Eds.), *The art of critical making: Rhode Island School of Design on creative practice* (pp. 230–243). Hoboken, NJ: Wiley.

Sheeran, P., Webb, T. L., & Gollwitzer, P. M. (2005). The interplay between goal intentions and implementation intentions. *Personality and Social Psychology Bulletin, 31*, 87–98.

Shenhav, A., Botvinick, M. M., & Cohen, J. D. (2013). The expected value of control: An integrative theory of anterior cingulate cortex function. *Neuron, 79*, 217–240.

Shiff, R. (1986). *Cézanne and the end of impressionism: A study of the theory, technique, and critical evaluation of modern art.* Chicago: University of Chicago Press.

Shirouzu, H., Miyake, N., & Masukawa, H. (2002). Cognitively active externalization for situated reflection. *Cognitive Science, 26*, 469–501.

Shoda, Y., Mischel, W., & Peake, P. K. (1990). Predicting adolescent cognitive and self-regulatory competencies from preschool delay of gratification: Identifying diagnostic conditions. *Developmental Psychology, 26*, 978–986.

Shrira, A., Palgi, Y., Wolf, J. J., Haber, Y., Goldray, O., Shacham-Shmueli, E., & Ben-Ezra, M. (2011). The positivity ratio and functioning under stress. *Stress and Health, 27*, 265–271.

Shu, L. H., Ueda, K., Chiu, I., & Cheong, H. (2011). Biologically inspired design. *CIRP Annals: Manufacturing Technology, 60*, 673–693.

Siegler, R. S. (2007). Cognitive variability. *Developmental Science, 10*, 104–109.

Silbey, J. (2011). Harvesting intellectual property: Inspired beginnings and "work-makes-work," Two stages in the creative processes of artists and innovators. *Notre Dame Law Review, 86*, 2091–2132.

Simon, H. (1973). The structure of ill structured problems. *Artificial Intelligence, 4*, 181–201.

Simons, J. S., Koutstaal, W., Prince, S., Wagner, A. D., & Schacter, D. L. (2003). Neural mechanisms of visual object priming: Evidence for perceptual and semantic distinctions in fusiform cortex. *NeuroImage, 19*, 613–626.

Sio, U. N., & Ormerod, T. C. (2009). Does incubation enhance problem solving? A meta-analytic review. *Psychological Bulletin, 135*, 94–120.

Smallwood, J., & Andrews-Hanna, J. (2013). Not all minds that wander are lost: The importance of a balanced perspective on the mind-wandering state. *Frontiers in Psychology, 4*, Article 441, 1–6.

Smallwood, J., Brown, K., Baird, B., & Schooler, J. W. (2012). Cooperation between the default mode network and the frontal-parietal network in the production of an internal train of thought. *Brain Research, 1428*, 60–70.

Smith, K. A., Huber, D. E., & Vul, E. (2013). Multiply-constrained semantic search in the remote associates test. *Cognition, 128*, 64–75.

Smith, P. (2010). *Just kids*. New York: HarperCollins.

Smith, R. (2008, January 25). David Smith: Sprays. *The New York Times*. Retrieved April 8, 2015, from www.nytimes.com/2008/01/25/arts/design/25gall.html

Smith, S. M., Ward, T. B., & Schumacher, J. S. (1993). Constraining effects of examples in a creative generation task. *Memory & Cognition, 21*, 837–845.

Snyder, M. (2009). In the footsteps of Kurt Lewin: Practical theorizing, action research, and the psychology of social action. *Journal of Social Issues, 65*, 225–245.

Sonnentag, S., & Volmer, J. (2010). What you do for your team comes back to you: A cross-level investigation of individual goal specification, team-goal clarity, and individual performance. *Human Performance, 23*, 116–130.

Sotomayor, S., & Greenhouse, L. (2014). A conversation with Justice Sotomayor. *Yale Law Journal Forum, 123*. Retrieved April 8, 2015, from http://yalelawjournal. org/forum/a-conversation-with-justice-sotomayor

Sowden, P. T., Pringle, A., & Gabora, L. (2015). The shifting sands of creative thinking: Connections to dual-process theory. *Thinking & Reasoning, 21*, 40–60.

Spreng, R. N., & Grady, C. L. (2010). Patterns of brain activity supporting autobiographical memory, prospection, and theory of mind, and their relationship to the default mode network. *Journal of Cognitive Neuroscience, 22*, 1112–1123.

Spreng, R. N., Stevens, W. D., Chamberlain, J. P., Gilmore, A. W., & Schacter, D. L. (2010). Default network activity, coupled with the frontoparietal control network, supports goal-directed cognition. *NeuroImage, 53*, 303–317.

Squyres, S. W., Arvidson, R. E., Bell, J. F. III, Brückner, J., Cabrol, N. A., Calvin, W., . . . Yen, A. (2004). The Opportunity Rover's Athena science investigation at Meridiani Planum, Mars. *Science, 306*, 1698–1703.

Sridharan, D., Levitin, D. J., & Menon, V. (2008). A critical role for the right fronto-insular cortex in switching between central-executive and default-mode networks. *Proceedings of the National Academy of Sciences, USA, 105*, 12569–12574.

Stickgold, R., & Walker, M. P. (2013). Sleep-dependent memory triage: Evolving generalization through selective processing. *Nature Neuroscience, 16*, 139–145.

Stigliani, I., & Ravasi, D. (2012). Organizing thoughts and connecting brains: Material practices and the transition from individual to group-level prospective sensemaking. *Academy of Management Journal, 55*, 1232–1259.

Stöber, J. (1998). Worry, problem solving, and the suppression of imagery: The role of concreteness. *Behaviour Research and Therapy, 36*, 751–756.

Stöber, J., Tepperwien, S., & Staak, M. (2000). Worrying leads to reduced concreteness of problem elaborations: Evidence for the avoidance theory of worry. *Anxiety, Stress, and Coping, 13*, 217–227.

Stokes, P. D. (2001). Variability, constraints, and creativity: Shedding light on Claude Monet. *American Psychologist, 56*, 355–359.

Stokes, P. D. (2007). Using constraints to generate and sustain novelty. *Psychology of Aesthetics, Creativity, and the Arts, 1*, 107–113.

Stokes, P. D. (2008). Creativity from constraints: What can we learn from Motherwell? From Mondrian? From Klee? *Journal of Creative Behavior, 42*, 223–236.

Stokes, P. D. (2009). Using constraints to create novelty: A case study. *Psychology of Aesthetics, Creativity, and the Arts, 3*, 174–180.

Stokes, P. D. (2014). Crossing disciplines: A constraint-based model of the creative/innovative process. *Journal of Product Innovation Management, 31*, 247–258.

Stratton, R., & Mann, D. (2003). Systematic innovation and the underlying principles behind TRIZ and TOC. *Journal of Materials Processing Technology, 139*, 120–126.

Stringaris, A., Medford, N., Giora, R., Giampietro, V. C., Brammer, M. J., & David, A. S. (2006). How metaphors influence semantic relatedness judgments: The role of right-frontal cortex. *NeuroImage, 33*, 784–793.

Stroebe, W., Nijstad, B. A., & Rietzschel, E. F. (2010). Beyond productivity loss in brainstorming groups: The evolution of a question. *Advances in Experimental Social Psychology, 43*, 157–203.

Su, L., Bowman, H., & Barnard, P. (2011). Glancing and then looking: On the role of body, affect, and meaning in cognitive control. *Frontiers in Psychology, 2*, Article 348, 1–23.

Subramaniam, K., Kounios, J., Parrish, T. B., & Jung-Beeman, M. (2009). A brain mechanism for facilitation of insight by positive affect. *Journal of Cognitive Neuroscience, 21*, 415–432.

Suddendorf, T., & Corballis, M. C. (1997). Mental time travel and the evolution of the human mind. *Genetic Social and General Psychology Monographs, 123*, 133–167.

Suddendorf, T., & Redshaw, J. (2013). The development of mental scenario building and episodic foresight. *Annals of the New York Academy of Sciences, 1296*, 135–153.

Sutton, E. (2013). Conversation: Critique. In R. Somerson and M. L. Hermano (Eds.), *The art of critical making: Rhode Island School of Design on creative practice* (pp. 210–229). Hoboken, NJ: Wiley.

Sutton, R. I., & Hargadon, A. (1996). Brainstorming groups in context: Effectiveness in a product design firm. *Administrative Science Quarterly, 41*, 685–716.

Sweeny, K., Carroll, P. J., & Shepperd, J. A. (2006). Is optimism always best? Future outlooks and preparedness. *Current Directions in Psychological Science, 15*, 302–306.

Sweeny, K., & Krizan, Z. (2013). Sobering up: A quantitative review of temporal declines in expectations. *Psychological Bulletin, 139*, 702–724.

Szpunar, K. K. (2010). Episodic future thought: An emerging concept. *Perspectives in Psychological Science, 5*, 142–162.

Taatgen, N. A., Juvina, I., Schipper, M., Borst, J. P., & Martens, S. (2009). Too much control can hurt: A threaded cognition model of the attentional blink. *Cognitive Psychology, 59*, 1–29.

Tadmor, C. T., Satterstrom, P., Jang, S., & Polzer, J. T. (2012). Beyond individual creativity: The superadditive benefits of multicultural experience for collective creativity in culturally diverse teams. *Journal of Cross-Cultural Psychology, 43*, 384–392.

Tang, Y. Y., Ma, Y., Fan, J., Feng, H., Wang, J., Feng, S., . . . Fan, M. (2009). Central and autonomic nervous system interaction is altered by short-term meditation. *Proceedings of the National Academy of Sciences, USA, 106*, 8865–8870.

Tang, Y. Y., Ma, Y., Wang, J., Fan, Y., Feng, S., Lu, Q., . . . Posner, M. I. (2007). Short-term meditation training improves attention and self-regulation. *Proceedings of the National Academy of Sciences, USA, 104*, 17152–17156.

Tangney, J. P., Baumeister, R. F., & Boone, A. L. (2004). High self-control predicts good adjustment, less pathology, better grades, and interpersonal success. *Journal of Personality, 72*, 271–324.

Taubert, M., Villringer, A., & Ragert, P. (2012). Learning-related gray and white matter changes in humans: An update. *The Neuroscientist, 18*, 320–325.

Taylor, S. E., Pham, L. B., Rivkin, I. D., & Armor, D. A. (1998). Harnessing the imagination: Mental simulation, self-regulation, and coping. *American Psychologist, 53*, 429–439.

Tellegen, A., & Atkinson, G. (1974). Openness to absorbing and self-altering experiences ("absorption"), a trait related to hypnotic susceptibility. *Journal of Abnormal Psychology, 83*, 268–277.

Terwiesch, C., & Xu, Y. (2008). Innovation contests, open innovation, and multiagent problem solving. *Management Science, 54*, 1529–1543.

Tharp, T. (2003). *The creative habit: Learn it, and use it for life.* (with M. Reiter). New York: Simon & Schuster.

Thibodeau, P. H., & Boroditsky, L. (2011). Metaphors we think by: The role of metaphor in reasoning. *PLoS ONE, 6*, Article e16782, 1–11.

Todorova, G., & Durisin, B. (2007). Absorptive capacity: Valuing a reconceptualization. *Academy of Management Review, 32*, 774–786.

Todorovic, N., & Petrovic, S. (2013). Bee colony optimization algorithm for nurse rostering. *IEEE Transactions on Systems, Man, and Cybernetics: Systems, 43*, 467–473.

Tranter, L. J., & Koutstaal, W. (2008). Age and flexible thinking: An experimental demonstration of the beneficial effects of increased cognitively stimulating activity on fluid intelligence in healthy older adults. *Aging, Neuropsychology, and Cognition, 15*, 184–207.

Trencher, G. Bai, X., Evans, J., McCormick, K., & Yarime, M. (2014). University partnerships for co-designing and co-producing urban sustainability. *Global Environmental Change, 28*, 153–165.

Trickett, S. B., Trafton, J. G., & Schunn, C. D. (2009). How do scientists respond to anomalies? Different strategies used in basic and applied science. *Topics in Cognitive Science, 1*, 711–729.

Trope, Y., & Liberman, N. (2003). Temporal construal. *Psychological Review, 110*, 403–421.

Trope, Y., & Liberman, N. (2010). Construal-level theory of psychological distance. *Psychological Review, 117*, 440–463.

Tseng, I., Moss, J., Cagan, J., & Kotovsky, K. (2008a). The role of timing in analogical similarity in the stimulation of idea generation in design. *Design Studies, 29*, 203–221.

Tseng, I., Moss, J., Cagan, J., & Kotovsky, K. (2008b). Overcoming blocks in conceptual design: The effects of open goals and analogical similarity on idea generation. *Proceedings of the 2008 ASME International Design Engineering Technical Conferences and Computers and Information in Engineering Conference.* New York.

Tsoukas, H. & Chia, R. (2002). On organizational becoming: Rethinking organization change. *Organization Science, 13*, 567–582.

Tucker, A. L., & Edmondson, A. C. (2003). Why hospitals don't learn from failures: Organizational and psychological dynamics that inhibit system change. *California Management Review, 45*, 55–72.

Tulving, E. (1983). *Elements of episodic memory.* New York: Oxford University Press.

Tulving, E., & Pearlstone, Z. (1966). Availability versus accessibility of information in memory for words. *Journal of Verbal Learning and Verbal Behavior, 5*, 381–391.

Tushman, M. L., & O'Reilly, C. A. III (1996). Ambidextrous organizations: Managing evolutionary and revolutionary change. *California Management Review, 38*, 8–30.

Ülkümen, G., & Cheema, A. (2013). Framing goals to influence personal savings: The role of specificity and construal level. *Journal of Marketing Research, 48*, 958–969.

Valentine, M. A., & Edmondson, A. C. (2015). Team scaffolds: How mesolevel structures support role-based coordination in temporary groups. *Organization Science, 26*, 405–422.

Vallacher, R. R., & Wegner, D. M. (1987). What do people think they're doing? Action identification and human behavior. *Psychological Review, 94*, 3–15.

Vallacher, R. R., & Wegner, D. M. (1989). Levels of personal agency: Individual variation in action identification. *Journal of Personality and Social Psychology, 57*, 660–671.

Van Daele, T., Van den Bergh, O., Van Aundenhove, C., Raes, F., & Hermans, D. (2013). Reduced memory specificity predicts the acquisition of problem solving skills in psychoeducation. *Journal of Behavior Therapy and Experimental Psychiatry, 44*, 135–140.

VanGundy, A. B. Jr. (1988). *Techniques of structured problem solving* (2nd ed.). New York: Van Nostrand Reinhold.

Van Wezel, W., & Jorna, R. (2009). Cognition, tasks and planning: Supporting the planning of shunting operations at the Netherlands Railways. *Cognition, Technology & Work, 11*, 165–176.

Vaquero, L. M., & Cebrian, M. (2013). The rich club phenomenon in the classroom. *Scientific Reports, 3*, Article 1174, 1–8.

Vartanian, O. (2012). Dissociable neural systems for analogy and metaphor: Implications for the neuroscience of creativity. *British Journal of Psychology, 103*, 302–316.

Vartanian, O. (2009). Variable attention facilitates creative problem solving. *Psychology of Aesthetics, Creativity, and the Arts, 3*, 57–59.

Vartanian, O., Martindale, C., & Kwiatkowski, J. (2007). Creative potential, attention, and speed of information processing. *Personality and Individual Differences, 43*, 1470–1480.

Vattam, S. S., Helms, M. E., & Goel, A. K. (2010). A content account of creative analogies in biologically inspired design. *AI for Engineering Design, Analysis and Manufacturing, 24*, 467–481.

Vera, D., & Crossan, M. (2005). Improvisation and innovative performance in teams. *Organization Science, 16*, 203–224.

Vincent J.F.V., & Mann D. L. (2002). Systematic technology transfer from biology to engineering. *Philosophical Transactions of the Royal Society of London, A, 360,* 159–173.

Viola, B. (2007, March 7). Presence and absence: Vision and the invisible in the media age. *The Tanner Lectures on Human Values,* delivered at the University of Utah.

Vosburg, S. K. (1998). The effects of positive and negative mood on divergent-thinking performance. *Creativity Research Journal, 11,* 165–172.

Voss, G. B., Sirdeshmukh, D., & Voss, Z. G. (2008). The effects of slack resources and environmental threat on product exploration and exploitation. *Academy of Management Journal, 51,* 147–164.

Voss, G. B., & Voss, Z. G. (2013). Strategic ambidexterity in small and medium-sized enterprises: Implementing exploration and exploitation in product and market domains. *Organization Science, 24,* 1459–1477.

Voss, Z. G., Cable, D. M., & Voss, G. B. (2006). Organizational identity and firm performance: What happens when leaders disagree about "who we are?" *Organization Science, 17,* 741–755.

Vukovic, N., & Williams, J. N. (2014). Automatic perceptual simulation of first language meanings during second language sentence processing in bilinguals. *Acta Psychologica, 145,* 98–103.

Wagner, U., Gals, S., Haider, H., Verleger, R., & Born, J. (2004). Sleep inspires insight. *Nature, 427,* 352–355.

Waks, L. J. (2001). Donald Schon's philosophy of design and design education. *International Journal of Technology and Design Education, 11,* 37–51.

Walker, C. O., Greene, B. A., & Mansell, R. A. (2006). Identification with academics, intrinsic/extrinsic motivation, and self-efficacy as predictors of cognitive engagement. *Learning and Individual Differences, 16,* 1–12.

Wallas, G. (1926). *The art of thought.* New York: Harcourt Brace.

Wang, M-Y., Chang, D-S., & Kao, C-H. (2010). Identifying technology trends for R&D planning using TRIZ and text mining. *R&D Management, 40,* 491–509.

Wang, X., Lu, Y., Zhao, Y., Gong, S., & Li, B. (2013). Organisational unlearning, organizational flexibility and innovation capability: An empirical study of SMEs in China. *International Journal of Technology Management, 61,* 132–155.

Wang, Z., & Wang, N. (2012). Knowledge sharing, innovation and firm performance. *Expert Systems with Applications, 39,* 8899–8908.

Ward, T. B., Patterson, M. J., Sifonis, C. M., Dodds, R. A., & Saunders, K. N. (2002). The role of graded category structure in imaginative thought. *Memory & Cognition, 30,* 199–216.

Watkins, E. (2011). Dysregulation in level of goal and action identification across psychological disorders. *Clinical Psychology Review, 31,* 260–278.

Weaver, J. M., Kuhr, R., Wang, D., Crawford, R. H., Wood, K. L., Jensen, D., & Linsey, J. S. (2009). Increasing innovation in multi-function systems: Evaluation and experimentation of two ideation methods for design. *Proceedings of the ASME 2009 International Design Engineering Technical Conferences & Computers and Information in Engineering Conference,* San Diego, CA, 1–19.

Webb, T. L., Sheeran, P., & Armitage, C. J. (2006). Implementation intentions: Strategic automatization of food choice. In R. Shepherd & M. Raats (Eds.), *The psychology of food choice* (pp. 329–343). Wallingford, UK: CABI.

Webster, J. D. (2011). A new measure of time perspective: Initial psychometric findings for the balanced time perspective scale (BTPS). *Canadian Journal of Behavioural Science, 43,* 111–118.

Wegner, D. M. (1986). Transactive memory: A contemporary analysis of the group mind. In B. Mullen & G. R. Goethals (Eds.), *Theories of group behavior* (pp. 185–208). New York: Springer.

Wei, D., Yang, J., Li, W., Wang, K., Zhang, Q., & Qiu, J. (2013). Increased resting functional connectivity of the medial prefrontal cortex in creativity by means of cognitive stimulation. *Cortex, 51,* 92–102.

Weick, K. E. (1998). Improvisation as a mindset for organizational analysis. *Organization Science, 9,* 543–555.

Weick, K. E., & Roberts, K. H. (1993). Collective mind in organizations: Heedful interrelating on flight decks. *Administrative Science Quarterly, 38,* 357–381.

Weick, K. E., Sutcliffe, K. M., & Obstfeld, D. (2005). Organizing and the process of sensemaking. *Organization Science, 16,* 409–421.

Weiss, A., & Neuringer, A. (2012). Reinforced variability enhances object exploration in shy and bold rats. *Physiology and Behavior, 107,* 451–457.

Weiss, M., Hoegl, M., & Gibbert, M. (2011). Making virtue of necessity: The role of team climate for innovation in resource-constrained innovation projects. *Journal of Product Innovation Management, 28,* 196–207.

Wen, M-C., Butler, L. T., & Koutstaal, W. (2013). Improving insight and noninsight problems with brief interventions. *British Journal of Psychology, 104,* 97–118.

Wendelken, C., Nakhabenko, D., Donohue, S. E., Carter, C. S., & Bunge, S. A. (2008). "Brain is to thought as stomach is to??" Investigating the role of rostrolateral prefrontal cortex in relational reasoning. *Journal of Cognitive Neuroscience, 20,* 682–693.

Wenk-Sormaz, H. (2005). Meditation can reduce habitual responding. *Alternative Therapies in Health and Medicine, 11,* 42–58.

Werfel, J., Petersen, K., & Nagpal, R. (2014). Designing collective behavior in a termite-inspired robot construction team. *Science, 343,* 754–758.

West, M. A. & Anderson, N. R. (1996). Innovation in top management teams. *Journal of Applied Psychology, 81,* 680–693.

Wetzel, B. (2014). Representation and reasoning for complex spatio-temporal problems: From humans to software agents. Ph.D. Dissertation, University of Minnesota.

Wetzel, B., Anderson, K., Gini, M., & Koutstaal, W. (in preparation). Thinking in action: A new affordances-based approach to complex spatiotemporal reasoning in humans and software agents.

Wetzein, A., & Hacker, W. (2004). Reflective verbalization improves solutions: The effects of question-based reflection in design problem solving. *Applied Cognitive Psychology, 18,* 145–156.

Wheeler, M. E., Petersen, S. E., & Buckner, R. L. (2000). Memory's echo: Vivid remembering reactivates sensory-specific cortex. *Proceedings of the National Academy of Sciences, USA, 97*, 11125–11129.

Wieber, F., Thürmer, J. L., & Gollwitzer, P. M. (2012). Collective action control by goals and plans: Applying a self-regulation perspective to group performance. *American Journal of Psychology, 125*, 275–290.

Wieth, M. B., & Zacks, R. T. (2011). Time of day effects on problem solving: When the non-optimal is optimal. *Thinking and Reasoning, 17*, 387–401.

Wilkin, K. (2006). David Smith, in *Grove art online*. Oxford, UK: Oxford University Press.

Williams, J.M.G., Barnhofer, T., Crane, C., Hermans, D., Raes, F., Watkins, E., & Dagleish, T. (2007). Autobiographical memory specificity and emotional disorder. *Psychological Bulletin, 133*, 122–148.

Wilson, J., Rosen, D., Nelson, B., & Yen, J. (2010). The effects of biological examples in idea generation. *Design Studies, 31*, 169–186.

Winkelmann, C., & Hacker, W. (2011). Generic non-technical procedures in design problem solving: Is there any benefit to the clarification of task requirements? *International Journal of Technology and Design Education, 21*, 395–407.

Winocur, G., Moscovitch, M., & Bontempi, B. (2010). Memory formation and long-term retention in humans and animals: Convergence towards a transformation account of hippocampal-neocortical interactions. *Neuropsychologia, 48*, 2339–2356.

Wodehouse, A., & Ion, W. (2012). Augmenting the 6-3-5 method with design information. *Research in Engineering Design, 23*, 5–15.

Woo, S. E., Chernyshenko, O. S., Longley, A., Zhang, Z.-X., Chiu, C.-Y., & Stark, S. E. (2014). Openness to experience: Its lower level structure, measurement, and cross-cultural equivalence. *Journal of Personality Assessment, 96*, 29–45.

Wood, W., & Neal, D. T. (2007). A new look at habits and the habit-goal interface. *Psychological Review, 114*, 843–863.

Wood, W., Tam, L., & Witt, M. G. (2005). Changing circumstances, disrupting habits. *Journal of Personality and Social Psychology, 88*, 918–933.

Woolley, A. W. (2009). Means vs. ends: Implications of process and outcome focus for team adaptation and performance. *Organization Science, 20*, 500–515.

Woolley, A. W., Chabris, C. F., Pentland, A. Hashmi, N., & Malone, T. W. (2010). Evidence for a collective intelligence factor in the performance of human groups. *Science, 330*, 686–688.

Woolley, A. W., Gerbasi, M. E., Chabris, C. F., Kosslyn, S. M., & Hackman, J. R. (2008). Bringing in the experts: How team composition and collaborative planning jointly shape analytic effectiveness. *Small Group Research, 39*, 352–371.

Woolley, A. W., Hackman, J. R., Jerde, T. E., Chabris, C. F., Bennett, S. L., & Kosslyn, S. M. (2007). Using brain-based measures to compose teams: How individual capabilities and team collaboration strategies jointly shape performance. *Social Neuroscience, 2*, 96–105.

Wrigley, W. J., & Emmerson, S. B. (2013). The experience of the flow state in live music performance. *Psychology of Music, 41*, 292–305.

Yamamoto, Y., & Nakakoji, K. (2005). Interaction design of tools for fostering creativity in the early stages of information design. *International Journal of Human-Computer Studies, 63*, 513–535.

Yang, J. (2014). The role of the right hemisphere in metaphor comprehension: A meta-analysis of functional magnetic resonance imaging studies. *Human Brain Mapping, 35*, 107–122.

Yaniv, I., & Meyer, D. E. (1987). Activation and metacognition of inaccessible stored information: Potential bases for incubation effects in problem solving. *Journal of Experimental Psychology: Learning, Memory, and Cognition, 13*, 187–205.

Ye, L., Cardwell, W., & Mark, L. S. (2009). Perceiving multiple affordances for objects. *Ecological Psychology, 21*, 185–217.

Yeager, D. S., & Dweck, C. S. (2012). Mindsets that promote resilience: When students believe that personal characteristics can be developed. *Educational Psychologist, 47*, 302–314.

Yilmaz, S., & Seifert, C. M. (2009). Cognitive heuristics employed by design experts. *Proceedings of the 3rd International Design Research Conference (IASDR '09)*, 1–11.

Yilmaz, S., Seifert, C. M., & Gonzalez, R. (2010). Cognitive heuristics in design: Instructional strategies to increase creativity in idea generation. *Artificial Intelligence for Engineering Design, Analysis and Manufacturing, 24*, 335–355.

Yokochi, S., & Okada, T. (2005). Creative cognitive process of art making: A field study of a traditional Chinese ink painter. *Creativity Research Journal, 17*, 241–255.

Youmans, R. J. (2011). The effects of physical prototyping and group work on the reduction of design fixation. *Design Studies, 32*, 115–138.

Yumer, M. E., & Kara, L. B. (2012). Co-abstraction of shape collections. *Proceedings of SIGGRAPH Asia, 2012, 31*, 1–11.

Zabelina, D. L., & Beeman, M. (2013). Short-term attentional perseveration associated with real-life creative achievement. *Frontiers in Psychology, 4*, Article 191, 1–8.

Zabelina, D. L., & Robinson, M. D. (2010). Creativity as flexible cognitive control. *Psychology of Aesthetics, Creativity, and the Arts, 4*, 136–143.

Zabelina, D. L., Robinson, M. D., & Anicha, C. L. (2007). The psychological tradeoffs of self-control: A multi-method investigation. *Personality and Individual Differences, 43*, 463–473.

Zaidel, D. W. (2013). Split-brain, the right hemisphere, and art: Fact and fiction. *Progress in Brain Research, 204*, 3–17.

Zatorre, R. J., Fields, R. D., & Johansen-Berg, H. (2012). Plasticity in gray and white: Neuroimaging changes in brain structure during learning. *Nature Neuroscience, 15*, 528–536.

Zenasni, F., Besançon, M., & Lubart, T. (2008). Creativity and tolerance of ambiguity: An empirical study. *Journal of Creative Behavior, 42*, 61–73.

Zeev-Wolf, M., Goldstein, A., Levkovitz, Y., & Faust, M. (2014). Fine-coarse semantic processing in schizophrenia: A reversed pattern of hemispheric dominance. *Neuropsychologia, 56*, 119–128.

Zhang, Y., & Fishbach, A. (2010). Counteracting obstacles with optimistic predictions. *Journal of Experimental Psychology: General, 139,* 16–31.

Zheng, Y., Venters, W., & Cornford, T. (2011). Collective agility, paradox and organizational improvisation: The development of a particle physics grid. *Information Systems Journal, 21,* 303–333.

Zhu, R., & Meyers-Levy, J. (2007). Exploring the cognitive mechanism that underlies regulatory focus effects. *Journal of Consumer Research, 34,* 89–96.

Ziegler, M., Danay, E., Heene, M., Asendorpf, J., & Bühner, M. (2012). Openness, fluid intelligence, and crystallized intelligence: Toward an integrative model. *Journal of Research in Personality, 46,* 173–183.

Zimbardo, P. G., & Boyd, J. N. (1999). Putting time in perspective: A valid, reliable individual-differences metric. *Journal of Personality and Social Psychology, 77,* 1271–1288.